PREPARING FOR THE NEXT GLOBAL OUTBREAK

PREPARING FOR THE NEXT GLOBAL OUTBREAK

A Guide to Planning from the Schoolhouse to the White House

DAVID C. PATE, MD, JD

AND

TED EPPERLY, MD

JOHNS HOPKINS UNIVERSITY PRESS | *Baltimore*

 Published 2023
Printed in the United States of America on acid-free paper
9 8 7 6 5 4 3 2 1

Johns Hopkins University Press
2715 North Charles Street
Baltimore, Maryland 21218
www.press.jhu.edu

Library of Congress Cataloging-in-Publication Data is available.

ISBN 978-1-4214-4575-5 (paperback)
ISBN 978-1-4214-4576-2 (ebook)

A catalog record for this book is available from the British Library.

Special discounts are available for bulk purchases of this book. For more information, please contact Special Sales at specialsales@jh.edu.

To my wife, Lynette, for what was supposed to be our first retirement year with wonderful travels full of memories but was instead a year spent mostly isolating ourselves from the threat of the SARS-CoV-2 virus and spending our fortieth wedding anniversary and Thanksgiving home alone. Thank you for your encouragement to write this book. To my daughters, Laurie and Lindsey, and my son-in-law Clif, each working respectively for local health systems in supply chain management, on a COVID-19 unit, and as a nursing administrator. I am so proud of each of you, and I thank you for what you did to care for our communities and those so unfortunate as to develop severe COVID-19. And, finally, to my grandchildren, David, Jax, Presley, Clif, and Dean. While I do not know if we will have another pandemic in my lifetime, I do not think it unlikely for the next one to occur during yours. I hope that we will have learned our lessons from this one. I will also never forget how, while adults struggled to follow public health guidance, I often found David wearing his mask, even when I told him he did not need to. I will remember Presley sitting in the backseat of her mother's car outside our home, while Lynette and I stood on the sidewalk, so that we could see each other and talk. Being hard of hearing, when I stepped forward to hear Lindsey, I got the biggest smile as my seven-year-old granddaughter told me (often dubbed the "King of Corona" by my wife) through her mother's car window: "Six feet please!" It is our youth, and particularly my grandchildren, who give me hope for the future.

And to Dave Jeppesen, Idaho's director of the Department of Health and Welfare, who led the state through this crisis with grace and patience that I can only aspire to; to Dr. Christine Hahn, the state medical director and epidemiologist who taught me so much and suffered my never-ending questions every week of the pandemic; and to all the amazing, dedicated, and hard-working experts in public health that work at the Idaho Department of Health and Welfare and the various Idaho public health departments who are among the unsung heroes of this pandemic.

DP

To all the countless physicians, nurses, and public health and other health care professionals who gave so much of themselves to serve our communities in a time of worldwide crisis—thank you! And to my wife Lindy, our two sons, Morgan and Avery, our daughter-in-law Jennifer, our three dogs, Star, Dart, and Luna, and our wonderful granddaughter Julie Hope, born during the pandemic, who all brought so much joy into the world. May we all "Hope" for a rapid and successful end to this pandemic and for meaningful learning that will prevent and lessen the next one!

TE

Those who cannot remember the past are condemned to repeat it.

George Santayana

[The COVID-19 pandemic] is historic. People will be talking about it decades and decades and decades from now.

Anthony S. Fauci, MD
DIRECTOR OF THE NATIONAL INSTITUTE
OF ALLERGY AND INFECTIOUS DISEASES
NATIONAL INSTITUTES OF HEALTH

CONTENTS

PREFACE

The authors are physician leaders in Idaho. Both have been on the tip of the spear in trying to educate and protect the public during the COVID-19 pandemic. They have worked together for more than a decade to transform health care in Idaho by leading their respective organizations and partnering with each other and, most recently, have served as co-chairs of the Healthcare Transformation Council of Idaho sponsored by the Idaho Department of Health and Welfare.

Dr. Pate, a specialist in internal medicine and a health care attorney, retired from his prior role as president and CEO of St. Luke's Health System based in Boise, Idaho, at the end of January 2020. He took a call from the governor of Idaho a couple of weeks later that brought an abrupt end to what he and his wife Lynette anticipated would be a relaxing time together, enjoying retirement. That call was a request for Dr. Pate to serve as a member of the governor's coronavirus working group to advise the governor on the public health issues associated with the threat of COVID-19. From that point on, Dr. Pate has attended weekly working group meetings, advised Idaho's largest school district on its pandemic plans, been active on Twitter (@drpatesblog) in commenting on COVID-19 and answering his followers' questions, written a blog (https://drpatesblog.com/), participated in numerous press and media interviews, and answered listeners' questions about the coronavirus on a weekly program on a local NPR radio station.

Dr. Epperly, a family physician who has committed his career to graduate medical education, developing future primary care physicians for Idaho and the nation, and caring for minority and poor populations of patients in Idaho, is the president and CEO of Full Circle Health, a large Federally Qualified Health Center with ten clinics, four family medicine residency programs, one pediatric residency program, and six fellowships. Idaho's public health system is divided into seven public health districts, and Dr. Epperly has served as a member of the board for Central District Health, the most populous health district in Idaho. During 2020, Dr. Epperly was an influential and outspoken board member, frequently advocating for the public health measures needed to protect Idahoans, influencing the district's board to take some of the strongest measures of any public health district in Idaho, often after being inundated with emails in opposition to any restrictions, and, regrettably, even after protestors showed up at his home in an effort to intimidate and harass him and his wife Lindy.

Dr. Pate's wife, Lynette, had urged him to write a book about the pandemic for months. It was, however, a call from Dr. Epperly to Dr. Pate, suggesting that the two consider coauthoring a book on the subject, that caused Pate to agree without hesitation. Both physicians have spent so much time and effort to combat the pandemic in Idaho that they agreed that, though an end is hopefully in sight given the COVID-19 vaccines, it is imperative that future US presidents and their administrations, the federal government and its health agencies, state governments and its leaders, public health leaders and health care leaders learn the lessons that this COVID-19 pandemic has to teach us. The authors know that there will be another pandemic; they just do not know when. Whenever it is, they pray that the country does not repeat the mistakes of this pandemic response and that, as a country, we can be better prepared for that future day so that there will be less loss of life, less serious illness, fewer long-term health consequences and health care costs, less economic devastation, less disruption to life, less impact on Americans' mental health, and fewer disparities in health care—and less politicization, less divisiveness, and more compassion as we come together as *one* Idaho, *one* nation, and *one* global community.

PREPARING FOR THE NEXT GLOBAL OUTBREAK

CHAPTER 1

The SARS-CoV-2 Virus and the COVID-19 Pandemic

The worst pandemic in modern history was the Spanish flu of 1918, which killed tens of millions of people. Today, with how interconnected the world is, it would spread faster.

BILL GATES

In March of 2020, President Donald J. Trump made several statements, including "Nobody knew there would be a pandemic or epidemic of this proportion . . . So, there's never been anything like this in history. There's never been." He also said, "And nobody's ever seen anything like this." On another occasion, he remarked, "I just think this is something . . . that you can never really think is going to happen."[1]

These remarks, of course, overlooked some facts: that there have been pandemics even more severe than COVID-19, such as the influenza pandemic in 1918–1919 (the Spanish flu), and that scientists have been monitoring the possibility of coming pandemics and alerting the public for decades. There have been numerous books written that project the chance of a future pandemic, and Bill Gates gave a TED talk in 2015 in which he warned of a coming global health threat. Hospital leaders have been doing pandemic planning for many years. The Obama administration had developed a pandemic plan and conducted a tabletop exercise with members of the incoming Trump administration before President Trump took office. Both SARS (severe acute respiratory syndrome) and MERS (Middle East respiratory syndrome) were caused by novel (previously unknown) coronaviruses, emerging within a decade of each other, so it is not all that shocking and unimaginable that we have a third novel coronavirus in less than a decade from the second one. What is surprising is how few are the lessons we remembered from what we should have learned from these previous outbreaks and how we still find ourselves unprepared.

Recommendation #1

Prepare for the Next Pandemic Now

The US government and its agencies must acknowledge the risk of future pandemics and plan for them.

Further hampering our efforts to recognize a newly emerging public health threat, and specifically this novel coronavirus, was the Trump administration's decision to make significant funding cuts to the US Centers for Disease Control and Prevention (CDC), the National Science Foundation, and the US Agency for International Development staff stationed in China.[2] The experts at these agencies work with foreign countries to assist them in identifying and containing disease outbreaks; notably, CDC staff have worked with their counterparts in China for the past three decades. Given that many of the emerging global health threats are from zoonotic diseases (infections transmitted by an animal to a human), it was unfortunate that before the SARS-CoV-2 virus outbreak, the Trump administration transferred the US Department of Agriculture manager of the animal disease monitoring program in China—who oversaw the animal disease monitoring program—out of China.[3]

The embedding of American scientists and epidemiologists in other countries is in the best interests of the United States because we are a connected world driven by global trade and because of the ease of international travel. Such travel allows a localized outbreak of a novel virus to be rapidly spread to people living elsewhere in the world, who will likely all be susceptible to the virus's effects. In 2018 alone, 41.77 million Americans traveled overseas for business or pleasure.[4] In that same year, approximately 80 million international visitors traveled to the United States (an average of almost 220,000 people per day).[5] These figures highlight the vulnerability of the United States to the introduction of new transmissible diseases from other countries, especially when that new disease does not make its host too ill too soon. Two factors that make a disease an even greater threat are (1) when the novel virus can be transmitted by respiratory droplets or aerosols, so that direct contact is not necessary, and (2) when the infected person can remain asymptomatic for a period of time while contagious, with a high viral load (the amount of virus in the person's nose or throat), and when transmission requires a low viral dose (the amount of virus necessary to infect someone else).

Recommendation #2

Establish a Public Health Presence in Foreign Countries

Future US presidential administrations should recommit and invest sufficiently in establishing a public health presence in certain foreign countries (developing countries without a sophisticated public health infrastructure; countries with closed societies that will allow our presence, which otherwise would be less forthcoming or less timely with information about an outbreak; countries where zoonotic diseases are a high risk or that have previously precipitated an epidemic or pandemic) to assist in the early identification of novel viruses and other pathogens, and their containment.

A note to readers: While we will refer to novel viruses throughout the book for simplicity and clarity, we do so because we believe that they are the biggest threat when it comes to future pandemics. However, we do not want readers to get the impression that viruses are the only potential pathogen that could lead to a future pandemic, nor do we suggest that the virus would necessarily have to be novel.

Given that we are writing this book during the pandemic, our description of the timeline and developments is incomplete. There is no doubt that we will continue to learn more about this virus and the disease it causes. It is entirely possible that the things we think we know will be proven wrong in the future. Regardless, it is unlikely that the technical aspects of this virus or the disease it causes will materially affect our recommendations. One day soon, we hope, SARS coronavirus-2

(SARS-CoV-2) will be behind us. We focus instead on what is ahead of us: likely another pandemic in the not-all-that-distant future. It is for *that* pandemic that we write this book. We believe that the lessons from the present situation may avert that future pandemic or at least lessen its impact.

How the Pandemic Unfolded

December 2019 through January 2020

On December 31, 2019, China publicly reported that a cluster of cases of pneumonia were noted in Wuhan and suggested a connection to the Huanan Seafood Wholesale Market in Wuhan.

On January 1, 2020, China reported that the seafood and animal market was closed and that samples retrieved from the market had tested positive for a novel coronavirus. By the next day, 41 patients had been admitted to a hospital in Wuhan, 32 percent of them requiring intensive care. Most patients (73 percent) were men, and the median age was 49 years. Only 32 percent had underlying health conditions. Twenty-nine percent developed acute respiratory distress syndrome, and 15 percent of the patients died.[5]

On January 10, 2020, Chinese scientists released the genetic sequence of this novel coronavirus, showing that it was a betacoronavirus and likely in the same family as the virus that had caused SARS, which was named the SARS-associated coronavirus (SARS-CoV). SARS was first reported in February 2003 in Asia. Initially, the new virus in Wuhan was named the 2019 novel coronavirus (2019-nCoV), but as the relationship to the first SARS virus became clear, the virus was renamed SARS-CoV-2. The disease it causes was called coronavirus disease 2019 (COVID-19, or simply COVID).

Live animal markets (wet markets) are common in Asian countries and sell live poultry, fish, reptiles, and mammals of all kinds. These animals are often caged in close quarters and less than sanitary conditions. The markets regularly cater to clientele who desire exotic animals as a culinary delicacy. Animals are typically butchered out in the open, with a significant potential to spread disease not only through direct contact but also by airborne particles. Cleaning throughout the day often involves spraying surfaces with hoses, which can aerosolize viruses from blood, urine, excrement, saliva, and other secretions. It is difficult to imagine a setting more conducive to the spread of disease from one animal species to another or from an animal to humans. Live poultry markets are believed to have been the source of the H5N1 avian influenza virus that infected people in Hong Kong, and the original SARS-CoV virus was thought to have been transmitted to humans in a wet market in China by civet cats infected by bats.[6] We cannot be certain that civet cats were the actual intermediary host because we cannot rule out the possibility that some civet cats were infected by the same source that infected humans.

In the study of the 41 patients admitted to the hospital in Wuhan in December 2019, it was noted that 66 percent had a potential exposure at the Huanan wet market. The animal source of infection has not yet been identified. It is conjectured by some—but it remains unclear and certainly not proven—that the animals that transmitted this virus to humans were pangolins, sometimes known as scaly anteaters, which were sold at the markets. Pangolins are known hosts for a number of betacoronaviruses. The molecular and phylogenetic analysis of a strain of coronavirus that had infected three Malayan pangolins showed that the virus was related to, but distinct from, SARS-CoV-2. While this proves that pangolins are natural and parallel hosts of betacoronaviruses, it fails to prove that pangolins were the intermediate host for and human source of SARS-CoV-2. There are other animals such as the raccoon dog, which are known to be host to coronaviruses that, to our knowledge, have yet to be tested and have been sold in various wet markets in Wuhan. It is also thought likely, but not proven, that if pangolins were the intermediary host, they were most likely infected by bats. Bats are a common reservoir for coronaviruses, and coronaviruses are commonly grown in culture from bat guano from bat caves in China.

A spillover event occurs when a virus found in one species of animal is transmitted to a new species; in this case, the SARS-CoV-2 virus was transmitted from one or more animals in the seafood market to humans. It is likely that there were multiple spillover events, just as there were for the first SARS virus back in 2002, as many of the wet markets in Wuhan and elsewhere use common suppliers that may have been the source of infected animals. But again, just as with the civet cats with SARS-CoV infection, we cannot rule out the alternative explanation that pangolins, should any be found to be infected with SARS-CoV-2, were infected by another source in the wet markets that also infected humans. The possibility certainly exists that there was no intermediate host, but rather the disease was directly transmitted to humans by bats.

While at this time it is widely believed in the scientific community that the SARS-CoV-2 virus emerged in China, and specifically in Wuhan, and that the Huanan seafood market is likely to have been the source of the first known outbreak of disease, it is not at all clear that the first isolated and sporadic cases did originate in Wuhan, or even necessarily in China. Researchers examined the throat swab of a 4-year-old boy in Milan, Italy, obtained on December 5, 2019, after the boy was suspected to have had measles but tested negative for the measles virus. His symptoms began on November 21, with cough and inflammation of his nasal passages. Nine days later, he was taken to the emergency room with respiratory symptoms and vomiting. On December 1, he developed a measles-like rash. The throat swab was tested by PCR (polymerase chain reaction) and genetic sequencing techniques and was confirmed to contain SARS-CoV-2 genetic material. Unfortunately, the quality of the sample did not allow for testing to identify the country of origin of the virus, neither proving nor disproving its relationship to the Wuhan strain of SARS-CoV-2.[7]

The SARS-CoV-2 virus has retrospectively been identified in wastewater samples taken on December 18, 2019, in the cities of Milan and Turin in Italy, even though Italy would not recognize its first confirmed case until mid-February 2020. The virus was also detected in samples from patients hospitalized in France at the end of December 2019. There have been studies of blood donations in the United States that tested positive for the SARS-CoV-2 virus in that same month.

Although uncertainty remains as to when, where, and how the SARS-CoV-2 virus first infected a human, the assessment of the World

Health Organization and the majority opinion of scientists and US intelligence services is that SARS-CoV-2 was transmitted to a human from an animal. Because an animal source has not yet been identified (which is not unusual for epidemics and pandemics), and because a virology laboratory in Wuhan is known to have been conducting coronavirus research, there is speculation as to whether the first humans infected were those working at the Wuhan Institute of Virology and whether those individuals may then have transmitted the virus outside of the laboratory—the so-called lab-leak theory. Unfortunately, a lack of cooperation and transparency from the Chinese government has only heightened this concern.[8] It should be noted that at this time, there is no evidence to support a lab leak. The Wuhan Institute of Virology has denied working with the SARS-CoV-2 virus and asserted that stored samples of blood from the scientists working in the lab do not show serologic conversion prior to the time of the outbreak of COVID-19 in Wuhan. There is currently no publicly available evidence to controvert these assertions. Furthermore, the fact that we have identified two lineages of the SARS-CoV-2 virus circulating in Wuhan in some of the earliest samples we have would seem to strongly favor multiple spillover events from animals to humans over a lab leak.

While at this time we cannot be certain when or where the virus originated, the outbreak in Wuhan, China, is nevertheless the first such event observed. Our recommendations below continue to apply, because the observation of a such a specific outbreak probably will be the earliest and only opportunity to detect and react to a future pandemic. Isolated and sporadic cases that often precede an outbreak typically are not identified, as these cases were, for many weeks or even months after the pandemic is underway.

Recommendation #3
Establish Infection Control Measures in Wet Markets

The United States and the world's leaders must place pressure on China and Asian countries that have wet markets to develop and enforce public health measures to prevent the high-risk activities that create significant threats for zoonotic infections and the transmission of novel viruses.

In early January 2020, China, the World Health Organization, and other public health experts indicated that there was no evidence of human-to-human spread, which unfortunately was not only wrong but also likely caused many of us to underestimate the threat of this disease outside China. In retrospect, one wonders whether the best approach would have been to automatically assume human-to-human transmission, given that while 66 percent of patients reported a connection to the wet market, 34 percent did not.

Recommendation #4

Presume Contagiousness Until Proven Otherwise

With a novel virus that causes respiratory illness, especially one belonging to a family of viruses known to be infectious, we should presume human-to-human transmission is possible until proven otherwise.

Furthermore, there were reported infections in at least one of the patients' families and later other families that certainly should have increased the suspicion of person-to-person transmission. Of course, human-to-human transmission was all but certain when we later learned that 3,387 health care workers in China had been infected as of February 24. A subsequent report by the Chinese Red Cross Foundation, the National Health Commission of the People's Republic of China, and the public media noted that as of April 3, 23 of those 3,387 health care workers had died from infections that were tied to patient care.

In looking at the characteristics of these 23 health care workers who died, a predominance of male patients was once again noted. The median age was 55 years, and only slightly more than 20 percent were known to have underlying health conditions. The median time from the onset of symptoms to hospitalization, for those for whom data was available, was six days. The median time from hospitalization to death was 19 days, with a range of one to 47 days. Alarmingly, a range of serious conditions was noted in those who went on to die: septic shock, multiple organ dysfunction, cardiac injury, hypercoagulability (a condition of increased blood clot formation), intracardiac thrombus (blood clot inside the heart), and secondary bacterial infections.[9]

Unfortunately, the timing of this outbreak in Wuhan was probably the worst possible. The Chinese New Year, or Spring Festival, took place on January 25 in 2020. It is customary for Chinese people to travel to be with family for this holiday, and every year, millions do. In fact, one of China's major international airports is in Wuhan. Chinese officials locked down Wuhan on January 23, restricting all travel in and out of the city. However, by January 20, there were already reports of confirmed cases of COVID-19 in three countries—Japan, South Korea, and Thailand—with exposures related to travel to China or to someone who had recently traveled from China.

Recommendation #5
Immediate Targeted Lockdowns

With an estimated 4 million international travelers per day, health officials must act swiftly to lock down travel in and out of any area of the world with an outbreak of a novel virus. We must seek agreement from the world's leaders to cooperate in instituting travel restrictions as soon an outbreak of a novel virus is detected.

China's National Health Commission did not announce confirmed person-to-person transmission until January 21.[10] By this time, many people had likely already traveled, were in the process of traveling or were planning travel very shortly and would not have wanted to cancel their trip in light of this important holiday. The CDC did not confirm human-to-human transmission of SARS-CoV-2 until January 30, 2020, when a man living in Chicago tested positive after his wife returned from Wuhan and she became symptomatic with COVID-19.

The first case of confirmed COVID-19 in the United States was on January 20, 2020. A 35-year-old man was evaluated at an urgent care center in Washington State on January 19 with a four-day history of cough and fever. He reported having returned home to Washington on January 15 from a trip to Wuhan to visit his family. Although there were abnormal breath sounds when the urgent care provider listened to the patient's lungs, the oxygen saturation (level of oxygen in the blood) and a chest X-ray were normal. A rapid flu test was negative. In consultation with the CDC, it was decided that, despite the man denying that he visited the Huanan seafood market or came into contact with anyone known to be ill in China, he would be tested for SARS-CoV-2. There was only one test for SARS-CoV-2 available in the United States at the time, and it required the samples to be sent to the CDC in Atlanta for testing. The test was reported to be positive on January 20, again providing significant evidence for human-to-human transmission.

As a precaution, the man was admitted to an isolation unit in a hospital following the test results. He reported cough, nausea, and vomiting, but no chest pain or shortness of breath. The patient had intermittent fever and accelerated heart rate. On the second day of hospitalization, he complained of abdominal pain and passed a loose stool. Testing of the stool came back positive for the virus.

Between the third and fifth day of hospitalization (the seventh and ninth days of illness), the patient's laboratory testing revealed a low white blood count and platelet count (3,120 and 122,000, respectively; normal levels are generally greater than 5,000 and 150,000, respectively). By the evening of hospital day 5 (illness day 9), the patient developed radiographic evidence of pneumonia in the left lower lobe of the lung, coincident with a drop in oxygen saturation to 90 percent on room air (normal generally being considered 95 percent or greater).

By the next day, the patient required low-flow oxygen, and the chest X-ray revealed the appearance of atypical pneumonia with streaky infiltrates (white lines on the X-rays within the lungs that suggest inflammation or infection) at the bases of both lungs. Given the progression of his disease and reports from China of severe pneumonia progressing to acute respiratory distress syndrome, or ARDS (a condition in which the air sacs of the lungs fill with fluid and become unable of adequately oxygenating the blood often necessitating assistance with breathing, including the use of a ventilator), the patient received Remdesivir (an antiviral medication) through the US Food and Drug Administration (FDA)'s compassionate use exception for the use of an investigational drug.

By hospital day 8 (illness day 12), the patient was much improved, with the ability to maintain normal oxygen saturation without the use of oxygen.[11]

The first recognized case of COVID-19 in Europe was reported in France on January 24, related to travel to China. On January 28, Germany reported cases of COVID-19 that were related to a person visiting from China.

On January 30, the World Health Organization (WHO) declared the outbreak of the novel coronavirus a "public health emergency of international concern." By this time, the WHO was reporting approximately 7,800 cases of COVID-19, with 98 cases confirmed in 18 countries outside of China, and confirmed person-to-person spread in four countries—Germany, Japan, the United States and Vietnam.[12] In comparison, the SARS outbreak of 2003 only infected 8,098 people in total.

While it can be argued that with the delay in halting travel out of Wuhan, there was little that the United States could do to prevent cases of COVID-19 being imported across its borders, it is clear that the United States' response was too late and not enough. On January 17, the United States began screening passengers at three major international airports for flights from Wuhan to the United States—JFK International, San Francisco International and Los Angeles International airports. However, as mentioned above, the first case of confirmed COVID-19 in the United States was a man who returned from Wuhan on January 15. Second, it would be learned in February that many people can be infected with SARS-CoV-2 and be infectious, but also asymptomatic or presymptomatic (will become symptomatic, but have not yet), thus undermining the efforts made in passenger screenings at airports.

February 2020

President Trump issued an executive order on January 31 that would go into effect on February 2, restricting entry to the United States for anyone who had been in China within the preceding two weeks. However, the travel restrictions would prove largely unsuccessful, since they excepted US citizens and residents and family members of US citizens or residents. Furthermore, with several days' advance notice of travel restrictions, many people accelerated their travel plans so as to arrive in the United States prior to the restrictions going into effect.

While there is controversy over the effectiveness of travel restrictions, that may be in large part related to their delay in being implemented. However, if they are going to be employed, it is important to understand that from a virologic standpoint, there is no reason to believe that US citizens and their families would be less likely to bring the virus into the United States than foreign nationals.

Recommendation #6

Travel Restrictions Must Apply to All

If a travel restriction is to be used, US citizens returning home from a country where there has been an outbreak of infection must either be tested prior to entry, if a reliable test is available, or they should be quarantined for an appropriate amount of time prior to returning to their homes, families, friends, and work.

On February 3, 2020, the Trump administration declared a public health emergency. Unfortunately, testing in the United States was very limited. The CDC was the only laboratory in the country that could perform SARS-CoV-2 testing; because of this, the criteria for who could be tested were limited to those who were ill and had symptoms typical of COVID-19, almost certainly causing health officials to underestimate the amount of disease transmission occurring in the United States.

On February 5, the CDC sent a limited number of test kits to state, county, and city public health labs so that testing could be performed locally—but again, due to the limitations in testing kits, criteria were in place to limit those who would qualify for testing. But before testing could even begin locally, the majority of labs experienced problems in the verification process whereby they test samples known to be positive and samples known to be negative to determine if they come out with the correct result. Attributing the errors to problems with the reagents, the CDC suspended plans for local public health labs to conduct testing and resumed being the only laboratory in the country that could perform testing until the problems with the reagents could be worked out.[13]

Regrettably, the very limited testing available confounded efforts at contact tracing and made it impossible to know the extent of the spread of COVID-19 in the United States. While private and academic labs were more than willing to develop tests, FDA regulations created a significant burden upon being able to do so.

On February 26, the FDA and CDC determined that testing could resume with the CDC's test if laboratories simply did not use one of the four vials of reagents. On February 29, a little more than five weeks following the first case in the United States, the FDA granted permission for any laboratory certified for high-complexity testing to perform the SARS-CoV-2 tests, which meant many large hospital labs and commercial labs could now begin testing.

Nevertheless, there were limitations on the volume of tests that could be run, and backlogs of testing occurred. At times, people reported waiting one to two weeks, or even longer, to get test results back, and naturally delays of this magnitude undermined the effectiveness of contact tracing, isolation of those testing positive and quarantine of those who were close contacts.

In dealing with an outbreak of a new contagious disease, testing is of paramount importance. It allows us to identify the extent of disease activity, which can then inform public health actions. Testing is also critical to determine who needs to isolate themselves, and consequently who among their close contacts needs to quarantine, which is essential to containing the spread of disease. Without adequate, widely available, timely and reasonably accurate testing, all efforts to manage an outbreak will be undermined.

Recommendation #7
Promote Rapid Test Development

The regulatory scheme must be modified to allow for rapid testing development in the private and academic setting under the direction of the CDC. If the WHO should develop a test prior to the CDC, we must be willing to employ the WHO's test until such time as we develop a test with greater sensitivity or specificity, with more rapid turnaround, or at lower cost.

Allowing for the rapid development of testing by private and academic institutions under the direction of the CDC will avoid our country's reliance on a single test that leaves us with no other viable alternatives in the event of unforeseen technical difficulties. Moreover, the simultaneous development of multiple tests can aid in the production and distribution of tests to facilitate availability to large areas of the country quickly to allow us to begin identifying the true spread of disease.

It is in the best interests of the United States and the world to ensure that poor and developing countries have sufficient access to testing in order to promote efforts to contain the spread of disease in those countries, which might in turn threaten containment efforts elsewhere across the world through travel and/or the development of variants. The United States and other wealthy countries should partner with the WHO to make this testing available.

The United States should also invest in the rapid development of high-sensitivity and high-specificity tests to identify novel pathogens ahead of a future epidemic or pandemic. There should likewise be a focus on developing tests that are low-cost and low-complexity, with a rapid turnaround time, which would assist with screening travelers, patients and health care providers, but could easily be scaled up in production for screening of the general public.

The United States and other countries of the world must increase their capabilities to conduct genetic sequencing of the pandemic virus infecting their populations. This is especially true in the case of RNA viruses because of the inherently greater frequency of mutations during their replication and the resulting increased risk for the development of variants. We must monitor the emergence and prevalence of variants of concern, as they may cause an increase in transmissibility, more severe disease and/or partial immune evasion.

In the case of COVID-19, the key to the successful testing of those with symptoms and their close contacts in order to minimize the spread of the disease was making testing low-cost or no-cost, easily accessible, convenient, in a safe environment and with rapid turnaround times. One way this was achieved was by setting up drive-through testing sites, where those needing testing could remain in their cars and insurance companies agreed to cover the cost of this testing. It is critical to have federal and/or state funding to cover testing for the uninsured.

Other intermittent constraints on testing were created by shortages of personal protective equipment (PPE) and testing machines, test collection kits (such as swabs), viral transport media, reagents, and even pipettes. This was particularly frustrating because these shortages were experienced early on in the pandemic and public health officials repeatedly warned the public that disease activity would increase in the fall. Despite more than six months given to the government for planning, shortages continued to occur.

We must anticipate ongoing supply chain challenges during a pandemic. These supply chain issues may be exacerbated by the sudden increase in demand for the same products worldwide and by the pandemic's impact on countries that account for a disproportionate amount of the production of supplies or their raw materials. Lockdowns or outbreaks can impact the workforce at manufacturing plants and the shipping, air, and trucking distribution channels.

Recommendation #8

Defense Production Act

The president should be prepared to implement the Defense Production Act to address supply shortages, realizing that the normal supply chains are not designed for a sudden worldwide sharp increase in demand and are likely not to function as needed if there is no government intervention.

Although person-to-person spread had already been confirmed in the United States on January 30 based on transmission within a family from one spouse to another, the first documentation of community spread was reported in California on February 26, when a person with confirmed COVID-19 had no history of travel to a COVID-19 hot spot or exposure to someone known to have COVID-19.

March 2020

New York City identified its first reported case of COVID-19 on February 29 and confirmed it on March 1, and then experienced a sharp rise in cases the following week and a sharp rise in deaths the week after. New York City became one of the world's hot spots of disease activity, with cases overwhelming hospitals. Field hospitals were set up, and volunteer and contract health care workers came from around the country to assist in the care of patients. The deaths from COVID-19 in New York City on a per capita basis greatly exceeded the death rates for many countries, including China.

On March 11, 2020, the World Health Organization declared the SARS-CoV-2 outbreak a pandemic, with the director-general reporting that in the prior two weeks, the number of cases outside of China had increased 13-fold and the number of countries with cases had increased threefold. Interestingly and appropriately (as the director-general specifically and the WHO generally has previously been reluctant to criticize member countries), the director-general also stated that the WHO was "deeply concerned both by the alarming levels of spread and severity and by the alarming levels of inaction," and he called on countries to take action immediately to contain the spread of the virus. "We should be more aggressive."

Recommendation #9

Improve Communication and Coordination

Safeguards against the transmission and spread of a novel virus require the coordination of efforts across the globe. There must be strong information sharing among the WHO member countries and the public health organizations of those countries, and strong mitigation measures must be put in place swiftly.

As the authors of this book, in continuing to review this timeline, we might now find it useful to focus on specific events occurring in Idaho, our own backyard. Events were changing rapidly across the country, and Idaho's experience during this time illustrates the challenges experienced by many across the nation—and, for that matter, around the world.

The Idaho Department of Health and Welfare announced the first confirmed case of COVID-19 in the state of Idaho on March 13—a woman over the age of 50 who contracted the virus while attending a conference in New York City. At the time of Idaho's first case, there were 1,629 confirmed cases in the United States and 41 Americans had died from COVID-19.

Also on March 13, Idaho Governor Brad Little signed an emergency declaration that allowed for the activation of the Idaho Emergency Operations Plan, freeing up funds for use in the Idaho Emergency Disaster Fund and allowing Idaho the ability to obtain critical supplies from the Strategic National Stockpile (SNS)—twelve secret locations throughout the United States that store medical supplies and equipment and medications in the event of a national disaster or emergency.

Community spread was first reported in Idaho in Twin Falls and Blaine Counties on March 18, 2020.

While many schools had already closed or switched to fully remote learning, on March 23, the Idaho State Board of Education ordered all schools closed for in-person classes until at least April 20, but—in the first of what would become a frequent recurring inconsistency among school boards—sports practices and games were allowed to resume on April 6. Idaho was one of the last four states in the United States to officially close its schools.[14]

On March 25, Governor Little issued a statewide stay-at-home order calling for the closure of non-essential businesses, a ban on all non-essential gatherings and for people to work from home when possible. Essential businesses that were permitted to remain open included grocery stores, health care facilities, all utilities, gas stations, financial institutions and residential and home-based care. Restaurants were permitted to offer curbside and delivery services. Citizens were instructed to physically distance themselves from others with whom they did not live except when walking outside. Non-essential travel was prohibited.

The first deaths in Idaho from COVID-19 were reported on March 26 and involved three unrelated males.

April 2020

Initially, public health officials discouraged the use of masks by the public, fearing that individuals would compete for a limited supply of surgical and N95 face masks needed by health care providers. At that time, while there were reported cases of asymptomatic or pre-symptomatic individuals transmitting SARS-CoV-2,[15] it was not initially appreciated how significant the role of transmission from asymptomatic individuals was (40 to 45 percent of individuals infected with COVID-19 may be contagious, though asymptomatic[16]) and, therefore, how important the role masks or face coverings would play in the containment of the spread of the virus. At that time, we also had little appreciation for the role that airborne transmission played in spreading SARS-CoV-2, and we did not fully realize how protective masks would be for both the wearer of the mask and the individuals that person came into contact with.

Unfortunately, when the CDC changed its position and began encouraging the widespread use of face coverings on April 3, for some people, this contributed to a lack of trust in public health guidance. For others who did not want mask wearing to be mandated, this change in position became a convenient excuse for not wearing a mask, with an argument along the lines of "Even health officials cannot agree or make up their minds about masks, so they should not be mandated."

The stay-at-home order in Idaho remained in effect through to the end of April. It was clearly effective in reducing cases of COVID-19 in Idaho (a process also referred to as "flattening the curve"). The peak number of cases by date of report to the state during this initial onset of the pandemic was on April 2, when 222 new cases were reported. By May 1, as seen in figure 1.1, the number of new cases reported was down to 20.

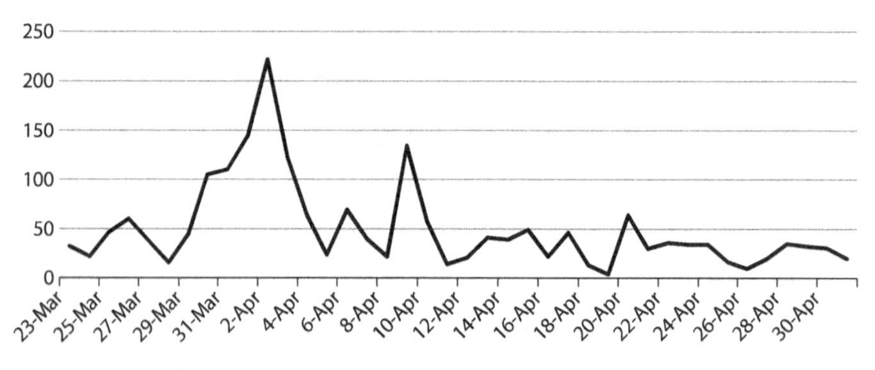

Figure 1.1. The fluctuations of new daily cases by date of report to the State of Idaho, from March 23, 2020, to April 30, 2020.

May 2020

It was on May 1 that Governor Little terminated the stay-at-home order and began moving the state of Idaho through four stages of what was called "Idaho Rebounds," through progressive "Stay Healthy" orders.

There is no doubt that the stay-at-home orders significantly diminished the spread of the coronavirus. However, it also led to a loss of employment and some businesses. Despite this, Idaho's economy has ranked among the top state economies, depending upon the measure selected. In a press release issued on September 18, 2020, Governor Little attributed Idaho's top rankings in economic prosperity to six factors:

1. "Idaho has responsibly managed the pandemic response.
2. Idaho has prioritized direct support for Idaho businesses and citizens in the allocation of federal coronavirus relief funds.
3. Idaho has cut red tape to ease the burden on businesses and strengthen the coronavirus response.
4. Idaho has demonstrated fiscal conservatism in the state budget.
5. Idaho has made historic investments in K–12 education during the pandemic to support students, families, and a strong economic rebound.
6. Idaho has prioritized transparency and has engaged the business community and experts in all aspects of the coronavirus response."[17]

No doubt the resilience of the Idaho economy was likely in part due to its strength going into the pandemic, with some giving Idaho the top spot among US states.[18]

Another consequence of the stay-at-home orders was what came to be known as "COVID fatigue," a yearning for a return to "normalcy" and defiance of public health advice that asked people to wash or sanitize their hands frequently, cover their coughs and sneezes, stay home when possible (especially if they were sick), clean frequently touched surfaces, avoid large gatherings and, if they were going indoors, maintain a physical distance of at least six feet from others with whom they did not live and wear a face covering when that was not possible. Over the course of 2020, we would see flagrant noncompliance with this advice—including parties, weddings, sleepovers, large numbers of people at sporting events standing shoulder-to-shoulder, and gatherings for backyard barbeques. People refused to wear face coverings altogether, alleging that their religious or Constitutional freedoms were being violated, that masks didn't work, that people were breathing in unsafe levels of carbon dioxide while wearing a mask, that there were various questionable medical reasons why they could not wear a mask, that people were passing out while wearing masks, and that COVID-19 was no worse than the flu. Additionally, the widespread dissemination of misleading and false information, especially through social media, significantly thwarted the efforts of doctors and public health officials to provide accurate information and education. In fact, in some cases, it was health care professionals themselves that contributed to the false or misleading information.

A commonly made suggestion was that the elderly should remain sequestered at home, since they are "high risk," and that younger people should be allowed to return to their normal lifestyles. In fact, it might be desirable—or so the argument went—for young and middle-aged adults to get infected to achieve "herd immunity." Arguments to this effect were even made by certain White House advisors. There were several flaws with this argument, but however often we pointed out these flaws, we were never able to persuade those who advocated for this strategy.

The first problem was the meaning of the phrase "high risk." Health care and public health officials tried to educate the public as to who was considered at high risk of severe illness and potentially death: namely, the elderly and those with chronic medical conditions, such as diabetes, obesity, cancer, chronic kidney disease, chronic obstructive pulmonary disease, various heart conditions, underlying immune disorders, and sickle cell disease, as well as those who were immunocompromised by medications.[19] What it appears that many heard was that people not in this group—young and middle-aged adults who were otherwise healthy—were not at significant risk of getting ill or being hospitalized with COVID-19. There was certainly some truth to this, but while most young, healthy people did have mild illness, for reasons that still elude us at the time we write this, there have been young adults who have ended up with severe illness and been hospitalized, requiring intensive care and, in some cases, mechanical ventilation. In some cases, they died. Furthermore, what started out as a virus that produced respiratory illness was soon discovered to be manifesting itself in a multitude of other ways that are quite concerning. More on this follows in the chapters below.

Second, throughout the pandemic, we saw how difficult it was to actually keep the elderly and those with multiple chronic illnesses in a "bubble"—the term used to describe the sequestering of people to avoid exposure to the SARS-CoV-2 virus. We saw time and time again that those in communal settings—long-term care facilities, prisons, and so forth—were exposed to the virus and became ill less often due to a new resident or prisoner being introduced to the facility and more often the young people who served as staff in these facilities, who would acquire the infection through activities outside of work and then expose the residents or prisoners when they came to work. Such staff members could often be contagious but not yet symptomatic, or infected and "pauci-symptomatic"—meaning that the symptoms were mild, perhaps overlooked, leading them to assume that they had overdone things or not gotten enough rest or that the symptoms were caused by something else, such as allergies.

Elderly people and people with multiple chronic illnesses who did not live in communal settings often felt the need to go to the grocery store, or their dentist's or doctor's office. There were varying degrees of compliance with mask mandates even in those cities or counties that had issued these requirements, but there were far more cities and counties that had no mandate.

Additionally, during the pandemic, in what has been described as an epidemic of isolation, loneliness, and mental health issues, elderly grandparents longed for the opportunities to visit with family and their grandchildren. In some cases, appropriate precautions were exercised, but in other situations—either through misunderstanding what precautions were needed or a common misperception that family members would be unlikely sources of the virus—many seniors were infected, even though they believed they were employing precautionary measures.

Time and time again, throughout the course of this pandemic, we would see surges in the numbers of cases, followed by increases in the number of hospitalizations and then finally an increase in the numbers of deaths. This was especially the case following holidays, where it is traditional for friends and family to come together, and many continued to meet up through the pandemic, despite pleas from public health officials not to do so.

The third problem with the argument was the belief of some that achieving herd immunity through natural infection would be a desirable way to bring an end to the pandemic. While there are disagreements as to whether this was or was not Sweden's attempted strategy, Sweden's approach most resembled what a country would do if this was the strategy, and we will discuss the outcome of that experiment in chapter 12.

There were many problems with this proposed strategy. First, in the modern era of vaccines, we could not come up with an example of another viral disease for which herd immunity has been achieved through natural infection. Certainly, neither the United States nor the world has ever achieved herd immunity with any other known coronavirus. Second, no one knows the level of population immunity required for herd immunity for this novel virus. Given that the R-naught (R_0 or reproduction number) was 2.2–2.7—and there are some that believe the true number could be almost double this due to instances of so-called super spreaders, who ended up infecting large numbers of people—at the beginning of the outbreak, with no one having preexisting immunity and no mitigation measures in place, a person infected with SARS-CoV-2 would be expected to infect 2.2 to 2.7 additional people. According to the mathematical model, herd immunity would thus require roughly 60 percent of the population to be immune to safeguard vulnerable individuals within the herd from infection. We note that while these data points were based upon the original SARS-CoV-2 virus circulating at that time, variants have arisen due to the uncontrolled transmission of the virus across the world. Some of these variants have enhanced transmissibility, and because of this biological advantage, they have become the dominant forms of the virus in many parts of the world. An increase in contagiousness or transmissibility means that the reproductive number has increased. The so-called Delta variant is currently rising in prevalence in the United States and is known to be considerably more transmissible, with a reproduction number estimated to be as high as 7 or 8. It is now anticipated that herd immunity may require up to 85 percent of the population to be immune, though there is increasing skepticism as to whether herd immunity can ever be achieved with this virus.

Though New York City became an epicenter of COVID-19 activity in March of 2020, with overwhelmed hospitals and health care workers and an excessive mortality rate compared to many other countries, including China, a seroprevalence study conducted in New York City at the end of March indicated that only 22.7 percent of the population had antibodies to the SARS-CoV-2 spike protein.[20] If the mathematical projections were anywhere near correct in the estimation of immunity required in the population for herd immunity, New York City was far from reaching it. Therefore, those who advocated for this strategy risked overwhelming the country's health care system and causing large numbers of deaths, not to mention incurring the health care costs that would be associated with such resource-intensive hospital care.

These arguments in support of herd immunity, some of which continued to be made in the White House, became even more outrageous and irresponsible as we entered into clinical trials for vaccines and two mRNA vaccines were shown to be safe and effective in phase 3 trials, ultimately receiving emergency use authorizations from the FDA before the end of 2020.

The fourth problem with the arguments in favor of achieving herd immunity through natural infection was a huge problem concerning the very foundation of herd immunity—individual immunity. In 2020, we simply did not know whether people who recovered from SARS-CoV-2 infection were immune; whether everyone was immune, including those with asymptomatic or mild infections, and if so, for how long; or whether natural immunity would be protective against the variants that would develop over time. We certainly could detect antibodies to the spike protein in most people following infection, but conveying to the public that the presence of antibodies does not necessarily mean immunity was a challenging task, the message being contrary to commonly held beliefs. Furthermore, with continued high levels of disease transmission around the globe, many new variants of concern have emerged, and no doubt more will continue to develop, some already demonstrating a degree of immune escape/evasion. Unless immunity to the wild-type virus or prior variants continues to protect the population from these new variants, any herd immunity developed by the population will be short-lived if new variants spread and have significant and effective immune evasion/escape capabilities.

Explaining to the public that not all antibodies are created equal and that the body produces a wide array of antibodies in response to an infection, not all of which may be protective against subsequent infection, was very difficult, especially at a time when others were promoting antibody tests as a way to determine whether a prior illness was a "cold" or COVID-19, whether they were now protected and as a way to be cleared to return to work. This was further complicated by the fact that due to many challenges with having adequate testing available, the FDA allowed several of these tests to enter the market without their authorization or approval. Many tests were available with widely varying sensitivity and specificity levels established by their manufacturers, which could not always be substantiated when tested by third parties.

Early studies showed that while most (but not all) persons mounted an IgG antibody response to infection, few people made high levels of neutralizing antibodies and most people made some, but lower levels. Furthermore, antibody titers tended to decline significantly over two to three months, with some people becoming seronegative. While these data were generally discouraging, we still did not know the indicators of immunity for this disease; therefore, while we suspected that any immunity gained from natural infection might be short-lived (on the order of perhaps three to six months, as is typical for other more common coronaviruses), declining levels of IgG antibodies would not necessarily imply a loss of immunity, especially given that we had little data on the cellular immune response to this disease. We would subsequently learn that the protection provided by the mRNA vaccines was far more robust than expected, with adequate protection maintained at one year and many speculating that protection may last for a number of years, and that in those persons who had COVID-19 and subsequently were vaccinated, there might even be lifetime protection.

Though it was difficult to document cases of reinfection, as testing was generally done through nucleic acid amplification methods (such as PCR testing), which did not preserve a sample of the virus for genetic sequencing, there have been, as of the time of this writing, 149 documented cases of reinfection worldwide, with three resulting in death, and 71,931 suspected cases of reinfection worldwide, with 277 resulting in death. Supporting our impressions that immunity from the SARS-CoV-2 virus infection may be short-lived, the average time interval between infection and reinfection for the confirmed cases was 115 days.[21] While with other infections, we often see that a reinfection is milder than the initial infection, that was not true in every case with COVID-19, including instances where the reinfection was serious enough to require hospitalization and three cases of documented reinfection in which the patient died as a consequence of the reinfection.

The fifth problem was that while many of those who advocated for a rush to herd immunity through natural infection considered the US case fatality rate at the time of 1.77 percent to be acceptably low, there was generally no consideration of or accounting given to the emerging evidence of morbidity associated with COVID-19.

It became clear with time that what initially appeared to be a respiratory virus was really a respiratory and vascular virus, one capable of creating havoc with the immune system, driving it into overdrive in certain individuals.

One feared complication of COVID-19 is the development of acute respiratory distress syndrome (ARDS) due to the high mortality rate. A segment of the population of those COVID-19 patients with ARDS that have an even higher mortality rate are those with an elevated D-dimer blood test (D-dimer is a protein that is released into the blood with the breakdown of blood clots; an elevated level of D-dimer in the blood suggests that the patient is forming abnormal blood clots, which the body's natural processes are then attempting to break down).

In one study, 94 percent of patients with ARDS and an elevated D-dimer blood test had evidence of bilateral thromboembolic disease (blood clots) in the lungs.[22] A study of the lungs in ten African American patients with COVID-19 revealed microvascular platelet-rich depositions in the small vessels of the lungs reminiscent of thrombotic microangiopathy. Most readers will have heard of people who have had blood clots in their lungs—pulmonary emboli. Those are large blood clots that travel to the lungs and land in large blood vessels of the lungs. In this case, these were small clots, mostly made up of platelets that clogged up very small blood vessels, likely due to abnormalities of those blood vessels themselves, and thus these clots formed in the lungs.[23]

Vascular complications that have developed in patients with COVID-19 have included acute limb ischemia (decreased blood flow, generally to the legs), abdominal and thoracic aortic thromboses (blood clots in the body's largest artery in the abdomen or in the chest coming off of the heart), mesenteric ischemia (reduced blood flow to the blood vessels that supply the gut), myocardial infarction (heart attack), deep venous thrombosis or thromboembolism (blood clots in the veins of the legs that in some cases may break off and travel to the lungs), and acute cerebrovascular accidents (strokes).[24]

We have also seen a peculiar illness in children two to four weeks following a COVID-19 illness that resembles a combination of Kawasaki disease and toxic shock syndrome. Signs and symptoms include fever, abdominal (stomach) pain, a rash, bloodshot eyes, vomiting, diarrhea, and profound weakness. It has been named multisystem inflammatory syndrome in children, MIS-C. As of the time of this writing, there have been at least 4,018 cases in the United States, resulting in 36 deaths. Most cases have occurred in male children (60 percent), with half of all cases occurring between the ages of 5 to 13, with an average age of 9 years. Curiously, it has disproportionately affected Hispanic, Latino, and Black children (62 percent of cases).[25] Since June of 2020, we have also seen a similar illness in a small number of adults. That illness has been named multisystem inflammatory syndrome in adults, or MIS-A.

Another complication of COVID-19 can be myocarditis (an inflammation of the heart muscle). The first case of COVID-19 infection noted to cause myocarditis was in a patient that resulted in fulminant myocarditis. The case was reported on April 10 in a 63-year-old man with no history of heart disease or underlying hypertension. This patient had elevated levels of the heart muscle protein, troponin, in his blood, enlargement of part of his heart, low pumping movement of his heart muscle and the pumping effectiveness of his heart was reduced by 40 to 50 percent (left ventricular ejection fraction 32 percent). In this particular case, the patient's heart function largely recovered; however, he died of secondary infection on the 33rd day of hospitalization.[26] Since then, numerous cases of clinical and subclinical myocarditis have been detected on cardiac MRIs of student and professional athletes, many of whom were undergoing return to sports evaluations. Currently, we do not know the duration or long-term implications of COVID-19 myocarditis; however, there have been cases of sudden death, likely due to associated arrhythmia (irregular or abnormal heartbeats).

Although many have raised concerns about the mental health impacts resulting from school closures, wearing masks, and isolation, very few of these discussions were balanced with considerations of psychiatric and neuropsychiatric complications resulting from COVID-19, not to mention the mental health consequences resulting from the loss of family members due to COVID-19, especially in those family members who learn that they were the likely source of exposure for that family member's illness and resulting death. While we still do not have an adequate understanding of the long-term psychiatric and neuropsychiatric sequelae resulting from the direct infection of brain cells by the SARS-CoV-2 virus or the indirect immunologic injury to brain cells resulting from infection, early studies suggest that 20 to 40 percent of COVID-19 cases may present with neuropsychiatric complications, including headache, dizziness, stroke, loss of smell and or taste, mood disturbances, or encephalopathy.[27] More recently, concern has been raised that some patients are displaying Parkinson's disease-like manifestations following infection as well as long-term neurocognitive deficits, including the potential for the development of dementia based upon findings of loss of grey matter in memory-related areas of the brain after infection in some patients.

It is not within the scope of this book to fully discuss all of the complications and long-term effects from COVID-19, but we do want to point out one more morbidity associated with COVID. It goes by various names, including long COVID, chronic COVID, post-acute COVID or long haulers' syndrome, but recently it has been given an official name of post-acute sequelae of SARS-CoV-2 infection, or PASC.

Many young, previously healthy, and active individuals have described disabling long-term effects of their COVID-19 infection, and a recent study estimated the prevalence of PASC among those infected with SARS-CoV-2 at 30.3 percent.[28] Even though many described their infections as mild and certainly not requiring hospitalization, these disabling symptoms lasted for months and, in many cases, have continued to persist.

These patients have not yet been systematically studied, and there are challenges to understanding what is going on because not everyone had confirmed infection; many were likely infected during the initial surge in cases when testing was difficult to obtain or when they had symptoms that were not on our early symptom lists, having only been recognized later. Furthermore, many of these patients do not have positive antibody tests either, which we know happens in some cases of infection and perhaps has some relationship to the symptoms these patients are experiencing. Interestingly, in a study of 1,400 long-haulers, two-thirds of those who underwent antibody testing had negative antibody tests, including some who had previously documented positive PCR tests.

The symptoms experienced by these patients are wide-ranging, and it seems as though no two patients are alike. However, what is common among many of these patients is what they describe as a marked change compared to their "pre-COVID" status, and oftentimes quite disabling symptoms. These have included:

- Anxiety, depression, and other psychiatric manifestations
- Awakening with shortness of breath
- Burning sensations in the tips of their fingers and/or toes
- Diarrhea

- Discomfort with taking a deep breath
- Extreme fatigue, with one patient describing it as too exhausting to take showers; some describe being unable to stand for long periods of time
- Hair loss
- Hand tremors
- Headaches, often throbbing
- Heavy menstrual periods or loss of menstrual periods
- Insomnia
- Memory loss—"brain fog"—a combination of short-term memory loss and inability to focus
- Nausea
- Night sweats
- Palpitations, tachycardia (rapid heartbeat)
- Persistent anosmia (loss of smell) and/or ageusia (loss of taste)
- Persistent fevers
- Seizures
- Sensitivity to light and/or sound
- Shortness of breath, getting winded walking up stairs
- Tendency toward bruising

It is hard to know exactly how many people have been affected by these "post-COVID" symptoms, as there is no standard definition for them and no central repository for reporting them, but it is believed that PASC affects more than 90,000 people in almost 100 countries, including the United States, United Kingdom, India, France, Finland, Senegal, and South Africa.

Interestingly, while most people consider those in their thirties and forties to be of "low risk" for severe COVID-19 and death, the average age of these long-haulers has been 38, and while men tend to have worse outcomes and more severe illness with COVID-19 infection, it is women who constitute the majority of recognized long-haulers. A recent study raises the possibility that Epstein-Barr virus (EBV) reactivation may play a role in the development of PASC, in that 66.7 percent of study subjects with PASC had serologic evidence of EBV reactivation (EBV early antigen-diffuse IgG or EBV viral capsid antigen IGM) compared to only 10 percent in the control group ($p < 0.001$).[29]

New York City's Mount Sinai Hospital is one of the first hospitals in the country to establish a post-COVID clinic. They have reported seeing this predominance of PASC in women, and the average age of their patients was reported as 44. Dr. David Putrino, who runs this clinic, has indicated that many long-haulers have symptoms that resemble dysautonomia, an umbrella term for disorders that disturb the autonomic nervous system, which controls bodily functions such as breathing, blood pressure, heart rate, and digestion. It remains unclear whether the virus itself causes damage that results in these long-term effects, or whether these long-term consequences are a result of an overactive or exaggerated immune response, despite the failure to develop an antibody response or the loss of antibodies once produced.

More than 90 percent of long-haulers whom Putrino has worked with also have "post-exertional malaise," in which even mild bouts of physical or mental exertion can trigger a severe physiological crash. "We're talking about walking up a flight of stairs and being out of commission for two days," Putrino said. This is the defining symptom of myalgic encephalomyelitis, or chronic fatigue syndrome. The CDC has had little to say on this subject, but it acknowledges that 35 percent of COVID-19 patients, even those with mild illness, do not recover even after three weeks.

There are few clinical studies on these patients. Here are results of some of the few studies that have been done.

1. One report is from patients themselves out of the United States. A patient-led research team conducted an open survey on Facebook and published the results.[32] The most common symptoms reported were (in descending order) fatigue, muscle or body aches, shortness of breath or difficulty breathing, difficulty concentrating or focusing, inability to exercise or be active and headaches.
2. A study out of Germany[30] examined the cardiac MRIs of 100 people who had recovered from COVID-19 and compared them to heart images from 100 people who were similar but not infected with the virus. The average age of the study group

was 49 and two-thirds of the patients had mild illness and recovered at home, while 33 percent were hospitalized. More than two months later (median time interval from diagnosis with infection to the MRI evaluation was 79 days), infected patients were more likely to have troubling cardiac signs than people in the control group: 78 patients showed structural changes to their hearts, 76 had evidence of a substance in their blood signaling cardiac injury typically found after a heart attack, and 60 had signs of ongoing inflammation of their heart muscle.

3. An Italian study[31] showed that 87.4 percent of hospitalized patients (mean age 56.5 years) still had at least one symptom, and often a variety of symptoms, after two months since the onset of their initial symptoms of infection. The most common symptoms were fatigue and shortness of breath.
4. A researcher from the Indiana University School of Medicine surveyed 1,500 long-haulers from Survivor Corps, an online COVID-19 support group, in July 2020. They reported almost 100 distinct symptoms, from anxiety and fatigue to muscle cramps and breathing problems.[32]

Recommendation #10

Avoid Strategies to Achieve Herd Immunity through Natural Infection

Communicate clearly to the public the unintended consequences of prematurely returning to normal activities with the intent of developing herd immunity through natural infection.

Strategies to achieve herd immunity through natural infection may not be attainable, and in fact may be very dangerous. At the very least, this has proved to be an unsuccessful strategy with a highly transmissible virus that led to severe illness and mortality in a substantial part of the population. Early on in an epidemic or pandemic with a novel virus, it may not yet be clear what the long-term health consequences of infection are. With COVID-19, many of the long-term consequences of infection remain unclear. A herd immunity strategy by promoting natural infection may result in tremendous morbidity, loss of employee productivity, and significant long-term health care costs. One must also consider the risks, especially with RNA viruses, of promoting the development of variants that may escape or partially escape immunity with uncontrolled disease transmission.

When people advocate for a strategy of achieving herd immunity through natural infection by promoting a loosening of restrictions on children and young and middle-aged adults, while sequestering the elderly and those with multiple chronic illnesses, we must consider not only the mortality rate, but also the morbidity that those who become infected may suffer. Furthermore, we must acknowledge our lack of success in keeping the elderly and other high-risk individuals in "bubbles" and the consequence that many of these higher-risk individuals will invariably end up infected. Meanwhile, the social isolation of the elderly may have many deleterious effects, including depression and delayed health care services accompanied by poorer outcomes.

We have experienced hospitals becoming overwhelmed in the United States, as well as a number of countries across the world, when disease transmission is unchecked. Overwhelmed hospitals are associated with increases in mortality rates not only for those infected, but also for those with other time-sensitive emergencies and critical conditions. Overwhelmed hospitals often care for patients in nontraditional care spaces and with additional staff that may not be as expert or experienced in critical care. When non-clinical spaces in hospitals are converted into patient care space for an overflow of critically ill patients, there may not be ideal visualization of all patients and these spaces may not have the same patient alarms as traditional spaces, or else those alarms may not be monitored or easily heard throughout the expanded area, which may lead to a patient's sudden deterioration not being recognized in a timely fashion. It is also important to keep in mind that uncontrolled disease transmission will result in many health care workers being infected early on in the pandemic in hospital settings, but as the pandemic progresses, these staff are more often infected in their communities and families. Absences of staff due to illness (isolation) or exposure (quarantine) further exacerbate the ability of hospitals to care for a large influx of patients.

Finally, we must consider the complications and long-term health effects from infection in terms of the attendant increase in health care costs, potential loss of insurability, decreased productivity in the workplace, and potential increased need for disability benefits, especially in young and middle-aged adults who may be at the peak of their workplace productivity and contributions, as well as the impact this may have on their families.

If a herd immunity through natural infection strategy is going to be considered, it is important to understand not only the mortality of the novel pathogen, but also the morbidity. Such a strategy should not be undertaken unless (1) it is clear that natural infection produces an effective and durable immune response in those who have become infected; (2) effective therapeutics have been identified or developed; and (3) it is clear that a safe and effective vaccine is not likely within a reasonable amount of time. In the event that these conditions are met and a decision is made to pursue herd immunity, it is critical to engage in this process in a stepwise fashion while closely monitoring the rate of new cases and the impact on the health care system, in order to temporarily pull back and reinstate restrictions if cases accelerate too quickly and either excessive numbers of health care workers are being infected or hospital capacity is being strained.

Recommendation #11
Protect High-Risk Individuals

The communication of public health measures must also include additional guidance for those who are at high risk, including those who are immunocompromised. Messages to the general public must explain the importance of compliance with public health measures among those believed not to be at high risk in order to protect those who are at high risk.

Recommendation #12
Accelerate Trials of Therapeutics and the Development of Vaccines

Begin trials of convalescent plasma, monoclonal antibodies, and antivirals as soon as possible. Provide incentives for pharmaceutical companies to develop a wide variety of potential vaccines, and get those vaccines into clinical trials as soon as possible.

There are hundreds of ongoing clinical trials in search of effective treatments for COVID-19. There is currently only one drug approved by the FDA for the treatment of COVID-19 and six therapies authorized for use by the FDA pursuant to emergency use authorizations.

The only medication approved by the FDA for use in treating COVID-19 is an antiviral drug, Remdesivir, and this is limited to adults and children over the age of 12 who are hospitalized (there is an authorization for children younger than 12 years old who weigh at least 3.5 kilograms). You may recall that this drug was used under a compassionate use exception in treating the first patient with COVID-19 in the United States. It is approved only for hospitalized adults and children of at least 12 years of age.

The six authorized treatments include the following:

- Convalescent plasma for use in hospitalized patients
- Bamlanivimab and Etesevimab (monoclonal antibodies), authorized for use together in mild to moderate COVID-19 in patients over the age of 12 years who are at high risk of progressing to severe disease or hospitalization, but who are not yet hospitalized or requiring supplemental oxygen
- Tocilizumab (monoclonal antibody), authorized for use in adults and children over the age of 2 who are receiving systemic corticosteroids and require supplemental oxygen, non-invasive mechanical ventilation or extracorporeal membrane oxygenation
- Sotrovimab (monoclonal antibody), authorized for the treatment of mild to moderate COVID-19 in adults and children over the age of 12 years who are at high risk of progression to severe disease
- Baricitinib (a Janus kinase inhibitor—this drug modulates the inflammatory process by interfering with a protein that contributes to inflammation by cytokines and other mediators of the inflammatory response), authorized for the treatment of patients over the age of 2 years who are hospitalized and require either supplemental oxygen, mechanical ventilation or extracorporeal membrane oxygenation

- Casirivimab plus Imdevimab (monoclonal antibodies), authorized for use in combination for the treatment of patients with mild to moderate COVID-19 who are over the age of 12 years who are not hospitalized but are determined to be at high risk of progressing to severe and/or hospitalization

In addition, studies have shown the significant benefits of dexamethasone for patients who are hospitalized with severe COVID-19.

An interesting and perplexing part of the story of the development of therapeutics was the touting of the use of hydroxychloroquine for prevention and treatment of COVID-19 by two of the world's leaders—the presidents of the United States and Brazil—with no scientific data to show the safety or efficacy of the drug for these purposes. Unfortunately, these sensational claims led to shortages of the drug (which has been in use for many years in treating patients with conditions like systemic lupus erythematosus and rheumatoid arthritis), compromising the availability of the medication for these patients and causing significant price hikes for the medication. There have also been reports of counterfeit drugs being sold on the black market. Subsequent clinical studies have not been able to show any benefits of hydroxychloroquine in preventing or treating COVID-19.

At one time, President Trump indicated that he was taking hydroxychloroquine as a measure to avoid contracting COVID-19. The president, as well as many in the White House, in his cabinet, and in the Republican Party, declined to follow public health advice. They were rarely seen wearing masks and often disregarded advice concerning physical distancing and limitations on the size of gatherings.

While non-pharmaceutical interventions (NPIs) may have been a new concept for many and were scoffed at by some, these measures, such as covering coughs and sneezes, wearing a mask or face covering, physical distancing, limiting the size of gatherings, and washing hands frequently, were interventions that were used with the 1918 Spanish flu pandemic and epidemics and pandemics since then, such as SARS in 2003—interventions known for more than 100 years to be effective in limiting the spread of respiratory infections and credited with bringing these pandemics and epidemics to an end. Thus, it was all the more surprising to see many of our leaders either forgetting these lessons learned from past pandemics or simply rejecting them out of hand. But both the failure to learn from these past pandemics and epidemics and the rejection of those lessons have consequences.

It was disclosed on October 1, 2020, that the president and First Lady had both tested positive for the SARS-CoV-2 virus. The president was subsequently flown to Walter Reed National Military Medical Center, where he was treated with Remdesivir and monoclonal antibodies. The president was subsequently reported to have made a full recovery. While the White House was frequently testing the president and reportedly testing all those who were coming in contact with him, and while many in the public advocated for a testing strategy that would allow life to return to "normal," the infection of the president served as an important reminder that testing can certainly be an important adjunct to our public health measures, but it is not a substitute for following the public health guidance. As one of us often informed the public, "We cannot test our way out of the pandemic."

It is not clear whether the president's illness convinced, or at least silenced, many of the so-called COVID deniers, who disavowed the reality of COVID-19. It is also not clear whether the president's illness caused more people to exercise precautions or whether his recovery, especially considering the president was in the "high risk" category, gave more credence to the arguments that COVID-19 was not serious—"It is no worse than the flu." Unfortunately, it would not be revealed to the public just how concerned President Trump's treating physicians were that he might require mechanical ventilation or might not survive until June 2021, when it was revealed by two *Washington Post* reporters in a book.[33]

Presumably, the president's illness had little effect on the population's adoption of public health measures, because cases continued to soar during the fall to the point that hospital capacity, particularly the availability of beds in intensive care units (ICUs), became strained across the country in November and December. Faced with the combination of record-setting numbers of patients hospitalized and large numbers of health care workers isolated due to infections that in most cases were acquired outside of the hospital and not related to patient care, or in quarantine due to close contacts, hospitals cancelled elective procedures, worked to repurpose areas of the hospital for use as intensive care units, hired agency staff, and prepared their plans for "crisis standards of care."

In Idaho, a committee of health care professionals set out crisis standards of care that would allow hospitals and physicians to prioritize limited resources—ration them to those that appeared more likely to survive. In the event that all of the hospitals of an entire region of the state or the entire state became overwhelmed, the director of the Department of Health and Welfare would make a declaration that these standards were in effect, providing liability protections to these overwhelmed hospitals and the physicians caring for these patients. The failure to provide these resources during normal times, when the resources could prove lifesaving, would be a breach of the standard of care that could serve as the basis for a liability claim. Therefore, the declaration by the state or the state's governor of "crisis standards of care," to modify this standard of care and provide liability protections, were critical in protecting health care providers who had to implement these new standards from liability in lawsuits filed by the families of those patients who could not receive needed resources under these dire circumstances.

We ended 2020 with the good news that two safe and effective COVID-19 vaccines had started to be distributed and administered, and that a third would be authorized in 2021. At that time, due to limitations of the supply of the vaccine, those being vaccinated were health care workers and residents of long-term care facilities, according to a vaccine prioritization system recommended by the Advisory Committee on Immunization Practices (ACIP) and refined and implemented by the states.

CHAPTER 2

Pandemic Surveillance and Early Response in the Future

Let us not look back in anger or forward in fear, but around in awareness.

JAMES THURBER

We have had many opportunities to learn throughout this pandemic that we live in a globalized and interconnected world. That it does not take long for a new threat emerging on the other side of the world, with oceans separating us, to infiltrate our own borders and penetrate every area of our country, including our rural communities, is a lesson we hope is learned from this pandemic. This is why we must improve our surveillance of potential threats and respond much earlier, if we are to have a chance of preventing a novel virus from spreading across the United States—or, if not preventing it, at least slowing it down to allow us more time to learn about it, prepare for it, protect ourselves from it, and begin the process of developing therapeutics and vaccines. Of course, we must also appreciate that while developing countries and countries that engage in high-risk interactions with animals are at the greatest risk of being the site of the world's next pandemic, we cannot rule out the possibility that a new infectious pathogen might originate in the United States.

There are devasting consequences for delayed reaction to a novel virus, including millions of infections across the world, potentially overwhelming our health care delivery systems, leading to excess deaths, creating shortages of supplies and medicines, causing disruptions to economies worldwide that lead to unemployment and bankrupt businesses, and fundamentally impairing the education of our children and grandchildren. Furthermore, delays in an adequate response to a novel virus threaten to accelerate isolation and the resulting aggravation of underlying mental health conditions, as well as increase the potential of complications and long-term health effects in those who have been infected. And finally, a delayed response to such a virus will result in soaring current and future health care costs.

We must also consider the disruption to the world's governments and the possible national security threats that occur when the leaders of those governments potentially become infected, require hospitalization, or even die. During this pandemic, presidents or prime ministers in at least 13 countries were diagnosed with COVID-19, including Brazil, France, the United Kingdom, and the United States.

So, what must we do to detect and perhaps prevent the next pandemic threat and to react more effectively and promptly?

First, we reiterate our first recommendation from chapter 1: the US government and its agencies must acknowledge the risk of future pandemics and plan for them. We do not know what pathogen will cause the next pandemic. We do not know when it will occur. But we must realize that as our population grows, as we expand the footprint of our population centers into forests and wilderness, as our international travels increase, as the climate changes, and as long as developing countries have weak public health infrastructures and poor sanitation and a dependence on killing and eating wild animals, we will be at an increasing risk for the next pandemic. And we must be prepared for the possibility that the next pandemic could be even more transmissible and even more deadly.

Second, we must address current threats to public health. Our third recommendation from chapter 1 is an urgent one: the United States' and the world's leaders must place pressure on China and those Asian countries that have wet markets to develop and enforce public health measures to prevent the high risk activities (such as the close enclosure of wild animals in cages, which promotes the exposure of animals to one another's secretions and excrements, and the killing and butchering of wild animals out in the open in the presence of many people crowded together nearby without adequate sanitation and ventilation) that create significant threats for zoonotic infections and the transmission of novel viruses. There is no time like the present to agree that this is not the first pandemic or epidemic with its origin traced to wet markets and that the risks of such establishments must be addressed. Wet markets are sites especially susceptible to the transmission of animal viruses to humans, but they are not the only risk for evolving zoonotic infections and novel viruses. We don't know for certain that SARS-CoV-2 originated in the Huanan seafood market, or elsewhere in Wuhan, or necessarily even in China. Nevertheless, these wet markets pose a significant risk, and we must address these risks before another novel virus makes the leap from an animal to a human.

Third, the policies, procedures, regulation, and oversight of all labs conducting research of highly communicable potential pathogens must be enhanced. The very fact that a lab leak was considered a possibility by some in the US government, prompting an investigation by the World Health Organization (WHO), calls for a review by the international community to ensure that all such labs have adopted and strictly maintain best practices, even though there is no evidence a lab leak played any role in this pandemic. As an international community, we must also commit to not blaming, shaming, or imposing financial liability on a country in the event of a laboratory accident or the outbreak of a novel virus from a spillover event, as we only put those countries on the defensive and provide no motivation for them to cooperate in an international investigation. We also have to understand that few countries, if any, are going to welcome scientists from rival nations into their highest-security laboratories. While many Americans criticize the Chinese government for not providing more access to the Wuhan Institute of Virology, we don't have to imagine what the US response would be to a request to provide access to the CDC or any of our highest-security laboratories by Chinese and/or Russian scientists as part of a WHO investigation; nearly every US president of the modern era, both Republican and Democrat, has indicated that they would not permit it. Thus, we must explore ways that allow for a disease outbreak investigation without compromising the security and proprietary interests of a country. That might call for mutually agreed-upon scientists and inspectors from friendly or allied nations, together with WHO staff, to conduct interviews and review data.

Third, we must think differently about how we conduct surveillance. Our second recommendation from chapter 1 calls for future administrations to recommit to and invest sufficiently in establishing a public health presence in foreign countries to assist in the early identification of novel viruses and their containment. These scientists and public health experts stationed in other countries can be thought of in the same terms as ambassadors. We set up embassies in foreign countries, and we appoint ambassadors to those countries. These ambassadors and their staff are critical to our understanding of the foreign country and to understanding the issues, challenges, and threats facing that country, and potentially threats to us. In an analogous manner, the opportunity to have public health experts on the ground in a foreign country, especially those countries that are most cut off from the rest of the world and that pose the greatest threats, allows us to understand those threats better, conduct studies of those threats, and be aware of developments of concern sooner than we would be from outside the country.

This is also the time to bring the surveillance methods of the CDC and WHO into the twenty-first century. As an example, we recognize that we do not have people stationed around the globe with binoculars waiting and watching for evidence of a missile attack. We have satellites that are watching for movements that might signify the building of nuclear capabilities or the movement of military forces or weapons. We have computers that can identify the launch of a potential attack, determine the likelihood that it is aimed at us, and estimate the time before the missile will hit its target. This is critical, because it is human nature to dismiss such threats or to look for other explanations, fearing that an inappropriate response from our country would be nightmarish. No one wants to be blamed for overreacting.

Similarly, in this pandemic, we have seen examples where leaders of countries and public health organizations were slow in appreciating the early signs of a potential pandemic threat. This is because, by their nature, early outbreaks are generally localized and there is often a delay between when cases are first detected, when patients end up hospitalized, and when deaths later begin to occur. Further, as suggested above, leaders are often reluctant to be seen as overreacting. In fact, the steps we propose leaders and public health officials take in response to an outbreak with a novel virus will necessarily appear to be drastic and unjustified, because to be done most effectively, they must be implemented very early in the outbreak when there will not appear to be enough cases, hospitalizations, or deaths to justify the actions.

Thus, we need an "early warning system" for infectious threats. We need to use machine learning (artificial intelligence) with natural language processing in as many languages of the world as possible to pour through news reports, medical reports, news casts, social media, and other sources to alert us to outbreaks that a government may not have identified themselves. We also need to recognize that governments may be intentionally deciding not to report to public health officials and the WHO yet. For example, the *South China Morning Post* published an article entitled "Hong Kong takes emergency measures as mystery 'pneumonia' infects dozens in China's Wuhan city" by Mandy Zuo, Lilian Cheng, Alice Yan, and Cannix Yau at 2:35 p.m. on December 31, 2019. There were other news reports as well. Computers could identify these reports, flag them, and bring them to the attention of public health leaders to make them aware of a possible outbreak. This would stimulate efforts at identification and containment of the virus, while working through the WHO to alert countries of the world to this risk.

Of course, the benefit of knowing about the risks earlier is only realized if we then take actions earlier. As it was, the first patient to be diagnosed in the United States with COVID-19 entered the country on a flight from Wuhan on January 15. We should have been alerted to the potential infectious risk two weeks earlier and to the epidemic or pandemic potential of the virus a week earlier. As it was, we began airport screenings of individuals arriving in the United States from Wuhan on January 17, two days after the index case had already arrived. That patient would become ill and be diagnosed with COVID-19 on January 21.

President Trump then issued an executive order on January 31 that would go into effect on February 1, restricting, but not halting, travel to the United States from Wuhan. This advance notice of the travel restriction caused many to accelerate their travel plans to reenter the United States before the restrictions would go into effect. This, of course, partially defeats the purpose of the travel restrictions.

As we pointed out in Recommendation #6 from chapter 1, while there is controversy over the effectiveness of travel restrictions, if they are going to be employed, it is important to understand that from a virologic standpoint, there was no reason to believe that US citizens and their families would be less likely to bring the virus into the United States than foreign nationals. Therefore, if a travel restriction is to be used, US citizens returning home from a country where there has been an outbreak of infection must either be tested prior to entry, if a reliable test is available, or be quarantined for an appropriate amount of time prior to returning to their homes, families, friends, and work, where they could spread the infection if they were exposed prior to their return home.

In retrospect, we made three fundamental errors with our travel mitigation measures. First, they were too late. We know from the first COVID-19 patient in the United States that he arrived two days before we began screenings. Second, screenings only detect people with signs and symptoms of disease. In the case of COVID-19, it is estimated that around 40 percent of persons infected with SARS-CoV-2 can be asymptomatic and contagious. Third, the travel restriction, once implemented, had too many exceptions that would allow too many persons into the United States without testing or quarantine.

Far more effective than trying to restrict travel arrivals from Wuhan would have been to restrict travel departures out of Wuhan. As we pointed out in Recommendation #5 from chapter 1, with an estimated 4 million international travelers per day, health officials must act swiftly to lock down travel in and out of any areas of the world in the event of a novel virus outbreak. We must seek agreement from the world's leaders to cooperate in instituting travel restrictions as soon as a novel virus outbreak is detected. These travel restrictions, at the location of the outbreak, can be implemented much more quickly, effectively, and easily than attempting to halt travel into all other countries. Given that people traveling out of Wuhan might make several other connections, it will not be easy to identify everyone who poses a risk, although this could be greatly enhanced with artificial intelligence and access to the data of airline companies. Further, we have seen how difficult it is to implement and maintain non-pharmaceutical interventions with the degree of compliance that would be needed to contain the spread of disease in many countries. Our best hope is to act so quickly at the site of the initial outbreak to lock it down that public health officials will be blamed for overreacting.

We sincerely hope that the world's current and future leaders have learned from this pandemic that hiding uncomfortable or embarrassing information is not a solution. The nature of viruses persists, whether we acknowledge it or not. Not acknowledging the threat, informing the public, mobilizing the public health and medical communities, or taking decisive action will merely increase the number of cases, put health care workers at increased risk, increase the likelihood that the outbreak will spread to other parts of the country and to other countries, result in avoidable loss of life, and make the magnitude of the outbreak and subsequent epidemic or pandemic greater. Any perceived public relations or political gains from not acknowledging the threat will be short-lived, because most viruses will be increasing the number of people infected exponentially and the costs and consequences will grow rapidly, making it impossible to hide.

Recommendation #13
Rapid, Coordinated Responses to a Novel Virus Are Necessary

The world's leaders must be quick to respond to an outbreak of a novel virus. Locking down travel into and out of the site of an outbreak of a novel viral infection is likely to be more effective than other countries implementing travel restrictions.

Although it may have previously been thought too overreaching to lock down all travel in and out of a city experiencing an outbreak, the impact on countries across the world from the current pandemic is likely to make leaders more amenable to this proposition. We just need to prevent travel out of the area until we have time to develop an understanding of how the novel virus is transmitted and a reliable test for the virus. We can more likely achieve agreement from all the world's leaders that we will lock down the town or city of an outbreak rather than the subsequent country-wide lockdowns that may then have to be implemented.

We would hope that an early lockdown, along with the now-familiar litany of instructions for those in the outbreak area—to wash or sanitize their hands frequently, to clean surfaces that are frequently touched, to cover their coughs and sneezes, to stay home and work from home when possible (especially if one is ill), to avoid gatherings, to keep a physical distance when you do have to go outside your home, to wear a face covering when you are out and unable to always maintain a physical distance—would keep the outbreak from spreading to other parts of the country or other countries. However, even if it does not, it is enough to buy us time, perhaps weeks, to study the virus, identify the virus, and begin the development of vaccines and studies of potential therapies.

Keep in mind that for a virus to propagate and cause an epidemic or pandemic, those it infects must in turn infect more than one other person. If one infected person only infects one other person, there will be no long-term growth in the number of cases. If one infected person infects less than one other person, on average, the spread will gradually decrease and die out. Thus, the viruses we worry about are those in which one infected person infects more than one additional person. As stated earlier, it was estimated that the number of persons infected by one person with COVID-19 at the beginning of the outbreak (the R-naught, as seen in chapter 1) was around 2.5, on average. Therefore, there will be exponential growth in the number of cases if we cannot intervene to decrease exposures to others. Imposing a lockdown and having those in the lockdown area take the proper public health measures mentioned above is intended to break the chain of transmission, or at least slow it down. Obviously, with exponential growth—especially with exponential growth, in fact—if even one infected person slips through and enters the United States but we prevent a thousand others from entering, the cumulative rate of growth in cases will be far slower, buying us more time to prepare, take action, put public health guidance into effect, and learn more about the virus.

As stated in chapter 1, it is essential that the United States develops quality tests rapidly, deploys them widely to detect the extent of disease transmission, and has sufficient lab capabilities and capacity to turn around tests quickly in order for the testing to be an effective method of identifying and isolating those with infection, as well as identifying those who may have been infected because of close contact through contact tracing so that they can be quarantined. Similarly, we must ensure that developing countries also have this capability so that we can monitor disease activity and potential travel risks. Further, testing becomes even more useful when point of care or rapid tests can be made available that allow for testing within minutes and without having to send the sample to a lab. However, keep in mind that the problem with rapid tests available to the public is that this will interfere with the reporting of cases and data from which we can calculate the test positivity rate since laboratories are required by law to report results to state health departments, but the general public is not.

World Health Organization

The World Health Organization (WHO) is an agency established under the auspices of the United Nations with its own constitution that was adopted in 1946 and began operations in April 1948. There are 194 member states, or countries. All countries that are members of the United Nations may accept membership in the WHO by agreeing to the terms of its constitution. Countries that are not members of the United Nations may apply for membership to the WHO and can be admitted by a vote in favor from the member countries.

What should the role of the World Health Organization (WHO) be in preventing, identifying, and responding to potential pandemic threats?

First, the independence of the WHO needs to be established. The WHO is put in a difficult position when its member countries are world leaders and also a funding source. The WHO needs to be able to investigate outbreaks promptly without fear of retribution from a member country. Currently, the WHO must be invited to visit and conduct an investigation on-site by the country with an outbreak. Obviously, WHO visits and investigations need to be coordinated with the host country, but the WHO needs the authority to initiate a visit and investigation on its own. Some allege that the WHO deferred more than it should have to China, due to China's importance as a member. On the other hand, the United States was very willing for the WHO to be its scapegoat for its own delayed response to the pandemic, and President Trump indicated that the United States would terminate its membership in the WHO. (This decision was rescinded by the Biden administration.)

Political pressures should have no place in the investigation and development of public health recommendations in an outbreak, epidemic, or pandemic. The WHO must have the latitude to come in immediately following an outbreak, conduct interviews, investigations, and testing, and put out public guidance and warnings free of intimidation or the impression that they must sugarcoat findings in order to save a member country from embarrassment or economic hardship.

The participation of most or all the world's countries is critical to the proper prevention, identification, and containment of infectious outbreaks. Therefore, there needs to be a mechanism to prevent a country from immediately withdrawing from the WHO in retaliation, particularly during a pandemic, or threatening the termination of its membership to influence the WHO.

Recommendation #14
Expand the WHO's Authority

The organizational documents of the WHO should be amended to allow the WHO to initiate a request for a site visit and investigation in coordination with the host country.

In addition to expanding the WHO's authority to be able to initiate a site visit to investigate an outbreak of disease, there should be a prolonged cooling off period—five years, to give an example—before a member country can terminate its membership in the WHO. This cooling-off period will help eliminate the ability of countries to threaten the WHO for its actions in investigating an outbreak. Another suggestion is to require a member nation that wishes to terminate its membership within that cooling-off period to show good cause and a justification as to why that country will be harmed by having to wait for the cooling-off period to expire to a panel of member nations that must vote in some supermajority, such as greater than 60 percent of its members, in order to approve early termination from the WHO.

The WHO should develop, revise, and update pandemic planning guidance for all nations, but particularly developing nations, considering what we have experienced during and learned from this pandemic. Part of the planning must be directed at options to increase disease surveillance for early identification of a novel organism and the expansion of testing capabilities in many of these countries to not only identify communicable diseases, but to assist in the containment efforts during an outbreak by prompt identification of individuals who are infected who need to be isolated and contacts that need to be quarantined.

In the event of an outbreak, the WHO should assist the country having the outbreak with its investigation, identification of the pathogen, and recommendations for containment. The WHO should also alert all countries of the outbreak and assess the risks associated with the outbreak. If the pathogen is a novel virus, the WHO should work with the country involved to institute an immediate travel restriction in and out of the area and quickly develop testing and quarantine strategies to assist persons visiting the area to safely return home.

The WHO should then monitor the outbreak and if it does become an epidemic or pandemic, monitor the cases, hospitalizations, deaths and complications from each member country and report those results to the rest of the world. At the same time, the WHO should update the world about medical and scientific information about the pathogen as it is learned, developing guidance for public health strategies.

The WHO should also partner with the CDC and the European Centre for Disease Prevention and Control to share information, learn from each other, and coordinate public health preparedness, guidance and responses.

Finally, the WHO must lead the exploration of options as to how we can significantly increase the manufacturing capabilities and capacity around the world to allow for the rapid production and distribution of tests and billions of doses of vaccines once authorized in order to quickly vaccinate the world in response to a novel organism.

Centers for Disease Control and Prevention

What is the role for the CDC with respect to future pandemics?

First and most importantly, the CDC must win back the public's trust. The CDC has been one of the most trusted organizations in the country, but the appearance of political pressure has compromised that trust. Future leaders of the CDC must speak out emphatically and often, using science as their compass, even when their guidance or predictions are at odds with the president and his or her administration. Although the CDC's director is appointed by the president, the director must provide accurate information to the public and all the information needed by state and local health departments without undue influence. The director must correct inaccurate or incorrect information that is made public by federal or state governments and their leaders.

Recommendation #15

The CDC Must Be the Independent, Trusted Voice of Science

The CDC must regain the public's trust. It must be the voice of science, and its leaders must speak out often and with clarity during a public health emergency, even when the information, guidance, and predictions conflict with the president and his or her administration.

It is surprising in retrospect that in February of 2020, the World Economic Forum released the results of its study of the countries best prepared for a pandemic, with the United States taking the top spot. Despite being ranked as the best prepared, the United States experienced the third-highest number of COVID-19 cases per capita and the highest number of COVID-19 deaths per capita of any country in the world. Obviously, the criteria by which we judged preparedness in the past do not reflect the capabilities and resources needed today.

The skill sets needed for the CDC's success in this new environment of the internet, social media, and disinformation campaigns are different. All too often, in an unsettling time of uncertainty, people tend to believe what they hear first that is reinforced by others, especially their trusted sources or people "like them." Social media has a tremendous amplifying effect on misinformation and disinformation. Therefore, it is important that the CDC maintains a significant presence on social media to get messages out faster and more clearly.

The CDC of the future will need social scientists, science communications experts, political scientists, experts in combating misinformation and disinformation, cultural anthropologists, and social media experts. It is no longer enough to get the science right (which unfortunately, was even an issue at times); the CDC must communicate it better and faster, and at the same time refute false information. We coauthors certainly did not anticipate politics entering into the management of a pandemic. While we believe that there should be bipartisan disdain for misinformation, disinformation, and political interference with the CDC and public health agencies, nevertheless, we must confront and adapt to this new reality.

Secondly, the CDC must conduct a full, multi-agency, retrospective review of mistakes and lessons from the pandemic. One mistake was the delay in announcing that there is person-to-person transmission with this novel virus. As we recommended in chapter 1's Recommendation #4, with a novel virus that causes respiratory illness, especially one belonging to a family of viruses known to be infectious, we should presume human-to-human transmission is possible until proven otherwise. Another mistake was the nearly year-long delay in acknowledging that airborne (aerosol) transmission is an important mode of transmission for this virus.

Recommendation #16

Multi-agency Review of the Pandemic Response

The CDC must conduct a full, multi-agency, retrospective review of mistakes and lessons from the pandemic.

Another problem was the failed rollout of testing. As we indicated in Recommendation #7 in chapter 1, in dealing with an outbreak of a contagious new disease, testing is of paramount importance. It allows us to identify the extent of disease activity, which can then inform public health actions, and is critical in determining who needs to isolate and which close contacts need to quarantine, which is essential in containing the spread of disease. Without adequate, widely available, timely, and reasonably accurate testing, efforts to manage an outbreak will be undermined. Therefore, the regulatory scheme must be modified to allow for accelerated testing development in the private and academic setting under the direction of the CDC. This is so as not to rely only on the development, production, and distribution of a single test that does not leave us with viable alternatives in the event of any unforeseen technical difficulties.

After completing the retrospective review, the CDC should revise and update its pandemic plans based on these new lessons. This planning should include:

- Investments in public health infrastructure
- The positioning of CDC staff in other countries, especially those that are closed societies, those that have presented pandemic threats in the past, and developing countries where the lack of public health measures may place the world at risk for zoonotic infections
- The adoption of artificial intelligence/machine learning, as discussed above, to enhance disease surveillance
- New strategies for containment of a novel virus that emphasize restrictions on travel in and out of the area of the outbreak
- The strengthening of disease reporting in the United States to facilitate standardized reporting with common definitions on a timely basis; data was critical to the public health response during the COVID-19 pandemic, but it also became clear that the public desired this information and has come to expect this data now and in the future

Recommendation #17

Revisions to Pandemic Plans and CDC Competencies

The CDC should revise and update its pandemic plans based on the lessons from this pandemic to include, at a minimum, needed investments in public health infrastructure, the positioning of CDC staff in certain foreign countries, the adoption of machine learning for enhanced surveillance, new strategies focusing on containment, and the strengthening of disease reporting in the United States. The CDC of the future will need social scientists, science communications experts, political scientists, experts in combating misinformation and disinformation, cultural anthropologists, and social media experts.

Disease reporting has had its challenges. A lack of clear definitions created an overstatement of the number of COVID-19 tests being performed in the United States, especially when some states were reporting antibody tests performed in their total testing numbers. Antibody tests give us little useful information in determining the current disease activity and levels of community spread. Furthermore, data was often not reported by all laboratories and all hospitals over weekends and holidays, which could mislead the public into believing there was a drop in the numbers of cases or deaths when there was not. It is important for the CDC to explore ways to make such data reporting less onerous, more consistent and, when possible, more automated.

This reporting strategy also meant that the early public release of the number of people "recovered" from COVID-19 since the beginning of the pandemic became somewhat misleading, since we lacked full information about complications and long-term effects. This straightforward designation of those who developed COVID-19, who completed their period of isolation, and who did not die during that period of time unintentionally resulted in an incomplete assessment, since a significant percentage of these patients did not fully recover. Perhaps "survived" would be a better description.

Looking back, after the threat of the original SARS coronavirus was over, much of the funding for continued research on SARS and potential therapies and vaccines was terminated. Obviously, in retrospect, that was unfortunate. We must not make the same mistake this time. Yes, research is costly, but consider that the United States spent 4.4 trillion dollars on just the first two economic stimulus packages to deal with the economic effects of SARS-CoV-2 on businesses and individuals, and is now considering another $1.9 trillion dollar relief bill. This $4.4 trillion expense does not even include the purchase of medical supplies, the payments to vaccine manufacturers as part of Operation Warp Speed, or the costs to government health programs for the treatment of patients with COVID-19. We can obviously afford to spend significant amounts of money on research, given that the cost of a pandemic is so extraordinarily high.

One of the bright spots of the pandemic was the singular resolve of the medical and scientific community all across the world to engage in clinical research and quickly and broadly share their findings that might help in our collective war against this novel coronavirus. We could potentially develop a consortium of countries that would fund and continue this important research after this pandemic comes to an end.

Regardless of the potential for international collaboration, the National Institutes of Health, the National Center for Biotechnology Information (NCBI), and the CDC should put forth a research agenda and funding request that would allow for continued research on those viruses that we believe are the prime candidates for the next pandemic, such as influenza viruses, coronaviruses, flaviviruses, and paramyxoviruses.[1] Part of this research would be the surveillance of novel organisms by obtaining samples and cultures of viruses from the habitats of animals (such as bat caves) that we believe are most likely to be sources or intermediaries for a future spread of a novel virus, focusing on wild animals that humans are increasingly encroaching upon or using as a food source. We must learn as much as we can about these viruses, including utilizing artificial intelligence to assist us in identifying medications that are most likely to be effective in the prevention or treatment of infection. Given the large number of genetic differences between virus strains even within the same family, we should particularly focus our research on medications and therapies that can disrupt the basic reproductive machinery of entire classes of viruses and would be safe, effective, and able to be readily and inexpensively manufactured in sufficient quantities for distribution around the world.

We must also continue our research into the SARS-CoV-2 virus and the disease it causes. We still have many questions without answers or only partial answers. Finding the answers to these questions can help us understand future viruses and the risks they might pose. Some of the questions remaining include these:

- Why does SARS-CoV-2 cause severe disease or even death in some persons of the same age and with the same risk factors and not others?
- Why do men appear to have more severe illness than women and why do women seem to have a higher incidence of long-term effects?
- In children and young adults, why are so many persons infected with SARS-CoV-2 asymptomatic, while others have mild or moderate disease?
- What is the full immune response to SARS-CoV-2 infection? Does everyone who is infected develop immunity? What are the markers of immunity and how long does the immunity last?
- How long-lasting is the immunity conferred by vaccination?
- Why do some people who are reinfected suffer more severe illness with the second infection?
- What predisposes some children to develop MIS-C?
- Is severe disease the result of overwhelming direct viral invasion or an exaggerated immune response?
- What is the pathophysiology of PASC (long COVID or long-haulers syndrome)? What predisposes people to develop these long-term effects? Are there any effective treatments?

In addition to these specific questions about the SARS-CoV-2 virus and COVID-19, we need much more research into airborne transmission and effective measures to mitigate this route of transmission.

Recommendation #18

Increase in Research Funding

We must increase our investment in research of novel organisms that are candidates for future pandemics. This should at least be a collaboration among our US medical and public health research agencies, if not a collaboration among the international community.

The CDC, WHO, and NCBI should also evaluate how to provide the medical community with daily or weekly updates, podcasts, and summaries of important new information about the next novel pathogen that is causing an epidemic or pandemic. Physicians and nurses on the front lines of fighting an outbreak are working most days, if not every day, and these days are long. With this pandemic, it was very difficult to keep up with the large volume of new data, studies, and guidance in competition with all the time commitments physicians have in their care of patients. Unfortunately, on occasion, it was health care professionals that were providing their communities with misguided and incorrect information, some of which could have posed a threat to patients.

CHAPTER 3

The Intersection of COVID-19 and Society

The microbe is nothing. The terrain is everything.

LOUIS PASTEUR

Personal Story: Forewarning in the "Strangest of Snowstorms"

Ted Epperly, one of the book's coauthors, tells the following story.

On January 1, 2020, I greeted the new year with an annual ski trip to a wonderful ski hill just outside of Boise, Idaho. After my seventh ski run of the morning, an ominous, rolling black wall of clouds swooped in from the northwest. With it came lightning, pellets of hail, and torrents and torrents of snow. In all my years of living in Idaho, I had never seen a lightning storm within a snowstorm!

The ski mountain was closed immediately with an eerie wailing siren as thunder shook the mountain and lightning struck dangerously close to the metal ski lifts where people sat captive to the storm's fury. Two feet of snow fell in one hour.

As I sat outside at the base of the mountain, which was being buried in snow, I could not help but think how bizarre this storm truly was. My mind wandered to an article I had read the previous day about a new virus identified in Wuhan, China, which had sickened many people and health care workers. I was worried about what this might mean for the world. But little did I know in that moment beside the ski hill, in the midst of the strangest of snowstorms, that I had a forewarning of just how shocking the year 2020 was going to be.

There is much that can be said regarding the intersection of COVID-19 and society. The story of the COVID-19 pandemic and its impact on the world and our nation is really the story of two interrelated pandemics. The first is the story of the SARS coronavirus-2 (SARS-CoV-2) pandemic itself. The second is the story of our societal and cultural response to it. The microbiology and pathophysiology of infectious diseases make clear that the host organism in which an infection occurs makes a big difference as to the severity of the infection. Similarly, the severity of the COVID-19 pandemic was profoundly affected by the fertile culture—the politics and ideologies of our human societies.

A large part of what made COVID-19 such a major pandemic was the nature of our human population, producing the conditions that promoted the jump of a novel virus from animals to humans followed by further transmission from person to person. Our society was not only fertile ground; it created an environment that accelerated the spread of the virus, an environment that was to have a dominant impact on our country and the world.

To be clear, SARS-CoV-2 had an impact on the world beyond just its effect on human beings. Not only did it likely originate in bats and spread to human beings, but it also affected other animals, including ferrets, minks, and other mammals. But the largest impact of SARS-CoV-2 by far was on human beings. There were several reasons why the United States was such fertile ground for the SARS coronavirus-2 in 2020:

1. Our society has become much more densely packed. Of the more than seven billion people who live on our planet, most are clustered in large cities and very close living conditions.[1]
2. Transportation across the planet, between countries and within states and provinces, has never been easier. The amount of traffic by air, car, train, cruise ship, and bus allow for rapid

transportation of pathogens across our globe, as well as the infection of fellow travelers along the way.

3. We have clusters of people within each of our communities who live in proximity with each other. Congregant living facilities such as nursing homes, jails, prisons, and homeless shelters allow easy spread among closely quartered people.
4. The average age of our nation's and the world's population has never been older.[2] People are living longer and are, on average, older in industrialized countries.
5. Because we are older, we have more chronic diseases. Elderly people who have more chronic diseases are more susceptible to viral illness.
6. Pandemics, epidemics, and major outbreaks of infectious disease have much more fertile ground among people of color and those with lower incomes within our societies. They are, as a group, often socioeconomically depressed and have less access to resources such as food, housing, readily available transportation and health care. They are also far less likely to be able to work remotely from home, and often their workplaces have inadequate protections to fully guard against the risk of exposure. This was seen throughout the pandemic, with high infection rates observed in Black, Latino, and American Indian and Native Alaskan populations living in socioeconomically depressed areas and reservations.
7. Many people throughout this pandemic chose to simply deny its existence or minimize its presence. In short, they chose to be ignorant of the potential danger and impact of COVID-19. This, of course, was magnified in the echo chambers of both their preferred media and social media platforms. Whatever you wanted to believe about SARS-CoV-2 and its infectivity of human beings could be supported by some news or media source and some "expert."
8. There was a tremendous lack of leadership early on in the pandemic. Effective leadership could have made a big difference in the spread of SARS-CoV-2 and how many lives were lost. This was especially true in the United States, where a lack of strong

leadership that otherwise could have helped mitigate the potential dangers of the pandemic and helped bring society together around our common defense simply did not occur. This failure of leadership was not only from the president, vice president, and others in the Trump administration, but also, at times, from the Department of Health and Human Services and the Centers for Disease Control and Prevention (CDC), made all the worse by the slow response from the World Health Organization (WHO) in the early days of this pandemic.

9. If all these factors were not enough, then the political polarization that had been brewing in American society for the last 20 years came to a boiling point during this pandemic.

SARS-CoV-2 did not care if it was infecting Republicans or Democrats, men or women, whites, Blacks, Hispanics, American Indians, Native Alaskans, Asians, or Pacific Islanders; it just knew it had a wide open field to run around in. Sadly, the polarization of our political system made this an issue of Democrat versus Republican. It became a symbol of your political party affiliation to either wear a face mask or not, allowing the infection to have a field day in our country.

Let us take a deeper dive and look specifically at some of the societal issues and organizations that provided so much gasoline to the fire of this pandemic.

National Leaders

President Trump and Vice President Mike Pence downplayed the seriousness of SARS-CoV-2 and the COVID-19 pandemic from the beginning. Not only was President Trump slow in closing our borders, but his administration was delayed in producing and distributing testing and unable to provide adequate personal protective equipment (PPE).

The president made many statements such as "You have 15 people, and the 15 within a couple of days is going to be down to close to zero."[3] Another refrain was, "We're opening up this incredible country. Because we have to do that. I would love to have it open by Easter."[4] We can only speculate as to whether these comments were meant to reassure the public, reassure the stock markets, or deflect blame from himself and his administration. Ironically, the president would later blame China for not being transparent and forthcoming about the outbreak. The most damage that occurred from the president "downplaying" the pandemic was due to his statements playing a significant factor in convincing some people that COVID-19 was a hoax, not actually a pandemic, or not even as bad as the flu. This in turn fueled resistance to adopting public health guidance and following local or state restrictions.

Recommendation #19

The Administration Must Promote Public Health

The role of the president, vice president and senior administration officials during a pandemic is to give accurate and timely information to the public and to stress the importance of public health measures to thwart the pandemic's spread. These leaders need to provide a "call to action" to motivate the populace to actively participate for the "good of the country" and for fellow citizens.

Not only did President Trump not understand the pandemic, he refused to listen to advice from experts who did. This was a particularly toxic combination from the top, as there were mixed messages on the importance of mask wearing both from himself and certain members of his administration. This led to a vital mistake made early in the pandemic, affecting the willingness of people to recognize the urgency of appropriate public health measures, including face masking, physical distancing, group size limits on gatherings, and handwashing. Millions of potential future cases and hundreds of thousands of later deaths could have been prevented with accurate messaging and action from our national leaders.

State Leaders

President Trump largely delegated the management of the pandemic to the states to implement their own plans. But in a pandemic as widespread as this was, there needed to be a federally led effort to organize responses. Because of this lack of national focus, we saw a patchwork of different state responses.

There were states that took this very seriously and did quite a bit of work around public health and the education of their citizens, and there were states that downplayed this and did little to address the threat. Sadly, the states' responses were broken down into different political camps, with blue states often having a more aggressive response to the pandemic and red states often having a more hands-off approach.

As an example, in Idaho, we had many members of the state legislature, including our lieutenant governor, Janice K. McGeachin, who actively campaigned in opposition to an organized statewide approach and failed to support our Republican governor during this time of public health emergency. Idaho never did implement a mask mandate, and the decentralized public health system set up by the legislature in 1970 only amplified the confusion and chaos of a failed federal approach to the problem. This promoted a patchwork of different approaches and health orders across different counties and public health districts, and it is not uncommon for Idahoans to live in one county and work in the adjacent one.

Recommendation #20

State Leaders Must Promote Public Health Measures

In a public health emergency, such as a pandemic, the governor, lieutenant governor, and legislative leaders must put partisan politics aside and speak together as one voice to support public health measures to address the emergency. During a public health emergency that threatens the welfare and lives of people, there is no political base to be played to; these leaders must protect all of their state's citizens.

Mayors and City Councils

As elected leaders of their cities, the pandemic challenged many mayors and city councils. They were torn between the health and well-being of their citizens and the economy of their cities and towns—and perhaps, in some cases, their political futures.

Depending on their mindset, their access to news sources, their social media interaction, and which groups had exerted the most influence on them, these leaders invariably had difficult decisions to make. In some cases, we saw mayors and city councils make the difficult decisions to protect the citizens they were charged with serving. In many cases, we saw leaders simply avoid making a decision or having a thoughtful debate and discussion. In at least one case, we saw reckless behavior, where the mayor and council defied public health orders in order to have a tree-lighting ceremony in anticipation of Christmas, when hospitals were already alerting the public to the concern that they were being strained in their capacity.[5]

Recommendation #21

Public Health Is Good for Business

During a public health emergency, especially a pandemic, elected leaders must lead, even when the public is divided and there is no politically safe decision. Educating their citizens about the importance of public health measures to contain the spread of the virus and protect the lives and welfare of their communities and citizens is paramount, but it is also the way to keep businesses open, people employed, and schools open.

The thinking that this was a decision between health or the economy was a false dichotomy. By advocating for face masks, limitations on the size of gatherings, and appropriate distancing, both individual citizens and the community could be protected, and businesses, schools, and economies could be continued with the least disruption. In fact, those communities, businesses, and schools that failed to implement the public health guidance often were the same ones that later faced significant disruption or closure due to uncontrolled disease transmission. This did not need to be an "either/or" proposition, but rather an "and" proposition.

Social Media

Social media was a new tool for public health organizations, doctors, and scientists to get good information out to the public, but it was also a tool for some to spread disinformation and conspiracy theories. It had a large impact on the confusion and chaos that occurred, not only across the nation, but in individual states. Facebook, Twitter, and other social media websites work off of algorithm-driven newsfeeds. The more you look at certain sources of information, the more you will get fed with data and information that supports those views.

What we saw play out in 2020 was a tremendous amount of misinformation, disinformation, lies, myths, and half-truths that got amplified by social media, more than with prior public health issues, creating much larger audiences than those espousing this information could have achieved on their own. To spread information, one no longer needed education, experience, or expertise, but simply followers—especially followers that are then willing to further propagate the misleading or untrue information to their own networks of followers. The public does not know at this time to what extent there were disinformation efforts through social media by foreign governments who sought to sow the seeds of division and hate in the United States. Discouragingly, many Americans seemed receptive to embracing conspiracy theories that undermined public health efforts and perhaps furthered the interests of our adversaries.

As a result of conflicting information being promoted, some people believed the doctors and scientists regarding the importance of face masks, physical distancing in public, and avoiding large gatherings, while others believed that face masks could kill you, cause cancer, give you toxic amounts of re-inhaled carbon dioxide, or cause you to pass out. It becomes a major challenge to get the public to stay calm and act in an organized manner for the good of the public when this happens. Why people believed that face masks could harm you when we have had surgeons, nurses, and others wearing them in operating rooms for over 100 years without harmful consequences was both surprising and difficult to understand.

National Media

The national media also found itself starting to polarize its messages and articles according to its readership or viewership. Instead of reporting factual information and data, some outlets tailored their messages based on the views of their subscribers. This, again, led to much misinformation and confusion at a time when we needed clarity and focus. What ensued was a tremendous amount of disharmony, discordance, and noise, inflicted on an already chaotic, anxiety-ridden, and concerned public—a public that was trying to sort out what was real and what was not. This loss of trust based on which camp you were in only drove people further apart when we needed people to come together.

During a national public health emergency, the press and media need to be a source of truth for a public that needs to understand what is happening and what actions they need to take. This does not mean that we should put debates about policy aside. It means that we should all agree on the facts and present the facts. Legitimate debates and discussions about how to address and respond to the facts are fair game, and we encourage the press and media to fairly represent both sides of and arguments surrounding proposed policy decisions.

Recommendation #22

Disinformation

The CDC and National Institutes of Health (NIH) must combat disinformation that is gaining traction on social media or cable networks. They should use experts in science communication to explain clearly why these messages are incorrect.

Recommendation #23

Critical Thinking and Assessing Reliability

Schools, colleges, and universities should teach students digital media literacy, how to distinguish high-quality information sources from low-quality sources and how to develop critical thinking. For adults who have already completed school, Facebook's "Tips to Spot False News" can be a useful resource. The public should also be directed to websites that end with .gov, .edu, and .org as likely trustworthy sites.

Hospitals

Hospitals were clearly under pressure during this time, trying to ensure that they had the capacity to keep the public served. The United States already has one of the lowest bed capacities as a percentage of the population of any of the industrialized nations.[6] What can happen in a pandemic, especially if there are not effective public health measures being introduced and adopted, is that hospitals can get overrun. In this current pandemic, hospital spokespersons were repeatedly faced with the challenge of how to forecast the potential for hospital capacity to be exceeded without appearing to be exaggerating or inciting panic if this outcome did not come to pass.

When a hospital's resources are stretched too thin, they have no beds, they have insufficient staffing, and they do not have the capacity to care for more patients. It is important for the public to understand that when a hospital is under severe pressure, it results in not only the inability to help those with COVID-19, but also the inability to handle all the other medical issues that come up in their community, such as heart attacks, strokes, bowel obstructions, car accidents, broken bones, appendicitis, and so on.

To make matters worse, President Trump and some state legislators made the irresponsible and reckless allegations that hospitals and physicians were inflating the numbers of patients with COVID-19 they were treating in order to be paid more.[7] Nothing could be further from the truth, and no evidence to support these outlandish claims was ever produced. It was unconscionable that these elected leaders would try to sow the seeds of doubt and distrust in these valiant heroes of this pandemic at a time when health care providers most needed the public's trust. What hospitals and physicians wanted was to have people take good care of themselves and avoid getting infected and ending up in their care.

The pandemic has revealed people's fundamental characters. It has brought out the best in people, and it has brought out the worst in people. The accusation that hospitals, health care workers, and physicians were profiteering during the pandemic was misguided and brought out anger, frustration, and distrust on all sides.

Hospital leaders, physicians, and nurses understandably do not want to unnecessarily scare the public. On the other hand, if they do not send clear messages to state and local leaders and the public about the potential for the hospital to be overwhelmed—and what that would mean for the people of that community—they lose the opportunity to engage the public in taking greater precautions in support of their hospitals. If they fail to communicate this message to the public, as well as define the steps they have taken to prevent this situation, they also risk being blamed for the consequences of rationing decisions that would have to be made in the event of overwhelmed resources.

Recommendation #24

Hospitals

Hospitals must leverage their websites, social media, newsletters, and spokespersons to communicate public health guidance, any capacity constraints, and any resource limitations to the public.

States that report hospital bed capacity generally report the number of beds or the percent occupancy. These are misleading numbers that tend to overstate hospital capacity because they do not account for limitations in staffing, which may be particularly acute during a pandemic with a highly contagious virus. The numbers also often include beds that cannot be used for adult patients, such as when neonatal or pediatric intensive care beds are included in the numbers of intensive care unit (ICU) beds. Therefore, hospitals or hospital associations need to work with their states to understand these limitations in the data and to come up with appropriate language to explain this on the state's website, where bed capacity is reported, so as not to mislead the public.

Recommendation #25

State Pandemic Reporting

Hospitals and hospital associations should work with their states to simplify and, where possible, automate hospital reporting to the state. Data elements need to be defined and standardized across all reporting hospitals, and states should add these data element definitions on their websites.

Physicians and Other Health Care Providers

To be clear, the vast majority of physicians rose to the occasion of this crisis, made great sacrifices to serve their patients, and made their communities and colleagues proud. Sadly, as we witnessed here in Idaho and in other parts of the country, some physicians actively opposed face masks and believed that they were a detriment to not only their patients but to the community, or promoted unsubstantiated cures and debunked treatments. We heard stories from patients who related that their chiropractor or podiatrist and their staff were not wearing masks when seeing patients, explaining to these patients that it was their way of contributing to the development of herd immunity, which was not only faulty but also irresponsible reasoning. The failure to embrace evidence-based medicine and science by health care professionals was shocking and unacceptable in the time of a pandemic, when it is our collective responsibility to educate and protect the public.

The Oregon Medical Board took emergency action to suspend the license of a physician who was, according to the board's findings of fact, not only violating the orders of the board but also engaging in extremely reckless behavior, endangering his staff (by not wearing masks in the office while seeing patients) and his patients (by urging patients who were wearing masks to remove them) and providing dangerous instructions to his patients. According to the order, a patient was told that asymptomatic individuals should not be tested, that wearing masks does not prevent the transmission of COVID-19, and that they should not self-isolate because being around other people would provide the patient with immunity to COVID-19. The order additionally states that the "Licensee regularly advises, particularly for his elderly and pediatric patients, that it is 'very dangerous' to wear masks because masks exacerbate COPD and asthma and cause or contribute to multiple serious health conditions, including but not limited to heart attacks, strokes, collapsed lungs, MRSA [a drug-resistant bacterium], pneumonia, and hypertension. Licensee asserts masks are likely to harm patients by increasing the body's carbon dioxide content through rebreathing of gas trapped behind a mask."[8]

Health care professionals of all types have the great privilege to care for patients, but also the weighty responsibility to ensure their health, safety, and welfare. They have an obligation to study the science of disease and provide their patients with the best recommendations available based on the science. Health care professionals can do special harm to patients when they disregard the standard of care and the prevailing authoritative guidance due to the special trust patients place in their caregivers. Licensing boards should establish expectations for the behavior and practices of their licensees and then discipline those licensees that disregard the rules, the practices, and the science and place the public at risk.

Recommendation #26

Disciplinary Action

State licensing boards should investigate licensees who are accused of intentionally spreading misinformation, and discipline those who have done so.

First Responders (Police, Fire, Emergency Medical Services)

First responders were put in a very difficult situation during the pandemic. Many of them found themselves going into situations with potentially COVID-infected people, in which they put themselves at great risk. Early on, many did not have adequate personal protective equipment (PPE). The very nature of their jobs meant that they often had to be in close proximity to people who were not wearing masks; they would have no idea, at least in their initial interactions, whether the person or people they were dealing with might be infected with SARS-CoV-2. Like everyone else on the front lines of interacting with or treating COVID-19 patients, these professionals were afraid less for their own safety and health and more of inadvertently taking the virus home with them and infecting a family member.

Dr. David Pate, coauthor of this book, has a sister—Dr. Jennifer Pate—who is a transplant psychiatrist. She tells the story of speaking to one of her neighborhood constables early in the pandemic and learning of his concerns that they did not have basic supplies of masks, gloves, hand sanitizer, or face shields. She pulled together some of her own stock of PPE and called for the constable. When he came by and she handed him the supplies, he wept, overwhelmed with gratitude and the demonstration of one human being caring for another.

Recommendation #27

Personal Protective Equipment and Supplies

The federal government and states need a plan to be able to provide PPE to first responders promptly at the very beginning of a public health emergency with a contagious pathogen.

First responders, too, were heroes of the pandemic. They struggled at times not only with a lack of adequate PPE but also with staffing, as members of their station or squad would be isolated with COVID-19 or quarantined due to an exposure.

There were many protests, demonstrations, and marches during the pandemic for many reasons—demonstrations against public health restrictions, protests by parents against remote learning or hybrid school schedules, demonstrations concerning the presidential election, marches for Black Lives Matter, and protests for and against defunding the police. In at least one demonstration at the Idaho legislature,[9] and one at a public health district,[10] crowds rushed the police, attempting to enter the buildings or rooms within the buildings, causing protesters to be in extremely close contact with officers. As we now know from the recent attack on the US Capitol in Washington, DC, this sort of risk to law enforcement officers during a pandemic can escalate quickly and with dire consequences. It is too early to know the full psychological impact on law enforcement officers and what such events will mean for the interest of young people in pursuing careers in law enforcement. Similarly, what effect will the pandemic have on young people deciding to go into the professions of medicine, nursing, social work, and public health?

First responders work under stressful conditions in normal times. There can be little doubt that the pandemic and the intense societal divisions it induces are greatly contributing to that stress.

Recommendation #28

Emotional and Psychological Support for First Responders

We urge cities, counties, and states to consider options to provide necessary emotional and psychological support to first responders.

As the community spread of SARS-CoV-2 reached alarming levels throughout most of the country in the fall and winter of 2020, the number of calls to transport extremely ill patients, likely with COVID-19, grew at rates that stressed emergency medical service providers. Ambulance and rescue squads also faced staffing shortages when paramedics had to quarantine. At times, some towns, cities, and counties faced delays in response times owing to the sheer volume of calls. At the end of 2020, this would be further worsened by hospitals themselves becoming overwhelmed and having to go on diversion. Sometimes this meant a longer ambulance ride to get to a hospital with capacity, which would take the ambulance out of service for other calls for a longer period of time. At other times, patients had to wait in ambulances or on gurneys in the hallways of the hospital when emergency rooms were filled beyond capacity.

Police forces have additional challenges, and theirs are particularly difficult. While most often they follow the best path, sometimes there is an unwanted detour. There can be a legitimate debate about whether mask mandates can be effective in the absence of enforcement. There can also be a legitimate debate as to whether mask mandates, in areas where there is significant resistance to such restrictions on the basis of an infringement on one's civil liberties or government overreach, will actually backfire and cause some people that would have worn masks without the mandate to now refuse to do so in defiance of this perceived encroachment on their personal freedoms. Nevertheless, an unexpected development that hampered at least one public health district's ability to implement a mandate was the county sheriff coming out publicly and indicating that the sheriff's office would not enforce the mandate.

It is critical that towns, cities, counties, and state governments meet with law enforcement agencies to discuss their role in a public health emergency. The whole of government must provide a common voice and a common message to the public during times of health crises. If it becomes necessary for public health officials to put health orders in place for the protection of the public, there needs to be an enforcement mechanism. This does not mean that we should remove the discretion that law enforcement officers have always had, but there needs to be an agreement that in the case of repeated violations or vocalized refusals to comply, especially in situations where the violators pose a risk to others, there will be consequences to the violators.

Recommendation #29

Enforcement of Public Health Orders

It is a best practice for public health officials to consult with law enforcement leaders about the penalties and enforcement of a public health order before issuing that order.

Schools and School Boards

Schools and school boards were put in a very tough situation. They wanted to do the right thing in regard to keeping students, staff members, and teachers safe, but also knew the limitations of remote learning and their own technology and the importance of ongoing in-person education and socialization that school provides students, as well as the inability to provide certain services to children remotely, particularly their special needs students. One of the most practical challenges was that school funding is, in large part, tied to in-person attendance. Another one of the largest obstacles to implementing infection control measures in high schools was the fact that sports would not only be of great emotional importance to students and parents, bringing the sense of normalcy that everyone craved, but also great academic importance to high school student athletes wishing to pursue sports in college, for which the loss of the season might mean not being recruited to a higher-ranked program or the potential loss of a scholarship opportunity.

All these considerations are important, and there were also discussions concerning the impact on students if schools were closed with regards to food insecurity and child abuse. Few, if any, school superintendents or school board members had medical or public health expertise, yet in many cases, decisions about whether and how to operate schools during the pandemic were left to these superintendents and boards. And yet, in our view, this was not the biggest challenge for school boards. After all, in most school districts, there were physicians and public health experts willing to provide consultative services to the schools.

The biggest problem we witnessed was the lack of good governance practices and how little many boards knew about the practices that could help them navigate complex, high-risk situations. What school boards needed to do, in addition to reaching out to physicians and public health experts, was to reach out to leaders of large, complicated, high-risk industries to help them implement good governance practices. If these had been initiated in March 2020, it would have put school boards in a better place for the fall.

The lack of these processes was demonstrated by lengthy meetings; rambling, directionless discussions; indecisiveness and frequent postponing of decisions; infighting among board members; decisions that were not internally consistent; the inability of most board members and stakeholders to be able to articulate the basis for the board's decisions; and loss of trust of stakeholders. We saw this play out over and over again with our local school districts.

So, how should school boards have handled this differently? While it is beyond the scope of this book to engage in a deep dive into board governance, some principles and practices may be useful to our readers that we preview here and go into more detail in chapter 14.

First, as emphasized above, the school boards should have engaged physicians, public health experts, and business or governance leaders early—back in March 2020, when schools closed. They also needed to engage stakeholders. All too often, parents felt that they had no say and teachers experienced a lack of communication and understanding as to what decisions were being made and why.

Second, the boards needed a decision framework. How would they make decisions about schools reopening and school closures? What factors should be considered? We certainly heard many issues being raised, but few school board members had any strategy for weighing these various factors against one another to assist in their decision-making. One of us coauthors often heard the concern raised that, if children were not in school, some would go hungry and others would suffer child abuse. Those are serious and important concerns, but how is a board member to weigh these concerns involving a portion of the student population versus the health threats posed to all children and their teachers by being in school? It also was never made clear why these concerns applied to students at home during the fall or winter but not during the summer, when school is out.

March and April were the proper time to identify the issues, even though we did not have most of the answers. For example:

- **Medical/public health**: Are children less likely to become infected? Are they less likely to spread the virus? What role do they play in the transmission of the virus? Does it vary by age or grade level? What are the outcomes of infection in children? Are there effective mitigation measures? What have we learned from schools in other states and countries? How many of our students live with high-risk family members at home? What is the risk to these family members if students are in school? How many of our teachers and staff are high-risk individuals? How many of them live with high-risk family members? Are students likely to transmit the virus to teachers? Are teachers likely to transmit the virus to students and to each other? How can we protect teachers? Does special education pose additional and specific risks? If so, how do we address those? What are the risks of extracurricular events? Can those risks be mitigated, or should the activities be postponed?
- **Education**: What is our experience with remote learning? What are our capabilities? Would all students have tablets or laptops and internet access? How will we assess learning and whether students are falling behind with remote learning? How would we execute hybrid learning? Is a hybrid program too disruptive

to parents and students? Should we take a different approach to different ages and grade levels? How can we meet the needs of special education students and those students who require special accommodations?

- **Sports, physical education, and extracurricular activities**: What programs do our schools have? What, if any, are the special risks associated with these programs? How can we mitigate those risks? Can physical education and certain sports be conducted with masks and physical distancing? Are there some extracurricular activities that are amenable to being held virtually? If we proceed with some or all activities, should those activities be suspended if school is remote? How would a hybrid schedule impact these activities?
- **Social issues such as food insecurity and child abuse**: How much of our school populations are impacted by these issues? How do we deal with these concerns when school normally is not in session—holiday breaks, summer break, and so on? Are there ways to provide meals to children when school is fully remote or in a hybrid schedule? Are there ways to identify children at risk for abuse and conduct family check-ins, evaluations, or counselling when school is fully remote? In a hybrid schedule?

There are likely other issues, but the above are examples of the thought process the boards and staff should have gone through that spring. Then, once the issues and questions were identified, work groups that included teachers, parents, and experts could have been constituted to research and think through these issues and questions during the summer. We were getting quite a bit of new information about the SARS-CoV-2 virus and COVID-19 over the summer, and these work groups could have been updated with information as it became available.

Then, midway through the summer, a virtual or distanced retreat with masks could have been held, during which time work groups could have made reports and updates on their thinking. This session could have been opened to teachers and parents on a virtual platform or by recording and posting the session online for their viewing. One common approach would then be to identify all the factors that should weigh in on the board's decision to reopen or close schools. These could have been put up on a board, and then participants could have been given a certain number of Post-it notes to place under the issues they thought were of most importance to the decision-making to influence the ultimate weighting of the issues for the board. Alternatively, there are online voting methods that can be used if people are meeting virtually.

With a decision framework and the weighting of criteria, the board and staff could then work to create dashboards of metrics or indicators for those things that can be measured or quantified to provide a constant update to the board to be used at their meetings as they decide and vote on issues.

Although this process takes time and effort on many people's part, it is a way to streamline decision-making for complex and high-risk decisions. It would have relieved a great deal of stress on boards and it would have provided transparency to and engagement for stakeholders that, in turn, would have dialed down the pressure and rhetoric board members were subjected to.

Many schools, through their school boards and state boards of education, tried to set up formulas for case counts per 100,000. The thought was that this approach would place schools in either a green, yellow, or red category that would then dictate what conditions the schools would operate under. While we anticipated that the rate of infections among students resulting from in-school transmission would be less than that of the greater community, we did anticipate that it would increase with a commensurate increase in community spread and likewise decrease with a corresponding decrease in community spread. Instead, what we found was that in schools with universal masking in place and good efforts made at physical distancing, there was very little in-school transmission regardless of the level of community spread. However, more students and teachers were identified as infected when community spread was higher. Most in-school transmission that did occur was associated with extracurricular activities, particularly sports and cheerleading. While there were significant numbers of students and teachers infected, the vast majority of infections, on contact tracing, were determined to have occurred outside of school. Parties, sleepovers, carpooling, and getting together after school were commonly identified risks for how the exposures occurred.

Recommendation #30

School Boards Must Begin Planning Early

School boards and superintendents need to engage physicians, public health experts, and business leaders or governance experts early on in a public health crisis to assist them with planning and mitigation efforts. That planning should include clear, frequent, and transparent communications with stakeholders and provide for their engagement in the planning process.

Recommendation #31

School Boards Need a Decision-Making Framework

School boards need a structured process with a decision framework and dashboard to guide their decision making so that board discussions are focused, objective, transparent, and internally consistent.

Public Health Department, Boards, and County Commissioners

Another major issue that occurred in many parts of the nation, and certainly in our state of Idaho, was what happened within the public health districts, and with the public health boards of our state and county commissioners.

According to legislation enacted in 1970, Idaho is divided into seven public health districts, with each of the public health districts having one physician assigned to them by state law. The other members, for the most part, are all elected officials that are either county commissioners (realtors, lawyers, businessmen, farmers, ranchers, and so forth) or other elected representatives. There is no requirement that board members understand anything about public health, that they accept basic established principles of public health, or that they defer to public health experts as to the facts of a health threat.

Of course, in 1970, state legislators were likely not contemplating a pandemic or a health emergency that would impact our very geographically diverse state all at once. In normal times, these boards' business was liable to be mundane, many of their decisions involving choices as to priorities for public health investments and funding. Therefore, significant public health knowledge may have been less important, and it might make sense to have the boards mostly made up of elected officials who were familiar with allocating state and county funding.

But in the time of a pandemic, with a significant health threat facing the citizens these boards are charged with protecting, this structure was a mistake and caused great disarray. Despite the executive director being knowledgeable and bringing in outside medical and public health experts to the board meetings, many of the public health district boards became more focused on the economic impact of the pandemic, on businesses, on schools, on the freedom of individual rights not to wear masks and politics, evidenced in at least one case by a board member calling the pandemic a hoax.[11] As another example, a board implemented a mask mandate for their district, but at a subsequent meeting—at which the local hospital leaders were reporting a dangerous strain on hospital capacity—voted to repeal the mask mandate, a decision that notably drew a rebuke from the governor of a state that borders that district.[12] The focus on the public's health got lost in the process. Those that spoke the loudest and most forcefully seemed to carry the day.

In some cases, there was a lack of understanding that public health and medical guidance should come from scientific evidence, where we can compare the outcomes of large numbers of study participants who receive an intervention against a control group that does not. At least one board member seemed to have little appreciation that just because something did or did not happen in one anecdotal case, with a virus that produces very different effects among those it infects, it would be irresponsible to apply that one observation to guidance for all. In fact, studies that were contrary to that anecdotal observation were often dismissed, as was guidance from the CDC and WHO. In this specific case, the board member proposed guidance that those who had confirmed infections but were asymptomatic should not have to isolate, but could return to work and risk exposing other people because she knew of one individual who did return to work under these conditions and did not infect anyone.[13]

In our Health District Number Four, the Central District Health, on which Dr. Epperly was a physician board member, we saw the political pressure play out. Not only did those board members get well over 7,000 emails through the course of the pandemic up to the point of writing this book, but most of them actually were in support of the public health measures, such as masking, distancing, and gathering size limitations. In fact, the data from email traffic showed that more than 60 percent of people were in favor of these efforts. However, some board members indicated that they received many emails from constituents who were strongly opposed to mask mandates. It seems likely that the Idaho Freedom Foundation, Health Freedom Idaho and other vocal groups, whose message was that "this was an absolute infringement of people's personal liberties and life," were more influential with some board members, particularly those who would face reelection in the future.

"Who was the Public Health Department to tell people that they had to wear face masks?" was a common refrain. It became very apparent that the tail was wagging the dog. The minority of vocal citizenry upset by what they saw as governmental and public health overreach started to override the public's good with their protests. Because of this, county commissioners buckled under the weight of such decision-making and subsequently took either no action or, at best, just made recommendations. As a consequence, they punted their responsibility and accountability to a confused public who did not know what to do or, worse, decided their course of action based on misinformation. All of this represented a failure of leadership and a failure of our government in action. As Winston Churchill has famously said about our country, "You can always count on the Americans to do the right thing—after they have tried everything else."

Consideration should also be given to whether and what decision-making should be centralized with the state versus decentralized with the public health districts, especially in a public health emergency that impacts or is likely to impact the entire state.

Recommendation #32
Reevaluate State Public Health Structures and Infrastructure
Each state should reevaluate their public health structure and infrastructure to determine what worked and what didn't work, and what changes should be made for the future, anticipating that we will go through more epidemics and pandemics in the future.

Significant deference should be made by public health board members to the recommendations of career public health experts and leaders in the public health department. It is unfair to subjugate members of these boards to political pressures that might influence decisions that should be made in the best interests of those citizens the public health organization is charged with serving. For this reason, public health board members should not be elected, and if a legislator is going to be appointed to a public health board, it may be best that the legislator has decided not to run for reelection or retired from the legislature. Political pressures have no place in developing public health guidance in response to an emerging health threat.

Recommendation #33
Reevaluate Public Health Board Member Qualifications
A best practice would be to require board members to have at least a basic understanding of public health and a commitment to its fundamental principles.

Churches, Temples, Mosques, and Synagogues

Another group that had mixed reviews during the pandemic were our places of worship and their leaders. Certain church leaders took the pandemic seriously and had virtual online services or very physically distanced worship services, and others did not. We know from case reports that singing in choirs can forcefully expel the SARS-CoV-2 virus into the air in an aerosolized fashion that can infect others in the room. Some churches blatantly ignored the advice from public health departments around these issues—and worse, some pastors undermined the public health messages.

There were several court challenges to the restrictions states placed on worship services, with rulings typically supporting reasonable restrictions. Appeals to the US Supreme Court were turned down by a divided court that left in place decisions by lower courts, ruling that these restrictions were not unconstitutional. This should not be taken as a suggestion that courts should permit any and all restrictions on worship services, but certainly there seems to be a consensus that a serious public health emergency may require certain restrictions that are not greater than necessary to control the spread of disease and not in effect longer than necessary to accomplish these aims.

Religious leaders hold a position of trust and great influence with their congregations. With that trust and influence comes a responsibility to exercise great care not to abuse that trust and harm their followers. In times of public health emergencies, a consistent message is critical to the well-being of the public.

Recommendation #34

The Role of Religious Leaders

We urge religious leaders to work more closely with public health experts to understand health threats, minimize risks to their congregants, and amplify the public health messages that will help protect members of their faith.

Citizens

Ultimately, it is the responsibility and accountability of each of us as a citizen to determine what we think is the right thing to do in a pandemic environment, but it is also our responsibility as a member of a community and society to take actions that will protect others. To do so requires one to keep an open mind and look at multiple newsfeeds and media sources to try to get the best information one can get. Obviously, we should give great deference to the advice of our local and state public health officials and the CDC.

What became clear in this pandemic is that the citizens of our society received mixed messaging from the president, the vice president, the CDC, other top administrative officials, schools, school boards, physicians, public health departments, governors, lieutenant governors, legislators, mayors, first responders, television news editors, Facebook, Twitter, and countless other sources. Often, one's political party affiliation influenced which messages were given the most credence. As Louis Pasteur said: "The microbe is nothing, the terrain is everything."

We had a tremendously chaotic backdrop that allowed SARS-CoV-2—which was extremely contagious and many times more lethal than influenza—to declare open season on the United States. These complex intersections of COVID-19 and society provide some insight into why the United States struggled so much with the pandemic. Even though the United States represents only 4 percent of the world's population, it represented approximately 20 percent of the world's cases and the world's deaths from the pandemic. All of these social elements above were the kindling upon which the fire of the pandemic burned.

Recommendation #35

Preparing Our Children for the Next Pandemic

In preparation for the next pandemic, educators must find ways to teach students methods for assessing the reliability and trustworthiness of news and information. We must also instill in our children that as members of a society, we must realize that in those situations where the consequences of our choices do not solely affect ourselves, but can harm others, we must make responsible actions that protect others.

Personal Story: "Rights Were Replaced by Duty"

The following story was related to Dr. Epperly by Jim Girvan, PhD, MPH.

On November 29, 1941, my parents were married in Portland, Oregon. They honeymooned on the Oregon coast. The second-to-last day of their honeymoon was December 7: the day Pearl Harbor was attacked. They were ordered off the beach, told to head home to Portland and to darken all windows at night. Dad recalled that the military expected a possible Japanese attack on the West Coast, so darkening windows reduced the "target light."

As you might imagine, Dad reported that some folks disobeyed and did not darken their windows because it interfered with "their rights." Sound familiar? As a national and state emergency had been declared, those who disobeyed were fined and told in no uncertain terms to darken their windows. They were also told that their individual rights were "out the window," so to speak, in a state of emergency for the health and safety of others. Dad went on to become a B-17 pilot in the European theater of operations.

Fast-forward 27 years to the fall of 1968. A young graduate student in chemistry at Washington State University heard on the news that President Johnson was canceling most graduate student deferments immediately. I was drafted within one week of that announcement. The draft made young men's lives very unpredictable—our rights for a time were owned by the government. I did not protest—that is the way it was. Rights were replaced by duty, and ultimately I was sent to serve in Vietnam as a medical technologist in small clinics and a surgical hospital in Phu Bai Combat Base near Huế. It was there that I saw firsthand the effects of weapons on the human body. Weapons fire projectiles that do great harm. Bullets simply ate up portions of, if not all of, the limbs or organs that were impacted. Mines, booby traps, and trip wires were even more devastating.

Fast-forward again to 2020. A respiratory virus has invaded the human species. We learn that the virus is largely spread through droplets that easily transfer from one person to another when talking and in close contact if the person emitting the droplets is infected with the virus. To me, this is analogous to the soldier's situation, with one exception. The soldier knew who the target was when he fired the weapon, and the results were immediately visible.

The weapon, in the case of the virus, is a human—most likely an unsuspecting human who has been infected but has no symptoms—and the bullet is the infected droplet. The unintended target is another unsuspecting human, who may get seriously ill and even die. But we have a low-tech preventive measure against the "viral bullets" that is highly effective and inexpensive: a mask. Much more effective than a flak jacket for a real bullet.

And yet, we still have people who claim their rights are being trampled on when they are asked or mandated to wear a mask. If an emergency had not been declared, they might have had a point, but their viral bullets might well find an unsuspecting human target that is vulnerable to infection. Much like wartime situations, our individual rights have partly been paused during a public health emergency for the benefit of others' health and safety.

After all, if we all have these fundamental rights, then one person's fundamental rights cannot be said to trump another person's fundamental rights. Yet when someone is unwilling to wear a mask, that is exactly what happens. If legislators do not wear masks in the Capitol, then those who are at high risk if infected do not maintain their rights to attend in person to listen to the session or attend committee meetings, unless they are willing to risk their life to do so. When people claim it to be their "right" not to wear a mask in the grocery store, the pharmacy, or the hair salon, then the elderly who need these services and relish the opportunity to get out of their home once every few weeks may well decide that the risks are too high and feel that their right to attend these public places has been infringed.

But the problem is that it never was about fundamental rights. You do not have a fundamental right to go into a restaurant without a shirt and shoes on. You do not have a fundamental right to yell or sing during a movie. In society, we give up "rights" every day—you do not get to speed or run red lights on your way to work, you cannot park anywhere you please, you cannot have a loud party in our backyard until three in the morning. In society, we all agree to minor restrictions on our civil liberties or rights every day, because when we do, we also benefit from others agreeing to those minor inconveniences.

This was never about rights; it was about decency and caring for others. If I am sick and coughing, I don't go on a flight or go into work. Do I have the right to fly or go to the office? Probably. But because I have respect for others, I don't threaten their health by asserting my rights. If I get COVID, chances are I will be fine. But if I transmit it to someone else, maybe they won't be. In the end, it has never been about civil liberties; it has always been about our capacity to respect and care for others. The loss of life due to COVID-19 has been tragic. The loss of our humanity, our very souls, has been the greatest loss of all.

CHAPTER 4

The Haves and the Have-Nots

The Racial and Ethnic Disparities Revealed by COVID-19

Of all the forms of inequality, injustice in health care is the most shocking and inhumane.

MARTIN LUTHER KING JR.

To understand the racial and ethnic health disparities magnified by COVID-19, it is important to look at what systemically leads to these disparities and inequities. Let us start with the definition of health equity. "Health equity" means that everyone has the opportunity to be as healthy as possible. Equitable opportunity includes equal access to and distribution of resources.[1] It has become clear in the last several decades that only about 10 percent of a person's health is related to health care. Over 90 percent of a person's health comes from their behaviors, the environment in which they live, their genetics, and other factors.[2]

This recognition has placed an added emphasis on what have been called the social determinants of health. These social determinants have a greater impact on a person's health than the care provided by our existing health care system and can be lumped into several large categories that, when taken as a whole, can be foundational to understanding why racial and ethnic groups and people of color are more disadvantaged and have higher risks of illness, hospitalization, and death from COVID-19.

Five of these categories, as noted by the Centers for Disease Control and Prevention (CDC), are as follows:

1. **Neighborhood and physical environment**: People of color from different racial and ethnic backgrounds often find themselves having trouble getting affordable, quality housing due to their socioeconomic status. They live in more crowded conditions and have problems with reliable transportation. These situations often contribute to a lack of access to nutritious, affordable foods. They are also more likely to have exposure to environmental pollution, such as the presence of lead and radon. Oftentimes, houses may contain family members from multiple generations, with elderly citizens living with school-aged children; the children may bring home illnesses from school that can threaten their older relatives. Multigenerational living is also often associated with poor health of elderly family members, requiring care and support from their relatives, and lower overall family income, where assisted living is an unaffordable option.
2. **Health and health care**: People from racial and ethnic minority groups often lack access to quality, timely health care and health insurance. Physician offices are frequently not located in their neighborhoods.
3. **Occupation and job conditions**: Many socioeconomically disadvantaged people have jobs that are in an essential work setting. There is disproportionately more of that work in health care facilities, farms, factories, food production and processing, grocery stores, and public transportation.[3]
4. **Wealth**: Ethnic and racial minority groups often have lower income and greater debt. All of this leads to not being able to obtain affordable, quality housing, nutritious food, health care, and reliable childcare.[4]
5. **Education**: Similarly, people in these groups often struggle to find opportunities to achieve higher-quality education. This struggle decreases literacy and results in lower high school

completion rates, which present barriers to college entrance. These groups thus have limited future job options, which lead to lower paying and less stable jobs.

These social determinants of health disproportionately place racial and ethnic minority groups in harm's way when it comes to a pandemic like COVID-19. They exist in an environment that makes them easier prey for the virus, and data bears this out.

Let us now look at how the social determinants of health have recently played out, driven by SARS-CoV-2 exposure risks, disparities in COVID-related illness, disparities of COVID-associated hospitalizations, and disparities in COVID-related deaths.

Risk of Exposure to COVID-19

The environment one lives in has a direct link to potential exposure to COVID-19. The neighborhood and physical environment associated with poor quality housing, population density, and multi-generational households increases exposure risk. This has also been demonstrated in correctional facilities, homeless shelters, and long-term care facilities, which are often referred to as shared or congregate living and housing.[5]

The risk of exposure to COVID-19 also varies by occupation. Many racial and ethnic minorities are in essential jobs, such as health care, transportation, food service, farms, factories, warehouses, food processing, and grocery store workers. Since they are working close to the public, and to each other, their rates of exposure are increased. During April to May 2020, over 16,233 meat and poultry processing facility personnel were infected with COVID-19.[6] Among infected workers tracked by race and ethnicity, 87 percent were racial or ethnic minorities.[7] Not only do people in these jobs find themselves at greater risk of exposure, but they have more limited job options that allow them time away from work. If they miss work, they do not get paid and may lose their jobs. If they do not get paid, they cannot pay for child care, and without child care they cannot go to work, so they go to work sick.

In essence, they are locked into being at increased risk of exposure and then exposing others.

Other aspects of the social determinants of health reduce access to timely COVID-19 testing. Testing was a major problem for the United States in the early phase of COVID-19. One study found that the median travel time to COVID-19 testing locations was twenty minutes.[8] Racial and ethnic minority groups and people located in rural areas had longer travel times, more challenges in arranging for transportation to testing sites and more difficulty getting time away from work to obtain testing services. Many also lacked health insurance and had a harder time being able to pay for home testing. All these delays in testing potentially had people working when ill or infected but asymptomatic. Because of this, there was increased spread of the virus to others.[9]

Risk of Severe Illness or Death from COVID-19

Race, ethnicity, and gender, along with certain underlying medical conditions, have been demonstrated to place people at increased risk of severe illness. Race, ethnicity, and lower income are strongly associated with increased morbidity and mortality. A recent study has found that people from racial and ethnic minority groups are more likely to have increased COVID-19 disease severity upon admission to the hospital.[10] Much of this came from delaying care for reasons that have been previously mentioned in this chapter. This delay led to more severe disease, which then led to an increased number of hospitalizations, people being admitted to the ICU, and deaths.[11] A study in Atlanta, Georgia, showed that Black patients with COVID-19 were more likely to be hospitalized due to severe cases of COVID-19 than white patients. The admission rates were 79 percent for Black people in this study, compared to 13 percent for white people.[12] This data derives from the fact that the health status of racial and ethnic minority people is often poorer than their white counterparts. Common underlying conditions such as diabetes, high blood pressure, obesity, chronic kidney disease, and congestive heart failure are higher for people in racial and ethnic minority groups.[13] These individuals also have a higher proportion of other health conditions, including various lung diseases, cancer, and stroke. This results in a toxic combination of delayed care, higher exposure, and sicker people with underlying medical conditions. This then leads to increased hospitalization rates, ending up more often in the intensive care unit, and, again, a greater percentage of people dying.

These effects are well-documented. A study from New York City showed a correlation between Black and Hispanic patients having higher obesity rates and suffering higher COVID-19 mortality rates.[14] Another study from Boston found that Black patients were more likely to have one or more underlying medical conditions than people from other racial groups. Such studies demonstrate that people with high blood pressure, diabetes, and higher body mass index were more likely to die.[15]

It must also be noted that the impact disproportionately borne by racial and ethnic minority groups was not only on their health, but also on their jobs and finances. As of August 2020, more Hispanic (53 percent) and Black people (43 percent) had lost a job or taken a pay cut compared to white people (38 percent).[16] Black people (40 percent) and Hispanic people (43 percent) had to use money from savings or retirement to pay bills, compared to 29 percent of white people.[17] In addition, 43 percent of Black people and 37 percent of Hispanic people had trouble paying their bills compared with white people (18 percent).[18]

All of this taken together demonstrates how the social determinants of health can play out in poorer communities that are primarily made up of people from racial and ethnic minorities, which not only exposes them to higher risk, but results in a toxic combination of health care conditions. All of this leads to a higher risk of severe illness and death from COVID-19.

Disparities in COVID-19 Illness

As can be seen in the pie chart (figure 4.1), white people represent a 60 percent majority of the United States' population. Hispanic or Latino people represent 18 percent; Black people represent 12 percent;

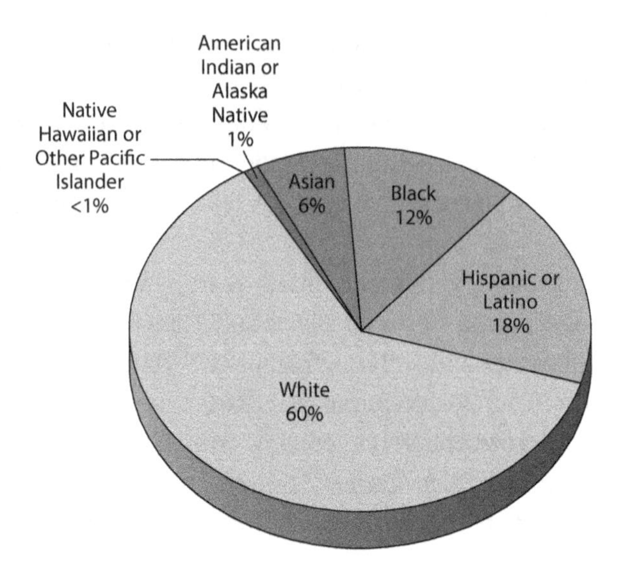

Figure 4.1. The percentage of racial and ethnic groups in the United States, with information drawn from the CDC.

Asian people represent 6 percent; people who identify with more than one race account for 3 percent (not shown); American Indian or Alaska Native people constitute approximately 1 percent, and Native Hawaiian or other Pacific Islander people represent less than 1 percent of the population.

The highest percentage of total COVID-19 cases are among white people because they represent the greatest number of people in the United States. However, people from racial and ethnic minority groups are disproportionately higher in their infection rate, hospitalization rate, and death rate than one would expect from their percentages of the general population.

The proportion of people who tested positive for COVID-19 is illuminating. This data revealed that, of white people who were tested, about 7 percent tested positive. Asians represented about 7.2 percent, Hispanic or Latino people 11.9 percent, and Black people 13.8 percent. Persons categorized otherwise tested positive at a rate of about 13.5 percent. This speaks to the fact that racial and ethnic minority groups often have a harder time accessing health care and are delayed in obtaining it. It is only when they become more ill from COVID-19 that they enter the health care system. The increase in positive percentage rate in a particular group represents a disproportionately high number of individuals who have become sick. As has been shown, when these racial and ethnic minority groups seek care because of more advanced illness, they then have increased risk of hospitalization, ICU admissions, being placed on ventilators, and death. COVID-19 cases, hospitalizations, and deaths by race and ethnicity are presented in table 4.1, which compares the rate ratios between various demographic groups and whites.[19]

As can be seen from the data, the rate ratios for Asian, Black, Hispanic, and American Indian or Alaskan Native people are much higher than that of white people. The relative risks of contracting COVID-19 for Black, Hispanic, American Indian, or Alaskan Native people are anywhere from 40 to 80 percent higher than that of white people. The risk of hospitalizations for Black, Hispanics, American Indians, or Alaska Natives are roughly four times higher than that for whites, and the risk of death is slightly less than three times higher for Black, Hispanic, and American Indian or Alaskan Native people compared to white people. In summary, there is a powerful connection and correlation between the various social determinants of health, such as housing, food security, good nutrition, good jobs, education, timely transportation, access to health care, and access to testing. This disparity then drives delays in obtaining care and the inevitable resultant outcomes.

Table 4.1. COVID-19 case, hospitalization, and death ratios by race and ethnicity compared with whites

Incidence	White	Asian	Black	Hispanic	American Indian or Alaska Native
Cases	1.0	0.6×	1.4×	1.7×	1.8×
Hospitalizations	1.0	1.2×	3.7×	4.1×	4.0×
Deaths	1.0	1.1×	2.8×	2.8×	2.6×

Source: Centers for Disease Control and Prevention, "Disparities in COVID-19 Illness: Racial and Ethnic Health Disparities," updated December 10, 2020, https://www.cdc.gov/coronavirus/2019-ncov/community/health-equity/racial-ethnic-disparities/increased-risk-illness.html

Disparities in COVID-19-Associated Hospitalizations

Racial and ethnic minority groups have disproportionately higher hospitalization rates among all age groups, including children younger than 18 years.

The age-adjusted COVID-19-associated hospitalization rates by race and ethnicity from March 1 through December 5, 2020, are shown in figure 4.2. The Hispanic, Native American, and Black populations represent significantly higher proportions than the white population, even though they represent smaller percentages of our society.

The rate ratios of hospitalization for COVID-19, with the rate for white people as the reference ratio, are given in table 4.2. As can be seen, people from racial and ethnic minority groups represent a disproportionately higher rate of people hospitalized.

Disparities in Death from COVID-19

As of December 31, 2020, there were 1.8 million deaths across the world and 342,743 deaths in the United States. The data on race and ethnicity in the United States gathered for more than 90 percent of all people

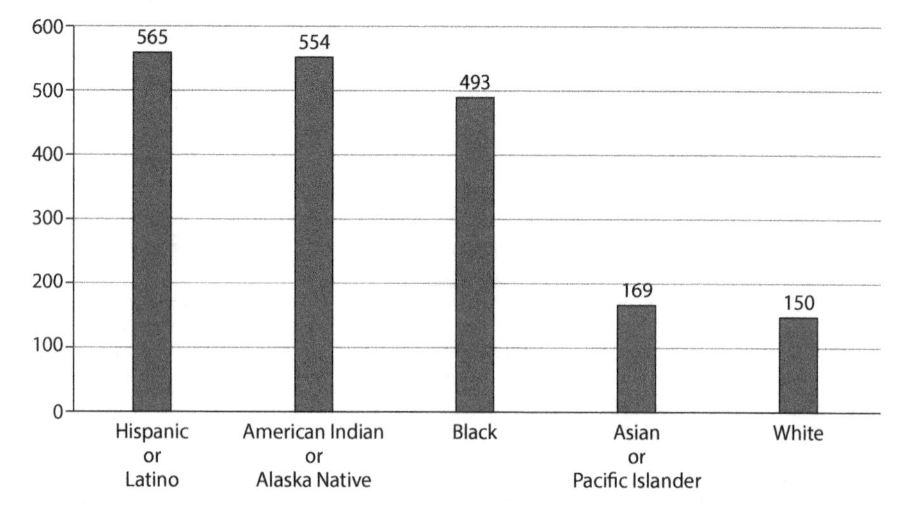

Figure 4.2. Age-adjusted COVID-19 hospitalization rates by race and ethnicity, with information drawn from the CDC.

Table 4.2. Hospitalization rate ratios per 100,000

Age Category	White	Asian or Pacific Islander	Hispanic or Latino	Black	American Indian or Alaska Native
0–17 Years	1.0	1.6×	5.3×	3.8×	3.1×
18–49 Years	1.0	1.4×	6.4×	4.4×	6.7×
50–64 Years	1.0	1.3×	4.7×	3.9×	4.6×
65+ Years	1.0	0.9×	2.4×	2.7×	2.2×
Overall Rate (Age Adjusted)	1.0	1.1×	3.8×	3.4×	3.7×

Source: Centers for Disease Control and Prevention, "COVID-NET: A Weekly Summary of COVID-19 Hospitalization Data," March 1 to November 28, 2020, https://www.cdc.gov/coronavirus/2019-ncov/covid-data/covid-net/purpose-methods.html

who have died from COVID-19 reveal that the percentage of Hispanic, Black, and Native American people who have died was higher than the percentage these racial and ethnic minority groups represent among the total US population. These excess death percentages follow the same higher trend lines in all racial and ethnic minority groups and for essentially all their age groups.

Death rate ratios among racial and ethnic minority groups compared to the number of deaths among white people are demonstrated in table 4.1. As with hospitalizations, there is a disproportionate number of deaths in Black, Hispanic, American Indian, and Alaska Native populations. When people live with more chronic illnesses and are adversely impacted by the social determinants of health, it is no wonder that they arrive for health care sicker and that their risk of hospitalization, ICU admission, ventilator usage, and subsequent death are higher.

Unintended Consequences of COVID-19 Mitigation Strategies

With the institution of public health measures to help control the COVID-19 pandemic, unintended consequences also developed. The public health measures that were used in the COVID-19 pandemic consisted of mask wearing, handwashing, physical distancing, limiting the group size of gatherings, restrictions on travel, closures of businesses and schools, and stay-at-home orders. These were all done in good faith to try to protect human life from COVID-19. What was not realized was that these measures would have a disproportionately negative impact on racial and ethnic minority groups and would cause an increased amount of difficulty in communities and populations with limited resources. These were communities that were already struggling with economic and financial survival. There were at least six areas in which this had an impact:

1. **Unemployment and loss of health insurance**: Black and Hispanic people were at particularly more risk than white people for losing jobs, losing insurance, or having reductions in pay.
2. **Food insecurity**: The loss of jobs and financial insecurity increase the risk for food insecurity. School closures decrease the number of kids getting school lunches. In 2016, 15.6 million US households were food insecure. Black families and households have nearly two times the rate of food insecurity (22.5 percent) versus the national average of 12.3 percent, while Hispanic families and households sit at 18.5 percent.[20] Based on a study done at Dr. Epperly's organization, overall food insecurity in our population was at 20 percent. Food insecurity is associated with poor health. Unfortunately, the mitigation strategies that were used to help fight COVID-19 disproportionately impacted the employment and health insurance coverage of racial and ethnic minority groups, placing them at greater risk.
3. **Housing instability**: Racial and ethnic minorities have been at greater risk of eviction and homelessness during the pandemic. Many have not been able to pay rent on time. The percent of adults who faced this challenge increased from April to July for all racial and ethnic groups, with the largest increase being in the Hispanic population.[21]
4. **Preventive health care services**: Health care providers through the pandemic saw a decrease in the number of people seeking health care services. This was marked in the first several months of the pandemic. However, decrements in

health care utilization existed throughout the time of the pandemic. Disruptions in providing routine preventive and other non-emergency care such as routine well-child visits, preventive dental care, and immunizations were observed. A recent survey estimated that 41 percent of US adults avoided medical care during the pandemic because of concerns surrounding COVID-19.[22] There was a substantial reduction in orders for vaccines for well-child visits that started after the pandemic, the week of March 13, 2020.

5. **Mental health care**: There is no doubt that the pandemic has had a major impact on mental health care. We are not sure we know the full depth of that impact yet. Fear and anxiety increased, which worsened their related disorders, as well the number of cases of depression and suicide. It is not clear what the impact of this is across racial lines. There is no question, however, that these conditions all worsened. Potential disruptions in getting timely medications for ongoing chronic mental diseases were an issue through the pandemic. The overall effect of COVID-19 on mental health is complicated. It lies at the intersection of age, income, employment, and other social factors, in addition to race and ethnicity.[23]
6. **Bereavement**: With close to 500,000 deaths in the United States as of this writing, there has been enormous grief and bereavement from the loss of loved ones. The pandemic has been particularly brutal in not allowing loved ones to be at the bedside to hold their family member's hand or say goodbye. This has had a disproportionate impact on racial and ethnic minority groups, primarily because they are overrepresented in the number of deaths that occurred from COVID-19. To be clear, this is a major issue for all people, not just racial or ethnic minority groups, but was particularly heightened in racial and ethnic minority populations because they were far more likely to have known someone who died from COVID-19.[24]

Summary

The COVID-19 pandemic has revealed many of the health inequities in the United States. These health and health care inequities put people in racial and ethnic minority groups at higher risk for being exposed to COVID-19, contracting COVID-19, getting sicker with the illness, presenting late for health care, being hospitalized, being admitted to the ICU, being placed on a ventilator, and ultimately dying from COVID-19. The data speaks powerfully to the racial and ethnic minority groups being disproportionately represented and exposed to COVID-19, having increased cases, hospitalizations, and deaths. The social determinants of health that impact low-income populations have a powerful, synergistic effect on morbidity and mortality.

The American health care delivery system, by the nature of its design, creates disparities in treatment and outcomes. These disparities become more apparent during a public health crisis. The country, its leaders, and the US Department of Health and Human Services must acknowledge these disparities and take actions to address them and improve the health and outcomes of care for those who are socioeconomically disadvantaged. We must address these disparities and inequities now in order to avoid unnecessary morbidity and mortality during the next pandemic.

Recommendation #36
Health Care Disparities

State and local public health agencies should partner with local social service organizations, schools, churches, libraries, and food banks to provide education relative to a public health crisis, screening, testing, and on-site or mobile health care services in a culturally sensitive manner.

Until such time as health care disparities have been successfully addressed, during an epidemic, pandemic, or other public health emergency, we must bring education, testing, and treatment to the worksites of disadvantaged parts of the population to help ensure adequate testing and care, while removing cost barriers. For example, delivering PPE to meat packing facilities, providing consultation as to how to reduce the risk of exposure, providing education to supervisors and employees, and making testing available would all help to minimize outbreaks. In addition, providing financial incentives to these companies to enable workers who are ill to remain home while preserving their jobs and pay should be explored.

Recommendation #37
Providing Personal Protective Equipment and Testing to Vulnerable Workers

We must identify those businesses with low-paid or skilled workers who must work in close proximity to each other and may not have access to PPE, so that we can deliver PPE to them. Further, we must make testing available on site, since these workers are likely unable to take time off to go to a testing center.

We must increase timely access to health care in racial and ethnic minority communities. This should be accomplished by having culturally appropriate health care clinics located in these neighborhoods with employees that reflect the diversity of the communities and who are able to take care of children, pregnant and nursing mothers, adults, and seniors. Arrangements must be in place to allow for a sliding-scale fee schedule according to the family's income, so that the care is affordable or provided at no cost.

Recommendation #38
Access to Care

We must increase timely access to health care in racial and ethnic minority communities, especially in times of a public health emergency. Lack of access will result in delayed diagnoses, the lack of ability to administer treatments designed to prevent severe disease (monoclonal antibodies and antivirals, for instance), patients presenting to hospitals with far more advanced disease, increased mortality, and increased exposures to others.

It is critical to remember that during an epidemic, pandemic, or other public health emergency, it will be very difficult to isolate those with infections and quarantine those with close contacts if these persons do not have housing and food security. Low-wage earners will often not have paid time-off benefits and will lose their income and potentially their jobs if they take time off to isolate or quarantine. With the loss of income, these people may be at risk for eviction for inability to pay their rent.

Recommendation #39

Protect Jobs, Pay, and Housing

During an epidemic, pandemic, or other public health emergency, we cannot expect low-wage workers to isolate and quarantine if there is no protection of their income and jobs. Congress must act quickly to provide for these protections, as well as preventing evictions.

CHAPTER 5

The Growing Fire

Public Health versus Public Protest

Be the change you wish to see in the world.

ANONYMOUS, OFTEN ATTRIBUTED TO MAHATMA GANDHI

One of the most incredible disconnects that occurred during the COVID-19 pandemic was the hostility and vitriol targeted at public health efforts trying to control the potential carnage of COVID-19 in our American communities. It is hard to believe that policies being done in good faith for the protection of the community and the community's health would be seen as infringements on people's personal liberties and freedom of choice. It was especially disturbing to us because these public health mitigation measures—so-called non-pharmaceutical interventions (NPIs) such as covering coughs and sneezes, wearing masks or face coverings, physical distancing, avoiding large gatherings, and washing hands frequently—are not novel or untested measures; rather, they are mainstays of containment strategies for respiratory viruses since the Spanish flu pandemic of 1918. These measures were critical to the success of limiting SARS in 2003 to an epidemic rather than the pandemic the virus threatened to become. Either we never learned the lessons from these past pandemics and epidemics, or we forgot them or disregarded them as we faced the COVID-19 pandemic. It is critical that we not forget or disregard the lessons of this pandemic as we prepare for the next.

We would agree that if this were not a public health emergency, there should not have been impositions on people's free will and personal choices. But the COVID-19 pandemic was, in fact, a public emergency, and we support science-based public health measures and restrictions, so long as those restrictions are the minimum necessary and for the minimum duration necessary to protect the public and so long as those actions taken are lawful and undertaken without putting others at unreasonable risk. Not only was COVID-19 declared a public health emergency of international concern by the World Health Organization on January 30, 2020, and a pandemic on March 11, 2020, but it was also declared a national public health emergency on March 13, 2020, by the United States.

This chapter examines the efforts made in public health across our nation to stem the transmission of this infection and how those efforts met with growing public resistance and pushback. These relationships are depicted in figure 5.1. On the x-axis (horizontal) are public health measures that increase in intensity as you go from left to right. On the y-axis (vertical) is growing public resistance as you go from the bottom to the top of the figure.

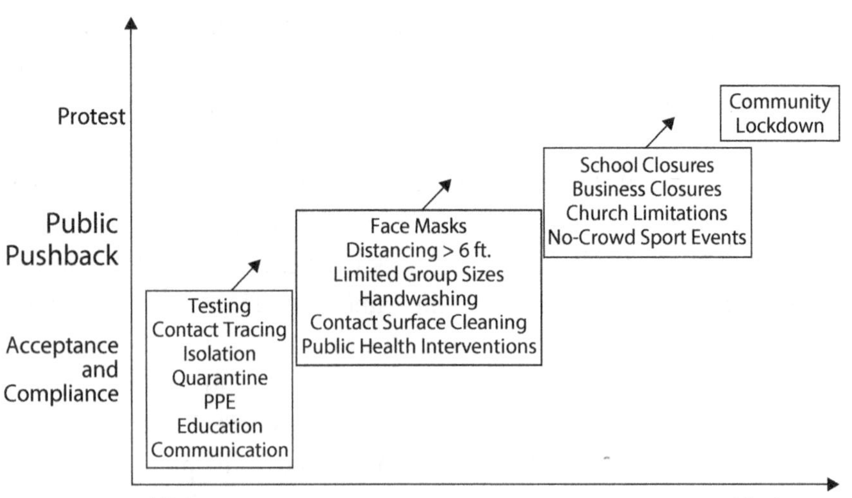

Figure 5.1. A comparison of public health non-pharmaceutical interventions by order of severity, on the x-axis, and the corresponding public pushback.

It would have been ideal if the United States had taken steps to corral and control the pandemic with the minimum amount of public health measures. Efforts such as widespread testing, contact tracing, isolation of sick individuals that tested positive, and quarantining of patients that are not yet sick but had been exposed to the virus would have made huge strides in stemming the rapid exponential spread of COVID-19 throughout the United States. However, the large number of cases that were due to asymptomatic spread of disease necessitated the additional measures of masks, physical distancing, and limitations on group sizes. These efforts, coupled with effective education and messaging campaigns using social media, TV, radio, and national media needed to be implemented early. Catchy messages like those other countries used, such as Austria and South Korea, could have helped early on in the COVID-19 outbreak in controlling the infection by encouraging public acceptance and compliance.

Recommendation #40

Act Early to Minimize the Severity and Duration of Non-pharmaceutical Public Health Interventions

For future pandemics or other public health emergencies, it is important to keep in mind that public health measures will be better embraced if implemented early, when they can be milder in terms of the restrictions imposed. Delays in efforts to contain the spread of illness will allow the threat to increase, and this may require more severe restrictions that are not only less likely to be adopted by the general public, but in fact may be met with organized resistance.

The United States failed in these early public health intervention efforts. Because there was an absence of widespread testing and an inability to conduct effective contact tracing due to the lack of testing, further exacerbated by insufficient amounts of personal protective equipment, it became inevitable that we could not get an early handle on controlling the spread of the infection. A nation as capable as the United States, which pumps nearly 18 percent of its gross domestic product into health care, should have been able to do more than we did.

The United States, through the CDC, has written the playbook on how to handle epidemics and pandemics in the past. However, with the weakening of the pandemic response resources, there was no clear plan or strategy. The United States, simply put, failed abysmally in controlling the COVID-19 epidemic effectively and efficiently in the months of March and April 2020—and, frankly, through the remainder of that year, at the end of which there was still no well-defined national plan.

Recommendation #41

Develop and Communicate the National Pandemic Response Plan

In a time of a pandemic or other public health emergency, it is critical that there is a national plan, and that plan must be clearly communicated to the states so that there is a clear understanding of what the federal government will do and what the states will need to do, with or without support from the federal government.

This then led to an escalation of public health measures across the nation needed to bring the infection under control. As noted in figure 5.1, some states, local governments, and public health districts then increased public health interventions. Ultimately, in a patchwork of uncoordinated responses, they then progressed to mandates that included face masking, distancing of greater than six feet, and group size limitations, while other states, local governments, and public health districts did not. All these interventions increased the amount of public involvement and individual responsibility and accountability required. This was met in some quarters with acceptance, compliance, and approval, but in other quarters with increased public anger, rejection, pushback, and protest.

The implementation of these public health measures to control the pandemic are by no means extraordinary. All of these had been used successfully in the 1918 Spanish flu pandemic, as well as with multiple epidemics that have occurred in Asia. In the face of both a global and nationally declared public health emergency, it was shocking that there was strong public protest and pushback around evidence-based public health measures. Measures that have demonstrated positive effects on flattening the curve and slowing the spread of COVID-19 in our society were met with considerable resistance. There is no doubt that it would have been best if we did not need to escalate to more restrictive public health measures. However, the failure of our federal response and its lack of a unified strategy to control the pandemic left states, local governments, and public health districts with a difficult decision to make: implement these restrictions with significant public backlash, take no action at all, or merely encourage the public to adopt the public health advice, the latter being the most common option taken.

Sadly, President Trump and Vice President Pence were not role models for mask wearing or speaking positively about these public health measures. In fact, they went out of their way to ignore the usage of face masks and repeatedly downplayed the seriousness of the pandemic. President Trump even said that "with the masks, it's going to be a really voluntary thing. You can do it; you don't have to do it. I'm choosing not to do it, but some people may want to do it, and that's okay."[1] This lack of role modeling and clear messaging only stirred up public confusion, anger, and resentment around these measures. The mixed messaging that came from the president, his administration, the CDC, and the surgeon general about whether the general public needed to wear face masks or whether they needed to leave those supplies for physicians, nurses, and other health care providers that needed them as part of their personal protection equipment only strengthened the public's perception that masks were unnecessary and not really that important.

As a result of the country's inability to gain control over the rapid spread of COVID-19 using public health measures in the March-April-May time frame, there needed to be an escalation of actions to try to increase control over the COVID-19 outbreak's impact on our nation's communities. This was particularly true with respect to outbreaks in long-term care facilities, prisons, and meat-packing plants. The rationale for this was so that we did not overwhelm hospital capacity in each of our communities that needed to care for not only COVID-19 patients, but also heart attack and stroke patients, trauma victims, and all the other patients we needed to care for even without a pandemic. This initially played out in New York City in March of 2020, where hospitals were overwhelmed. Field hospitals and morgue trailers had to be set up. Later, other cities such as Los Angeles would be overwhelmed, and in 2021, we would see entire states become overwhelmed, requiring the implementation of crisis standards of care.

The failure to successfully implement public health measures resulted in school closures, business closures, church closures, the cessation of sporting events, and more restrictions on group gathering sizes. All would agree that in an ideal situation, it would be best not to employ these measures. But in the March to May period of 2020, the impact of COVID-19 on the communities of our country made this necessary. Eventually, 94 percent of all schools closed across the country; at their peak, the closures impacted approximately 55.1 million students in 124,000 US public and private schools.[2] Almost every state either ordered or recommended that schools remain closed through the end of the 2019–2020 academic school year. Many businesses, including restaurants and movie theaters, voluntarily closed or closed because the reduction in customers meant not meeting overhead. With the passing of time, many businesses were mandated to close because of the growing and spreading infection. Gymnasiums, bars, and nightclubs fell into this category.

With the increase of these public health measures, public resentment, anger, pushback, and protests only grew. This was not helped by President Trump, who cavalierly said that he wanted schools to reopen and businesses not to close for the good of the economy. This mixed messaging only added fuel to the fire of public protest and pushback. "Which one is it?" the public angrily responded. "Are the schools supposed to close or stay open? If schools are to close, why are the bars open?"

We recognize that the most extreme form of public health intervention, community lockdowns, should only be done at the very beginning of the pandemic, when we don't yet understand a novel threat and need to buy time so that we can develop testing and employ isolation, contact tracing, and quarantines, or later in the pandemic, when all the measures that have preceded this have failed to stem disease transmission. But lockdowns became required widely across the United States for just this reason. Our failed efforts in planning, strategy, and implementation of more moderate public health measures or cooperation with those measures resulted in many communities having no choice but to implement some variation of a lockdown. State orders for a lockdown were issued across much of the United States in the early months of the pandemic. This resulted in an intensification of public resentment, anger, and protest. People were incredulous over the fact that such extreme measures were necessary when "COVID-19 was no more deadly than the flu," as they were repeatedly told by President Trump, conservative talk radio shows, and conservative TV networks. They were shocked that schools, businesses, bars, and restaurants were being shut down when the mortality rate was "less than 1 percent." Those advocating for fewer restrictions and a return to normal life would refer to other events with mortality rates of less than 1 percent and point out that we don't take these extraordinary precautions for those occurrences. But all of these arguments completely ignored the morbidity associated with infection and largely ignored the fact that the mortality rate was not uniform throughout the population. As the CDC would later report, using a reference age group of 18 to 29-year-olds as 1×, the relative mortality for those 40 to 49 years old was 10× (or 10 times) that of the reference group, those 50 to 64 years old was 30×, 65 to 74 years old was 90×, and those 75 to 84 years old was 220×.[3]

In the end, the lockdowns could not be sustained, partly due to the economic impact and partly due to public resistance. Terminating the lockdowns prematurely resulted in cases taking off again, but this time, few options remained.

Discussions about COVID-19 mortality likely confused the public. Those who wanted to minimize the mortality used the infection fatality rate, defined as the death rate among all who were infected. The denominator generally had to be projected to account for estimates of asymptomatic infections, since we did not have reliable numbers. In contrast, health professionals tended to use the case fatality rate, defined as the death rate using as the denominator only those persons with confirmed cases of COVID-19. Further, the public's assessment of risk based on the mortality rate was often inadequate because they would use the mortality rate averaged across all persons and ages, when in fact the risks for older adults were orders of magnitude greater than the mortality rate for children. As a result, the "average" mortality rate would greatly understate the mortality rate for older individuals. Worse, some would point to the extremely low rates of mortality in children and low rates in young adults to suggest that children should be back in school without precautions and young adults should return to work, while older individuals and those with underlying medical conditions that would face higher mortality if infected should remain home and sequestered. There often was little appreciation of or concern about the risks of these children and young adults transmitting the infection to others who would be at high risk for hospitalization and death.

Discussions of mortality also caused the public to largely overlook the risks of complications and long-term effects in those who survived COVID-19. Morbidity is the degree of suffering from a disease or medical condition, including the long-term health consequences, which for COVID-19 remained largely unknown at this point in the pandemic. The purpose of using the public health measures was not solely to try to prevent death, or mortality. The interventions were aimed at trying to ensure hospitals did not get overwhelmed and that they had enough staff, beds, and supplies to not only care for the sick, but also to make sure they had the bandwidth to care for all the heart attacks, strokes, appendicitis, bowel obstructions, and broken bones that inevitably happen even during a pandemic.

The public health interventions had less to do with deaths and more to do with the impact on people, both the effects related directly to the virus and the effects of other delayed care caused by people afraid to go to hospitals or emergency rooms for fear of exposure to the virus. They were also tied to COVID-19's impact on the economy, businesses, schools, and people's personal finances. And, as discussed in the preceding chapter, this impact was disproportionately felt in racial and ethnic minority groups and in those lower socioeconomic levels of our society.

All of this was magnified by COVID-19 having a very high asymptomatic rate. The studies show that up to 45 percent of people infected with the SARS-CoV-2 virus could be asymptomatic.[4] This could be as high as 79 percent in pediatric populations.[5] When you have a disease that can be unknowingly spread from person to person, it makes the usage of public health measures more important to control the disease's spread and eventual impact.

Why Did This Storm Grow Like It Did in the United States?

The United States has always been a nation that highly values individual rights and freedoms. This was apparent in our country's formation in 1776. Such statements as "give me liberty or give me death" and "don't tread on me" are iconic statements from our early years.

The United States, as a nation, is about 245 years old. This pales in comparison to our European and Asian counterparts, some of which are thousands of years old. Simply put, many of these nations are older, wiser, and more mature in their collective and societal approach to problems than the United States. They have gone through two major wars in the last 100 years in their own homelands. Many have gone through several epidemics and pandemics over the millennia and have learned lessons from them. The United States, conversely, has not had that much experience with wars on our own soil or with pandemics in our own land. Our response in comparison to that of many nations is one that is much more immature and inexperienced. In fact, if we use this comparison of the ages of these countries, the United States can be characterized as an angry adolescent versus older adults who have grown wiser and more mature by their own nation's life history.

It is of little surprise that the United States would struggle to accept increasing public health measures without a major overreaction, driven by our characteristic national focus on personal rights, freedoms, and perceived liberties. Since Donald J. Trump was elected as our 45th president, this struggle only intensified. President Trump has been the common denominator in stirring up antipathy among American citizens, doing much to divide and polarize our society to shore up his base and enhance his own power.

Unfortunately, the hyper partisan environment created the opportunity for politics to be injected into the response to a pandemic, and our nation's president can choose to promote or resist that. In our view, politics should never be a factor in the response to any national threat or emergency. Our criticisms of President Trump and his administration's handling of the pandemic are criticisms concerning leadership, not the Republican Party. One of us coauthors is a lifelong Republican. No doubt we would have had criticisms of a Democratic president were he or she in power at the time. At the same time, we praise President Trump and his administration for Operation Warp Speed elsewhere in this book, which in our view was the equivalent of President Kennedy's moonshot. Further, our criticism of President Trump's handling of the pandemic is only that, not an assessment of his presidency overall. The important point in preparing for our next pandemic is to acknowledge the failings and mistakes made throughout the world and the United States in the response to this pandemic, so that we learn from those and hopefully do not repeat them in responding to the next threat.

Why Did This Happen in Idaho?

Let us concentrate now for a while on our home state of Idaho. While each American state has its own circumstances, focusing on one example can be illustrative. Idaho has long been known, as are many of the intermountain western states, as a state that highly values personal liberties and freedom and disdains government intervention. We have a history in our state, from the Aryan Nations (1970) to Ruby Ridge (1992), of attracting protesters that are far-right extremists with political ideologies that are libertarian in thinking and anti-government in sentiment. This stems back to how Idaho was created. Throughout the 1800s, Idaho was known as being a wild western frontier territory. It promoted the rugged individualist. From fur trapping to forestry and logging to mining, it encouraged adventurous populations to come to the state and leave their "civilized" locations that were "too genteel," to get away from communities and states with perceived overreaching governments.

COVID-19, Black Lives Matter protests, and the 2020 elections have all factored in increased activity of paramilitary groups across the

United States, as well as growth in movements like Boogaloo and the elaborate anti-government conspiracy theory known as QAnon.[6] Protests against public safety measures during the pandemic created opportunities for joint activity by a variety of right-wing extremist groups such as the militias, the Three Percenters, Boogaloo, QAnon, Proud Boys and the Oath Keepers. These alliances continued throughout the pandemic as these groups protested the outcome of the 2020 presidential election.

There are three consistent themes that have been seen, most notably in right-wing groups, across this nation and that are perhaps even more pronounced in the state of Idaho because of its attraction to this type of rugged individualist. These three themes are anti-government sentiment, libertarian philosophies, and Christian identity politics.[7] This is observed particularly with the public protests around the public health interventions associated with the COVID-19 pandemic.

We should not be surprised that into this growing social and political storm and boiling cauldron of social unrest, a pandemic that forced escalating levels of public health actions needed to control a dangerous situation caused by a virus that is running in the community unchecked has caused such tension. Not unexpectedly, the result was public backlash and protests. All these issues only served to aggravate people with this mindset and activate them.

Of course, since most people are not looking to protest using armed violence, this expression of grievance-based political protesting based on personal beliefs was most often done in a way that did not escalate to armed violence. Most people were not intentionally looking to kill people as a protest against public health measures enacted in Idaho or in the nation, but they absolutely were looking to assert their personal freedoms, their personal liberties, and their Second Amendment rights to carry loaded automatic weapons. This is how it played out in the state of Idaho.

Literature supports that there is a neurotransmitter named dopamine that is released in the brains of individuals when they protest like this. In fact, brain imaging studies show that harboring a grievance (a perceived wrong or injustice, real or imagined) can activate the same neural circuitry as narcotics.[8]

Recent studies show that cues such as experiencing or being reminded of a perceived wrong or injustice activates these same sections of the brain, triggering pleasure and relief through retaliation. The retaliation doesn't need to be physical violence; it can be an unkind word or tweet and still generate similar gratification. People can become addicted to seeking retribution against those they consider their enemies. This has been called "revenge addiction," and explains why some people just can't "get over it" long after others feel they should have moved on.[9]

Not only are their needs and grievances being met as an individual, but collectively, as a social group, they feel the shared euphoria of this dopamine release. Indeed, their protests are probably not so much done as an individual action, but as a collective social activity as part of their perceived tribe. Herein lies the irony: even though they are protesting collectively against action being done for the public's good, they have now become part of a collective protest that potentially harms themselves individually. But beyond this, they also harm others in the community through their demand for their individual rights, unjustifiably setting aside the public's right to remain safe.

This dichotomy is frustrating. There is a significant disconnect between individuals who believe the government has no right to infringe upon their personal right and liberty not to wear a mask or to gather with a group of people, versus the government's collective role in protecting the public health of those among us who are most vulnerable. Instead of this being a collective response of maturity, calmness, and caring for our neighbors that requires us to make rather small self-sacrifices to our personal freedoms and liberties so that we can protect our neighbors and other members of our community, many angrily stomped their feet, as an immature child throwing a temper tantrum would, about their rights, without concern for others.

Was This Response More Extreme in Idaho?

This response, as described, occurred in every state across the United States. However, there was a spectrum of responses across states in regard to open protest. Older and larger states along the East and West Coasts of our nation showed a calmer, more mature, and collective approach to this issue, perhaps because they had already endured the impact of epidemics and pandemics on the public health of their communities, including the 1918 Spanish flu, smallpox, cholera, typhoid fever, and yellow fever. However, many of the younger states in the United States, including many in the intermountain west, as well as the Midwest and central part of our country, chafed under this bridle. We believe that Idaho serves as one of the most extreme examples of public protest and anger around public health interventions.

Part of this was because a large number of the citizens in Idaho embrace one or more of the three characteristics of the far-right movement. They embrace an anti-government sentiment, they espouse libertarian philosophies, and they have a right-leaning pseudo-Christian identity political viewpoint. Not only do these sentiments exist, especially in the rural areas of Idaho, but we also have several individuals and militia groups in Idaho that have led COVID-19 protests.

One such individual is Ammon Bundy. This is the Ammon Bundy who, with his father Cliven Bundy and another Bundy brother, along with a group of radical right extremists, took over the Malheur National Wildlife Refuge headquarters in Oregon in 2016. They held this station for 41 days while they conducted their protest against the American government for the perceived infringement of ranchers' rights by the Bureau of Land Management.

Ammon Bundy was later tried for this trespass and was acquitted for this crime because the prosecutors failed to prove conspiracy.[10] Ammon Bundy now lives in Idaho. His activity and direct engagement with protest in our community around an entire spectrum of perceived infringements on personal liberties and rights have been well-chronicled in multiple news articles about these protests. One such article is entitled "How Ammon Bundy Helped Foment an Anti-Masker Rebellion in Idaho."[11]

According to the article, Ammon Bundy began coordinating his first protests along with Health Freedom Idaho and the Idaho Freedom Foundation, which are other libertarian organizations in Idaho. Bundy has been quoted as melodramatically proclaiming, "If Idahoans complied with mask mandates and business shutdowns, then they will go further until we are lined up naked, facing a mass grave, being shot in the back of the head."[12]

Bundy, along with Health Freedom Idaho and the Idaho Second Amendment Alliance, have staged protests in Idaho as early as April 2020, with signs reading "Faith over Fear," "Liberty or Death," and that our governor is "non-essential."[13] These declarations, along with efforts by libertarian-leaning legislators in Idaho, have only intensified the political rhetoric and polarization around public protest. One Republican legislator in Idaho made outrageous statements, including that "The COVID-19 pandemic is a fraud perpetuated by a medical community that is enriching itself by misdiagnosing the rate of infection" and that "N95 masks are of no value."[14] These myths and untruths were amplified by President Trump months later on the national stage. There is a pastor in Idaho that is of libertarian leaning who suggested that the virus was not contagious as reported, and stated, "I've actually laid hands on people that have COVID and prayed for them. I never got COVID."[10]

A survey done by Carnegie Mellon University shows that Idaho is one of the least mask-compliant places in America.[15] It is no surprise, therefore, that in early July 2020, Idaho had the highest infection rate in the United States per capita, exceeding that of Florida. In fact, in the months of November and December, Idaho was in the top two states in the United States for its test positivity rate. The direct effect of the anti-mask protests has had a major impact on continuing to fuel the fire of COVID-19 in the state of Idaho.

Experts have warned that the right-wing embrace of conspiracy theories has become a mass radicalization.[16]

Leadership matters on such issues as these. Words also matter. When you have people like Ammon Bundy in the state of Idaho and a president like Donald Trump, who was a super spreader of conspiracies and disinformation from the White House, then you have an environment in which places like Idaho become the epicenter of a new epidemic: that of radicalization. When this type of thinking develops and is practiced by many people, exacerbated by a president eagerly stirring the pot of emotion and rhetoric, then it is not hard to imagine why people don't trust the government. They do not trust Congress. They do not trust the Supreme Court. They do not trust science. They do not trust medicine. They do not trust public health. They certainly do not trust the media. So, who do they trust? Well, they trust their tribe. They trust conspiracy theories that tell them what they want to hear.

What Lessons from the Public Health Protests Can Be Learned Going Forward?

This is a complicated array of issues that cannot be simply or easily solved. The steps necessary to help contain a viral pandemic with public health measures are the very same steps that only heighten the anger and resentment around the perceived personal loss of liberties in a nation and its states, whose citizens are used to having them. It is this resistance to non-pharmaceutical interventions that caused us to emphasize the need for quick action to lock down the area of an outbreak in hopes of containing it, or at least providing us with additional time to develop plans, testing, set up clinical trials for therapeutics, and begin work on vaccines, because once the virus is spreading to other countries, we have seen that containment efforts are often not complied with and difficult to enforce.

What needs to be remembered now and during future pandemics is that these public health interventions are short-term infringements on personal liberties. In fact, what we observed was when these vocal people promoted their own personal liberties, they infringed on others' liberties, making environments unsafe for all to enjoy. For example, when legislators and spectators insisted on their personal right to not to wear a mask in the Capitol during the legislative session, those who would have liked to participate in the legislative session or provide testimony but were older individuals with chronic medical conditions or disabilities no longer felt safe in attending the session. Further, in the case of Idaho, failure to employ non-pharmaceutical measures resulted in an outbreak among the legislature and staff that forced a recess for isolation and quarantine at public taxpayer expense.

Public health interventions are put in place so that we can all get through a viral pandemic as rapidly and efficiently as possible, with minimal loss of life, minimal morbidity, and avoiding overwhelming our health care delivery system while helping businesses, schools, and the economy function in this environment. If we all pitch in and do our parts during a pandemic, then society can function as best as it can until we get through the storm. That said, if this were a simple issue, we would have resolved it long ago. Really, what the pandemic is revealing is a more serious issue that is dividing our nation in regards to how we work and act with each other as a society in ways that are helpful, caring, and for the greater good. Therefore, some of the recommendations for what can be learned from this include the following:

1. **Provide education**: We need to have effective education, messaging, and communication around the pandemic as soon as possible in the earliest phases of an outbreak. By doing this, we hopefully will get as many people on board as is possible so that we can all pull in the same direction.

Recommendation #42

Communication and Education

Effective and timely education, communication, and messaging with the assistance of social scientists and professional communications and marketing experts are essential to help the public understand the threat, what they are being asked to do, and—most importantly—why it is critical to do it.

2. **Enhance civics education in elementary and secondary school curriculums**: We need to renew our emphasis on civics training to help growing children understand not only their role in society, but how in times of public health emergencies or mass crises, we need to pull together as a nation. Many people throughout the pandemic articulated a misunderstanding of the personal rights and liberties conferred by the US Constitution and failed to understand the limits on those rights and liberties. In fact, there was a complete misunderstanding by many that all

societies operate under norms and rules that govern behavior and necessarily involve some restrictions on rights in exchange for the benefits provided by that society or government. This can be effectively taught in school. Sadly, there will be some who will see this as indoctrination. Nothing could be further from the truth. We need to renew our covenant with each other and society about what each of us can do to help us all successfully navigate the next pandemic.

Recommendation #43

Civics and Social Responsibility

People of all ages need a better understanding of social contracts, particularly the US Constitution and the rights and liberties it confers, along with the limitations on those rights and liberties in the interest of promoting the well-being of our country's inhabitants. This education should begin in elementary school.

3. **Ensure that all people are heard, acknowledged, and respected**: America is a big place, full of a lot of different thoughts and ideas. We need to more effectively ensure that people have the right to be heard and the right to protest if they are not happy, in productive and respectful ways. However, we cannot let the right to be heard and the right to protest outweigh the collective right of the public to be kept safe in the time of a national pandemic or national emergency. At some point, we must rest on the principle that at times, but only temporarily, we all must sacrifice some of our personal rights for the greater good.

   We must embrace a culture where ideas are attacked, not people. Our leaders must try to determine and agree on the facts. Facts are facts. Our leaders should have a bipartisan disdain for untruths and misinformation. Once we agree on the facts, we can then begin to have productive discussions and debates as to how we, as a country, should respond to those facts. We must also acknowledge that no political party has a monopoly on all the best ideas.

The principle that we are all in this together and that we can all get through this together must be normalized and held as a personal and societal value.

Recommendation #44

Bipartisan Disdain for Misinformation and Disinformation

Misinformation and untruths must become a common enemy for all Americans, and especially our leaders. In a time of a pandemic or other public health crisis, leaders of all parties must determine and agree on facts and actively refute misinformation and untruths. We then should have vigorous debate on how the country should respond to those facts, by persuasive arguments rather than personal attacks.

4. **Elect effective leadership**: Leadership matters. It is critical to the successful management of a pandemic. We must have leadership at all levels from the president, vice president, senior administration officials, churches, schools, public health departments, governors, mayors, and others that are role modeling and educating the public on our best available public health guidance. These leaders must help effectively define and communicate our collective responsibilities in getting through this crisis together to the best of our abilities. Leaders must tell the public the truth, very clearly and without inciting panic. Leaders must communicate often, with empathy, but also projecting confidence and determination to contain the spread of infection. If we do this as a collective action, we will see a much better and effective response.

Recommendation #45

Communicating to the Public

Leaders should be clear as to the role we all play in protecting our families and neighbors and in containing the spread of the infection. When we learn new information that is in conflict with what we previously thought and communicated, we must be clear that we were mistaken and now have better information, explain why, and explain what we need the public to do with the information. Leaders must model the desired behaviors, or they will undermine them.

5. **Individual responsibility and accountability**: At the end of the day, each of us needs to ensure that we conduct ourselves with dignity, thoughtfulness, maturity, and respect in regard to our actions at the time of a crisis. This is particularly true in a public health emergency such as a pandemic or other natural disaster. If we all take that personal responsibility as a leader, as a parent, or as an individual person, helping our families, our neighbors and ourselves with our actions, then we collectively will do much better in our response as a nation. One quote often attributed to Mahatma Gandhi goes, "You must choose to be the change you want to see in the world." If we all could truly do that, we would make a huge positive impact on the next pandemic.

Recommendation #46

Personal Responsibility

We must stress the need for individual responsibility and accountability for our actions and the risks we pose to ourselves and others during the time of a pandemic. We must be clear about what is needed for each American and the consequences and risks posed by those who do not adopt our public health guidance. Furthermore, we must expect leaders to be role models for responsible behaviors.

Personal Story: "COVID-Crazy"

Dr. Epperly relates the following story.

Idaho is divided into seven public health districts, with approximately four to eight counties per health district. As the only physician member of the Central District Health (CDH) board of trustees, I was responsible for and accountable to a four-county region in the Boise metropolitan area. In this context, my role was to help set policy related to the medical and public health implications of the COVID-19 pandemic. As the pandemic surged in Idaho through the months of March, April and May of 2020, and into the summer and fall of that year, there was growing tension and pushback from within the four counties in our health district in response to public health measures we implemented, measures targeted at helping to control the pandemic's spread. CDH had received an increasing number of email responses and letters stating displeasure with face masking requirements and the closures of schools, bars, restaurants, and gymnasiums.

On December 8, 2020, we were contemplating moving from a public health advisory approach with no enforcement, which advised the use of face masks in all four counties and limits on group gatherings to less than ten persons, to instead issuing a public health order with enforcement provisions. Prior to that meeting, I had received well over 5,000 emails from disgruntled citizens stating their displeasure with us taking away their "personal freedoms, liberties and choices." They equated this to actual evil, maintaining that our public health board was power- and control-hungry, with board members who had lost touch with reality for a disease with a "mortality rate of less than one percent" and a medical condition "no worse than the flu."

On the evening of December 8, our board meeting was conducted virtually, as well as from the CDH's main office. I was at my home, the meeting having just started at 5:15 p.m., when I heard a tremendous clamor coming from outside the window from the street side of my home. I was shocked to see about 15 protesters, all without face masks, banging pails and buckets and crashing cymbals. They were pounding on pots and pans and shining strobe lights through my window. My wife had just come in from walking out of the garage and unexpectedly encountered the protesters, who yelled at her. She made a hasty retreat into the house to alert me.

Back at the main office, the CDH board chair had started the meeting, but additional protests were happening not only outside the CDH main office building in Boise, with well over 300 protesters, several with weapons, but also outside the home of one of my fellow board members. She herself was at her county commission office, but her 12-year-old son was home, completely alone. She left her office and the meeting in tears to hurry home to be with her son.

Several minutes later, the director of CDH, who was at the main building, informed us that the mayor and the police chief both advised that we stop the meeting, as police were concerned about their ability to control the crowds and feared for our personal safety. I was shocked.

I have no problems with people being upset and protesting, but I do have problems with what happened next. The protestors came up to my house twice, banged aggressively on my doors, and were shouting and screaming outside my windows.

This behavior was unacceptable. They were now trespassing on my property, and my wife and I had vowed that if there was a third such effort at disrupting our home, banging on the doors or trying to enter, we would immediately call the police, not realizing that my neighbors already had.

The group outside were blocking the street, not allowing our neighbors to pass and causing disruption. At one point after the meeting was adjourned, I peered out my window to look at the crowd and was surprised to see that it consisted of a wide range of ages, from older children to older adults. I thought: "Wow, what an example to set for your children!"

I was quite concerned that if they saw me peering out the window, it might incite them further. What has happened to our fellow countrymen and members of our community? Is this who we have become? Have we lost our minds?

The state song of Idaho is a lovely waltz titled "Here We Have Idaho." Its chorus begins, "Here we have Idaho, winning her way to fame." Based on the disturbing events described above, one might in retrospect worry that such words praising Idaho could be viewed as disappointingly sarcastic. But in fact, events like the ones I have recounted above, outbursts of unreasoning antagonism, and threats against honest efforts to control a foreboding pandemic have occurred many times across the entire nation. In the end, this is not an Idaho problem; it is an American one.

But I still wonder: Have we gone COVID-crazy?

CHAPTER 6

Man versus Virus

A Comparative View

Everything in your life is a reflection of a choice you have made. If you want a different result, make a different choice.

ANONYMOUS

One of the major stories of the COVID-19 pandemic is that there were really two pandemics happening simultaneously. The first was the pandemic of severe acute respiratory syndrome coronavirus-2 (SARS-CoV-2) progressing relentlessly across our planet. This was a novel (new) coronavirus, and, as such, it had the entire world's population as a playground. There was no natural immunity for this virus, so consequently SARS-CoV-2 had an open field on the earth in which to spread. It infected men, women, and children of all countries, of all nationalities, and of all races and ethnicities. It attacked the most vulnerable and the easiest to find, as naturally as water flows downhill.

At the same time, a second simultaneous pandemic was also occurring, which was the human reaction and response to SARS-CoV-2. It was a perfect example of cause and effect. SARS-CoV-2 (and its related disease, COVID-19) was the cause of the pandemic, but more important, it was society's response to this viral threat that was to determine the success or failure of countries, states, and counties to control its spread. The attributes of these two simultaneous pandemics are compared in table 6.1. The virus that caused COVID-19 was resilient, consis-

Table 6.1. A comparison of the two simultaneous pandemics, SARS-CoV-2 virus and the human pandemic response

Attribute	SARS-CoV-2 (virus)	Society (humans)
Fear	None	Minimal to excessive
Anger	None	Moderate to extreme
Lies/Myths	None	Some to excessive
Denial	None	Some to excessive
Agendas	None	Some to many
Blame	None	Some to extreme
Resilience	Much	Some to much
Anxiety	None	Moderate to excessive
Financial Impact	None	Significant
Consistency	Much	Minimal to none
Change	Some to much	Some to much
Discrimination	None	Moderate to significant
Logic	None	Minimal to much
Intelligence	None	Some to significant
Education	None	Some to significant
Economic Status	None	Poor to rich

tent, and nondiscriminatory. It was fearless, it was relentless, it did not play favorites, and it had no agendas. It simply just was.

The human and societal response, however, was anything but that. In fact, there was an incredible range of responses across various locales in how different groups handled this viral threat. As opposed to the steady and relentless march of the virus across the world, the human element was inconsistent, fearful, and unorganized. How this inconsistency, fear, anger, anxiety, and denial played out was best demonstrated by society's willingness (or lack thereof) to use public health measures known to combat the virus. Since we had not yet, in the early stages, developed antiviral therapies or vaccines for the virus, the only thing that stood between society and the virus was our coordinated public health efforts. This chapter will take a closer look at how different nations, different states, and different counties did or did not use effective public health initiatives. We will then take a deeper look at people's behaviors in these locations during their efforts to implement public health initiatives, which in the final analysis became the difference between successfully handling the pandemic and failing to do so.

A Comparison of Two Countries

Here we compare how two different countries, South Korea and the United States, handled the COVID-19 pandemic according to a number of attributes (table 6.2). Notably, the two countries had their first reported COVID-19 case within one day of each other, on January 20 and January 19, 2020, respectively.[1]

There was a marked difference, however, in the response of South Korea to the COVID-19 pandemic compared with the United States. Even though the population density of South Korea is higher and the median age older than that of the United States, South Korea had a significantly lower number of cases, infection rate, and deaths. Much of this had to do with the fact that South Korea was much more effective than the United States in both its messaging and its citizens obeying public health orders. As can be seen, Koreans' adherence rate with public health initiatives and wearing face masks was excellent, with higher than 90 percent compliance. Simply put, they took the pandemic more seriously.

South Korea's senior leaders made face masking mandatory for the nation. They communicated the importance of collective public health

Table 6.2. A comparison between sociocultural aspects of South Korea and the United States in the COVID-19 pandemic

Attribute	South Korea	United States
Population	51.2 million	331 million
Face Mask Mandate	Yes	No
Population Density	1,366/mile^2	93/mile^2
Number of COVID-19 Cases	80,131[a]	26,766,400[a]
Infection Rate	0.16%	8.1%
COVID-19 Deaths	1,459[a]	458,105[a]
Mortality/Death Rate	1.8%	1.7%
Compliance Rate with Public Health Guidance and Face Masks	Excellent (>90%)	Mixed (61%–94%)[b]
Education Level (% of Citizens with a Bachelor's Degree)	34%	34%
Median Yearly Income (US Dollars)	$42,285	$68,703
Median Age (Years)	43.7	38.1

[a] *Source*: Johns Hopkins University School of Medicine, "Coronavirus Resource Center," February 5, 2021, https://coronavirus.jhu.edu/map.html

[b] *Source*: Byron Spice, "COVIDcast Now Monitoring Daily U.S. Mask Use, COVID-19 Testing," Carnegie Mellon University, October 12, 2020, https://www.cmu.edu/news/stories/archives/2020/october/covidcast-mask-use.html

as the best way to keep everyone safe from the virus. The people of South Korea, from the start, responded with effective face mask coverings, social distancing, group size limitations, and handwashing. The country also immediately developed the capacity for high-volume testing so that infected individuals could appropriately quarantine. Because of this response, the virus was arrested in its tracks, minimizing its spread in the country.

This was much different than the response we saw in the United States. The United States failed in its leadership at almost all levels regarding messaging, testing, and quickly implementing appropriate public health measures. In fact, an inconsistency in messaging served to undermine potential compliance by American citizens. Our government's response, in contrast to South Korea's, polarized America and turned the pandemic into a political issue instead of a public health issue. Table 6.2 displays the consequences. The infection rate was over 50 times higher in the United States, and the death rate was similar between the countries, even though South Korea has an older population and lower per capita income. The United States is 6.5 times larger in population than South Korea, yet, disproportionately, it had 314 times the number of deaths.

A Comparison of Two States

We now compare two states in the United States that handled the pandemic differently: New Mexico and Idaho. We could have chosen among many states to make these comparisons, but we wanted two states of approximately the same size and geographic region but different in regard to outcomes. Therefore, we chose these two intermountain states for comparison. The results for these two states are itemized by attribute in table 6.3.

Although these states have similar population sizes and densities, they had different outcomes for infection rate, test positivity rate, and mortality rate. Their respective populations are relatively close to each other in median age, but they differ substantially with respect to education and economic levels. What stands out is their differing compliance with public health guidance. New Mexico implemented a statewide

Table 6.3. A comparison between New Mexico and Idaho on COVID's impact

Attribute	New Mexico	Idaho
Population	2 million	1.8 million
Population Density	17.2/miles^2	19.8/miles^2
Face Mask Mandate	Yes	No
COVID-19 Cases	179,000[a]	165,000[a]
Infection Rate / Test Positive Rate	8.8% / 7.2%[a]	9.2% / 26.8%[a]
COVID-19 Deaths	3,357[a]	1,749[a]
Mortality / Death Rate	1.9%	1.06%
Compliance Rate with Public Health Guidance and Face Masks	90.3%[b]	73.7%[b]
Education Level (% of Citizens with a Bachelor's Degree)	26%	12.8%
Median Yearly Income (US Dollars)	$39,811	$55,583
Median Age (Years)	38.1	36.8

[a] *Source*: Johns Hopkins University School of Medicine, "Coronavirus Resource Center," February 5, 2021, https://coronavirus.jhu.edu/map.html

[b] *Source*: Byron Spice, "COVIDcast Now Monitoring Daily U.S. Mask Use, COVID-19 Testing," Carnegie Mellon University, October 12, 2020, https://www.cmu.edu/news/stories/archives/2020/october/covidcast-mask-use.html

face mask mandate on May 16, 2020. Idaho did not. This led to over 90 percent compliance with public health initiatives and mask wearing in New Mexico, compared with 73.7 percent in Idaho. Because of this, New Mexico had a lower infection rate and test positivity rate than Idaho. Idaho's excessive test positivity rate (the highest or second highest in the United States at several points during the pandemic) was most likely the consequence of high infection rates coupled with low overall testing, resulting in higher overall test positivity.

The higher number of deaths and mortality rate in New Mexico most likely relates to how hard hit the Navajo Nation was during the pandemic. As we discuss later in this chapter, the behaviors of the people of New Mexico were much more aligned with public health guidelines for wearing face masks, social distancing, limiting group sizes, and handwashing. By doing so, the citizens of New Mexico not only protected themselves; they also protected their neighbors and families more effectively. This is similar to what was observed when comparing the citizenry of South Korea with that of the United States. We must point out that both New Mexico and Idaho, individually, had more deaths from COVID-19 than the entire country of South Korea, which is 25 times more populated.

A Comparison of Two Counties

Since both of us authors live in the state of Idaho, we next want to compare two counties adjacent to each other in the southwestern part of the state. Ada County is the largest county in Idaho and the home of our largest city and state capital, Boise. It is the home of a university (Boise State) and diverse urban businesses. Canyon County is its sister county, adjacent to the west, and is much more agrarian in its economy. The population, population density, age, education level, and economic levels of these two counties are compared in table 6.4.

Consider the two counties' infection rates, test positivity rates, and mortality rates. Even though these counties are contiguous, there is a measurable difference in infection rates and test positivity rates. This difference is graphically depicted in figure 6.1, which demonstrates the test positivity rate differences between Ada and Canyon Counties. Note that the test positivity rate is approximately 80 percent higher in the more rural Canyon County, where a face mask ordinance was not in place.

Table 6.4. A comparison between Ada County and Canyon County, Idaho, on COVID's impact

Attribute	Ada County	Canyon County
Population	481,587	229,849
Population Density	373/miles^2	322/miles^2
Face Mask Mandate	Yes	No
COVID-19 Cases	45,151[a]	24,056[a]
Infection Rate/Test Positivity Rate	9.35%/22%[b]	10.43%/35%[b]
COVID-19 Deaths	418[a]	261[a]
Mortality/Death Rate	0.92%	1.07%
Compliance Rate with Public Health Guidance and Face Masks	82.3%[c]	75.7%[c]
Education Level (% of Citizens with a Bachelor's Degree)	16.3%	7.7%
Median Yearly Income (US Dollars)	$66,405	$49,143
Median Age (Years)	37.4	33.6

[a] *Source*: Idaho Division of Public Health, "COVID-19 Vaccine Data Dashboard," last accessed July 14, 2022, https://public.tableau.com/app/profile/idaho.division.of.public.health/viz/COVID-19VaccineDataDashboard/LandingPage

[b] *Source*: Dr. David Peterman, CEO of Primary Health (Boise, Idaho), personal correspondence with author, December 28, 2020

[c] *Source*: Johns Hopkins University School of Medicine, "Coronavirus Resource Center," February 5, 2021, https://coronavirus.jhu.edu/map.html

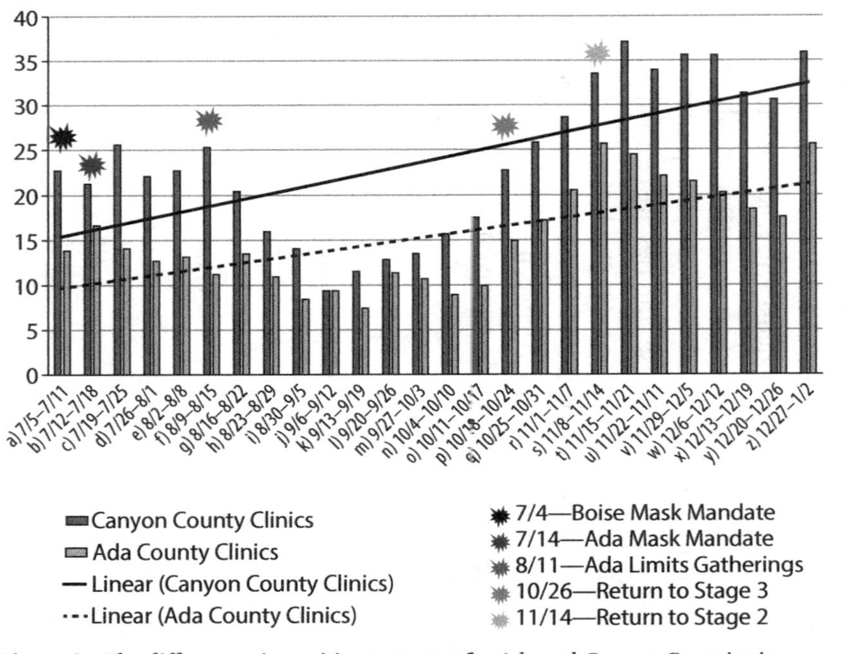

Figure 6.1. The differences in positive test rates for Ada and Canyon Counties in Idaho. The bursts mark weeks when public health measures were implemented.

The City of Boise and Ada County, early in the pandemic, adopted a mask requirement, as well as guidelines that restricted group gathering sizes and enforced social distancing. As was demonstrated previously by disparities between countries and states, the citizens of Ada County were more compliant than those of Canyon County in accepting public health guidelines, with 82.3 percent complying versus 75.7 percent.

These mandates, in a state like Idaho, were not put into place without controversy. There were many residents of Ada County who felt that this was government overreach and that the mandates infringed on their personal liberties. Idaho has a larger proportion of people with libertarian, anti-government, and Christian identity politics than do many other states. Public health interventions meant to stem the infection rate only served to galvanize Idahoans with this mindset. This in turn made public health efforts a more daunting educational and compliance feat.

Another difference between Ada County and Canyon County was that each had a different public health board. Ada County's Central District Health board enacted the public health mandates, while Canyon County's Southwest District Health board only opted to issue advisories. In the final analysis, it was the behaviors of the citizens of these two contiguous counties that ultimately became the determiner of each county's outcome.

The virus is the virus. It is relentless and nondiscriminatory. It will flow like water from the mountains to the oceans, to wherever it is easiest to find and infect people. If populations of people let it into their lives, their family homes, their jobs, and their social groups, it will mindlessly enter and infect them. If, on the other hand, individuals, families, workplaces, and communities opt to have an organized public health response to keep it out, it will be thwarted and bypass these groups as it moves relentlessly on to those who do not share this collective practice. The virus has no agenda; people do.

Why Are There Differences?

So why are there differences among these different populations? What leads groups of people on the same planet, in the same country, or in the same state to have different COVID-19 outcomes? In the final analysis, it boils down to differences in racial, ethnic, and socioeconomic status (discussed in chapter 4) and in people's behaviors and collective mindsets (the subject of this chapter). For the same reasons, there were drastically different outcomes for people's health across the nation prior to COVID-19. In this current pandemic, the biggest driver of an individual's health, other than their race, ethnicity, and socioeconomic status, is their individual health choices. Their behaviors drive outcomes. If people do not exercise enough, don't have good diets, choose to partake in harmful activities such as smoking and drug abuse, drink excessive amounts of alcohol, and engage in high-risk activities without appropriate precautions, they start to differentiate from others in terms of both quality and quantity of life lived.

Individual choices matter. It was therefore unavoidable that individual behaviors became key outcome differentiators during the COVID-19 viral pandemic. Ultimately, this came down to carefully following public health measures such as wearing face masks, physically distancing, and limiting group gathering sizes. Behavioral differences between those who follow public health guidance (such as wearing face masks, maintaining physical distancing and group size limitations, handwashing, and not going to work sick) and those who do not are broadly suggested by table 6.5.

There is no data that can precisely characterize these behaviors, but there is a range of responses that can serve as a comparison. Many of the attributes that become the differentiators between those who follow public health measures and those who do not are listed. This is not meant to be an exhaustive list but is meant to make the point that we all have a choice to make when it comes to what we can do to protect not only ourselves but others around us as well. It is nothing more than a choice. Do we choose to follow guidelines known to limit the transmission of COVID-19, or do we not? What drives this choice can be analyzed through the lens of these behaviors.

Many of these individual behavioral choices are, of course, made in the context of family, friends, and community. People are social creatures. People want to fit into their groups. But what became very

Table 6.5. Behavioral differences between face mask wearers and non–face mask wearers

Attribute	Face mask wearers	Non–face mask wearers
Empathy	More	Less
Kindness	More	Less
Cooperation	More	Less
Solidarity	Much	Much
Community-Minded	Much more	Less
Compassion for Others	More	Less
Education	More	Less
Economic Status	Skewing higher	Skewing lower
Political Ideology	Left and middle	Right
Compliance	More	Less
Individualism	Less	More
Self-Centered	Less	More
Maturity	More	Less
Responsibility	More	Less
Vanity	Less	More
Shared Identity	Much	Much
Altruism	More	Less

apparent early on during the pandemic was that there was an absolute polarization of these groups around these choices. There was a coalescence of groups, or "tribes," of people around the issues of accepting public health initiatives and guidance on wearing face masks.

The face mask became a political symbol of one's tribe. It no longer was a tool of public health; it became a symbol of one's political ideology. There were many people who absolutely wanted to do their part and be compliant with trying to keep themselves and others safe. There was another group who felt that this was a personal infringement on their liberties and their right to choose to not wear a mask. Their concern was not about the public's health and potentially keeping others healthy, but about their own needs and desires.

The problem with such a choice, in reality, was that it was not one that could effectively help protect their own group, their families, their community, and potentially the jobs in their communities, but instead laid the foundation for a less desirable set of outcomes. This single-minded focus on individualism—individual choice—undermined the very thing that could have prevented higher number of infections, kept schools open, kept businesses open, and protected vulnerable people. This led to the loss of a shared collective opportunity to utilize public health initiatives. Instead, we saw the rejection of these principles in single-minded favor of individual liberties to choose.

Words *do* matter. What people listen to as their news source and what their friends listen to as their news source matter. We had constant 24-7 news sources that were touting the benefits of both sides of this equation. There were news sources that made it absolutely clear that the public health initiatives were necessary and needed to be followed, and there were other news sources and echo chambers in which the initiatives were downplayed and derided through misinformation, lies, and myths as being unnecessary. More than once, we heard the refrain that we must prevent ourselves from "becoming sheep" by those who followed these latter news sources. In fact, in trying to prevent one from "becoming a sheep," they fell into their own flock of being fools. They were not exercising individual choices and behaviors based on data, science, and evidence, but ironically making their choices based upon their social group's thinking. They were not being individuals at all, but following their group's misinformed thinking.

Unfortunately, this led to more infections, hospitalizations, and deaths across those locations. Instead of focusing on long-term outcomes and the more rapid return of businesses, schools, the economy, and health, many ignored these for their own short-term convenience. Sadly, many people stopped listening to each other. Instead, they started talking over each other and then started shouting at each other. In a word, we stopped respecting one another.

Recommendation #47

Communication Must Be Customized

It is important to try to understand people's thought processes when it comes to their behaviors and choices. Effective communication, education, and messaging campaigns must be developed that will target different groups of people with messages that will resonate with their thinking. The goal should be to encourage them to make the right individual choices to protect the overall community's health, economy, schools, and businesses.

Recommendation #48

Utilize Trusted Spokespersons

It will be important to find appropriate individuals that are respected by each specific group so that they will be accepted messengers and spokespersons for these groups. These respected individuals would be charged with having an impact on these groups by helping them to trust the message. This would facilitate people pulling together in one direction instead of polarizing into factions.

CHAPTER 7

Needed Changes to the Federal Response

There are no secrets to success. It is the result of preparation, hard work, and learning from failure.

COLIN POWELL

Our country was founded on the principles of divided government (executive, legislative, and judicial branches) and also on limited government, where certain powers are enumerated in the Constitution and specifically granted to the federal government. Those enumerated powers are the only powers the federal government has. All other powers are reserved for the states.

Article I, Section 8, Clause 1 of the US Constitution states that "The Congress shall have Power To . . . provide for the common Defence and general Welfare of the United States." Similarly, the power to maintain a military and declare war rests with the federal government.

This makes sense. The framers realized that a military trained in a uniform fashion under a single command would be far more effective than each state maintaining a separate military force. Furthermore, we certainly would not want an individual state, such as Virginia or California, to declare war on a foreign country. There was an understanding that when it came to a military threat to the United States, or any part of it, the states would be better served by a unified, common defense.

President Trump compared the pandemic to a war and portrayed himself as a wartime president. In March 2020, he stated that our fight against the spread of COVID-19 is "our big war. It's a medical war. We have to win this war. It's very important." He went on to say, "I view it as a, in a sense, a wartime president."[1] However, his approach, in large part, was to have each state fight its own war with this viral invader.

During the transition between the Obama and Trump administrations, teams from both staff engaged in an eerily prescient tabletop exercise that dealt with a theoretical pandemic crisis. "The Trump team was told it could face specific challenges, such as shortages of ventilators, anti-viral drugs and other medical essentials, and that having a coordinated, unified national response was 'paramount,'" Nahal Toosi, Daniel Lippman, and Dan Diamond wrote in a Politico article.[2] Unfortunately, during the course of the pandemic, our national response was far from coordinated or unified.

Recommendation #49

Coordinated, Unified National Response

A coordinated, unified national response is essential to managing the next pandemic in order to ensure a successful rollout of testing, PPE, and vaccines.

Having previously gone through this tabletop what-if exercise, perhaps the Trump administration was not surprised by the shortages of basic medical supplies and equipment, but it was a big surprise to many of us across the country to find out how little help the Strategic National Stockpile (SNS) would turn out to be. Although the description has since been changed, until this pandemic, the website for the SNS defined it as the "nation's largest supply of life-saving pharmaceuticals and medical supplies for use in a public health emergency severe enough to cause local supplies to run out." But in reality, many of the SNS supplies were never restocked following the H1N1 virus pandemic of 2009, perhaps due to competing funding priorities in Congress or a sense that the pandemic was now behind us and no longer a significant concern for the foreseeable future.

One of the more surprising aspects of how the Trump administration dealt with the pandemic—and there were many—was the retreat from the notion that the federal government would provide for the common defense against this attack from a viral pandemic on the United States. In fact, the administration's decisions often both surprised and alarmed governors of both political parties.

In a completely unforeseen move, with health care providers facing shortages of personal protective equipment (PPE)—surgical masks, N95 masks, goggles, face shields, gowns, gloves, and hand sanitizer—across the country, the president, on a call with state governors, instructed them to try and buy their own supplies. He persisted in this position even when one governor indicated that this had resulted in bidding wars between the states and the federal government. Whether intentional or not, this meant that the federal government, perhaps in a belated effort to restock the SNS, was always winning out, leaving the states without the supplies and equipment they needed.

President Trump "repeated his belief that the onus should be on the states—and not the federal government—to obtain needed equipment to combat the pandemic, saying his administration is not a 'shipping clerk' for the supplies that could potentially save lives."[3] In an interview, when pressed by a reporter about PPE shortages that the states were facing, driven by the lack of a sufficient SNS to meet the states' needs, Jared Kushner, senior advisor to the president, replied: "The notion of the federal stockpile was it's supposed to be our stockpile. It's not supposed to be states' stockpiles that they then use." Needless to say, this was both unexpected and quite startling to many of us.

We would see this friction play out repeatedly during the pandemic. Great confusion reigned concerning the division of responsibilities between the federal government and state governments. The latest such conflict arose regarding vaccine distribution. The federal government indicated that it would procure the vaccine, but then it would be up to the states to determine how to distribute and administer it. However, with improved sanitation, better food processing and handling, and the advent of powerful antibiotics, many states, facing never-ending budgetary challenges, had cut back on their investments in public health infrastructure over the past decades. Not having the infrastructure in place to quickly vaccinate their entire state's population, and with many states already operating financially in the red due to the unforeseen costs associated with the pandemic, many governors pleaded with the administration to provide more funding directly to the states to give them the ability to implement a mass vaccination program. Congress finally included some funding to states in an end-of-the-year COVID-19 stimulus package, but many states feared it was too little, too late. Not only this, but the federal government initially promised the distribution of 100 million doses of vaccine through Operation Warp Speed. That commitment would subsequently have to be reduced twice—first to 40 million doses and then, in December 2020, to only 20 million doses.

So, what needs to change regarding the federal response to a future pandemic?

Communication

The communication from the Trump administration was at times purposefully misleading, if not outright lies. In taped interviews with Bob Woodward for his book, *Rage*, in February 2020, the president told Mr. Woodward that he knew that the virus was dangerous and could be spread through airborne transmission, something not generally known to the public at that time. On February 7, on a recorded phone call, President Trump told Mr. Woodward, "It goes through air. So that's a tricky one. That's a very delicate one. It's also more deadly than even your strenuous flus . . . maybe five times more deadly." At the same time, the president was telling the American people that we had very few cases, they were all getting better, and the novel coronavirus would go away "miraculously" when it became warmer.

In a subsequent interview on March 19, when Woodward asked the president why he was telling the public a different version of the facts than what he knew to be true, he responded, "I always wanted to play it down. I still like playing it down, because I don't want to create a panic."[4]

While not inciting panic or a sense of dread is a worthy communication goal for a president, we would argue that that goal should not come at the expense of being untruthful with the American people. To be clear, we do not believe that the president must always tell the whole truth. There may be information that is known or suspected by the president that would need to be kept secret due to national security concerns or not wishing to cause undue worry on the part of the public while not achieving any useful purpose, and that would be appropriate to withhold from the American people, but the president should not lie about the information he or she does share with the public.

As one of us coauthors, David Pate, told the school leaders he was advising, who by that point had lost the trust of both teachers and parents: "I have no idea how to lead through a crisis without trust. Earning and restoring trust must be a priority." This is why we do not believe that the president should ever intentionally lie to the public in an effort not to create panic. Lies oftentimes become uncovered, and the resulting damage to the public's trust takes an inordinate amount of time to repair—time that the leader of the country may not have when leading through a crisis.

As physicians, we have unfortunately had to share bad news with patients. It is part of the ethics of our profession that it is never appropriate to lie to patients. Obviously, when explaining a bad diagnosis to a patient, it is not necessary or helpful to tell the patient or her family everything we know about the course of the disease, depriving the patient of all hope, nor to engage in a discussion at that time about what the course of their illness will be like at the end of her life. But patients need to have all the information that is necessary for them to protect themselves, care for themselves, and understand what the treatment entails.

Similarly, the president should always be honest with the American people by informing them, without deception or equivocation, what they can do to protect themselves from the threat and what the government will do to combat it. "Downplaying" the COVID-19 threat, as the president put it, is likely to have contributed to many Americans underestimating its danger, thereby reducing the incentives for them to follow public health advice and increasing the risk to them and, in turn, their communities.

Recommendation #50

Communicate Truthfully to Establish and Maintain Trust

In a time of a national public health emergency, the president should be truthful with the American people. That does not mean that a president must tell the public all that he or she knows, but efforts to mislead the public or downplay the threat may give the public a false sense of reassurance and undermine efforts by public health officials to get the public to adopt their guidance. Maintaining the trust and confidence of the American people is critical to leading them through a crisis.

During an evolving pandemic, when we are learning at a very fast rate yet still have many unanswered questions, it is important for those speaking to the American public to be clear that our knowledge and understanding of the threat is evolving rapidly. It may very well be that something we believe to be true today may change with additional experience and research. It is important to convey to the public that as we get more data on and experience and understanding of this virus, leaders will keep the public updated with what we know and what we learn, but that with current experience, as of today, it is important that you do this and avoid that. Unfortunately, if dogmatic statements are made early on, followed by information or guidance that subsequently changes, it can erode trust, create doubt about whether the information the public is now being told is reliable, and provide an excuse for people who do not want to follow the guidance to blame others for their noncompliance.

This is what happened early on in the pandemic, when the American public at first was strongly dissuaded from wearing masks but then, within a short time (as we observed the significant percentage of infected persons who transmitted the virus while asymptomatic), public health officials began to plead with the public to wear them.

Recommendation #51

The Evolving Nature of Scientific Discovery

It is critical during briefings to the American people to emphasize that the information and guidance being provided to them is the best information that we know as of that time, but it is entirely possible as we gain more knowledge and experience with the virus and the disease it causes that this information or guidance may change.

It is also critical that the president, vice president, directors of health agencies, and physician leaders all reinforce and reiterate the messages of our top public health experts when dealing with a pandemic. Unfortunately, this did not happen. There were mixed messages and even infighting among members of the White House Coronavirus Task Force. To make matters worse, communications and recommendations to states from the White House Coronavirus Task Force conflicted with what the president was publicly saying.

Experienced leaders understand that they must model the behaviors they want from those they lead. Obviously, a middle school health education teacher's message to students that they should not smoke will be greatly undermined if students observe the teacher smoking during breaks. In the same fashion, the CDC and White House Coronavirus Task Force's recommendations to the public to wear masks or face coverings in public, physically distance, and avoid large gatherings were undermined when the president and vice president were frequently seen and photographed or filmed appearing before large gatherings while not wearing a mask.

Recommendation #52

Be a Role Model for Desired Behaviors

Leaders must model the desired behaviors they want the public to adopt. Even if the leaders have the benefit of additional protections not available to the general public, it is still important to reinforce these behaviors. The failure to do so will greatly undermine public health efforts.

The Strategic National Stockpile

The American health care delivery system relies primarily on private hospitals. Governmental (federal, state, and local) hospitals account for only about 19 percent of all hospital providers.[5]

Private hospitals are private businesses. While there are nonprofit hospitals that provide care to those without the ability to pay, and institutions that benefit from philanthropy, in most cases there are no other funding sources to subsidize a hospital's losses. Most hospitals depend on revenues they receive from delivering patient care. With the increase in costs of equipment, supplies, and pharmaceuticals and relatively flat payments from governmental payers, there has been tremendous pressure on private hospitals to cut costs over the past several decades.

This has resulted in a trend where hospitals have increasingly relied on group purchasing organizations to obtain volume discounts on equipment, supplies, and pharmaceuticals and have moved away from self-sourcing, warehousing, and distributing. This has also meant that hospitals have progressively relied on distributors to deliver equipment, supplies, and pharmaceuticals "just in time," while maintaining only days' worth of inventory on hand. Warehouses are expensive to build, operate, and maintain.

As such, most hospitals are ill prepared for a disaster—an unforeseen event that would dramatically increase their need for equipment, supplies, and medications. Medical practices and urgent care clinics have maintained even smaller inventories of any personal protective equipment, with most medical practices often having none.

In 1999 the SNS was created to serve as a backstop to states and locales in the event of a bioterrorist attack, pandemic, or other public health emergency. It consists of twelve secret locations throughout the United States that store medical supplies, equipment, and medications in the event of a disaster or emergency. It is funded by appropriations from Congress. It was initially overseen by the CDC, but is now managed by the Office of the Assistant Secretary of Preparedness and Response within the Department of Health and Human Services.

Unfortunately, funding for the SNS has waxed and waned, depending on how strong a case could be made to Congress to prioritize this funding over competing priorities. Pandemics and bioterrorism events have not generally been Congress' primary concerns.

Following the H1N1 influenza outbreak, the SNS did not replenish many of the supplies it had distributed to the states. Thus, early on in the COVID-19 pandemic, the federal government could provide little assistance to the states, and most often directed the majority of the resources to states that were being hit hardest. While the federal government went out to the market to buy more supplies, by this time, all the countries in the world were bidding on limited supplies and, predictably, prices skyrocketed.

Because the federal government could not provide supplies for the states, the president told state governors to go out and try to purchase what supplies they could. But this resulted in medical groups, hospitals, and states all bidding against other countries for these supplies, including their own federal government. Unsurprisingly, medical groups had no leverage, hospitals had little, and even states were frequently outbid by the federal government. This proved to be a more costly and limited path to getting badly needed supplies, and likely increased the costs for the federal government as well.

Recommendation #53

States Must Secure a Supply Source for a Future Pandemic

States must be able to count on a quickly accessible, dependable source of emergency supplies for their hospitals, long-term care facilities, medical practices, and first responders. Unless the federal government can commit to this with adequate funding by Congress, each state should consider whether it will rely on the SNS or create its own stockpile.

To make matters worse, because the president and his administration were relying on commercial supply chains and were reluctant to implement the Defense Production Act to require American companies to make these crucial supplies, there were instances where states, hospitals, and medical groups were in desperate need, while flights were leaving the United States with supplies going to another country that had outbid the United States and its states.

Recommendation #54

Federal Role in Procuring and Distributing Supplies

In the event of a public health emergency, the purchasing of supplies, equipment, and medications should be done by the federal government on behalf of the states and their health care infrastructure. This contrasts with creating an uncontrolled purchasing free-for-all within the marketplace between the federal government and the individual states and territories, hospitals, and medical practices. In the end, such an uncoordinated strategy, where the federal government does not take a leadership role, most often causes these lower-level entities to lose out to, or at the very least pay more than, other countries competing for the same supplies.

Recommendation #55
Defense Production Act
In a public health emergency that is expected to last for months, and where shortages of supplies and equipment are already being experienced, the president should be quick to implement the Defense Production Act to ensure that the United States' needs can be met by production within the country by US companies and, where the supply can be assured, to be distributed to meet US needs.

China is the major producer of many PPE items and ingredients for many medications. Interestingly, and ultimately fortunately, we had waged a trade war with China at the beginning of 2018 and had reached a trade deal on December 13, 2019, just a little more than two weeks before the outbreak in Wuhan began.[6] Because of this, we were able to get some supplies from China, even though the first major outbreak of COVID-19 occurred there, slowing or shutting down some manufacturing operations where large numbers of workers had become ill.

Recommendation #56
Create Redundancies in the Supply Chain
We must identify critical supplies, equipment, and medications to ensure that we are not overly reliant on any one country that would, in the case of a public health emergency, internal political instability, or a war, be challenged in their ability to maintain the supply of these critical resources or for which a sudden increase in world demand would threaten the supply to the United States.

Since many states' budgets are constrained, they may understandably be reluctant to create their own stockpiles. However, states have seen firsthand what happens to the availability and cost of supplies when there is a sudden global spike in the need for these supplies. One option that states may consider is working with the largest health systems in their state that have already moved to operating their own warehouses. If space is available or can be added at a lower cost than building a separate state warehouse, this would allow them to lease space from these health systems rather than having to build new facilities.

There is another cost in operating a warehouse, one which involves the stocking and storing of supplies, equipment, and medications that all have expiration dates. Upon reaching those expiration dates, these supplies, equipment, and medications must be discarded and new supplies, equipment, and medications purchased to replace them. But the state can lower these costs by rotating their inventory and distributing it to hospitals for their routine use. The hospitals can purchase these items from the state, rather than purchasing exclusively from their usual supply chains. This allows the state to maintain a refreshed inventory without having to discard so much expired supplies and without incurring unnecessary replacement costs.

Testing

When we found out what virus we were dealing with, the CDC began to develop its test to identify the presence of SARS-CoV-2 infection. FDA rules prohibited or made it extremely difficult for anyone else to develop a test.

Understandably, when a crisis occurs, there will always be those that try to capitalize on that crisis, and the FDA had legitimate concerns that public health would be threatened if hundreds of tests flooded the market, many with poor quality performance. However, this abundance of caution meant that we placed all of our eggs in the CDC basket, so to speak, and unfortunately, while the CDC is generally very good at creating diagnostic tests, this time there was a flaw.

There was a problem with one of the reagents, which caused a significant delay in the availability of testing in the United States. This was at a critical time when we really needed to understand what was going on with COVID-19 transmission, so that we could isolate infected individuals and conduct effective contact tracing.

Recommendation #57

Mobilize Academic and Private Partners to Develop Tests

The CDC should work with the FDA to modify existing rules, or, alternatively, propose legislation, if necessary, that would allow our large, trusted commercial laboratories and US academic laboratories, under the direction of the CDC, to develop tests for the detection of a new pathogen that poses a threat to the health and welfare of US citizens.

It was somewhat surreal that when Democratic governors expressed reasoned criticism of the Trump administration's pandemic effort and made pleas for more supplies or equipment, President Trump retaliated with petty responses. For example, President Trump said that he instructed Vice President Pence not to call governors that had not been "appreciative" enough of the administration's efforts to combat COVID-19.[7]

As events unfolded, Governor Andrew Cuomo of the state of New York then announced that because of the politicization of the vaccine and because of many people's distrust of the process, his administration would conduct an independent review of the safety and efficacy of any vaccines that received emergency use authorization (EUA) from the FDA. Outraged, when the first successful vaccine did receive an EUA, President Trump loudly declared that the government would distribute the vaccine across the United States, except to the state of New York. "As soon as April, the vaccine will be available to the entire general population with the exception of places like New York state where, for political reasons, the governor decided to say—and I don't think it's good politically, I think it's very bad from a health standpoint—but he wants to take his time with a vaccine."[8]

While politics should have no place in the management of a national crisis or emergency, as in these examples, we have seen nearly every aspect of the pandemic politicized, much to the chagrin and disappointment of those of us in health care.

CHAPTER 8

The Future Role of the States

You hit home runs not by chance but by preparation.

ROGER MARIS

Pandemic Plans

The pandemic has been a wake-up call for the states. They learned early on that, at least under the then-current administration, they were often left to their own devices. They discovered that they were unable to depend on the federal government for a prompt rollout of testing, for the distribution of supplies and equipment, or for adequate support in a massive vaccination campaign. It also became clear that Congressional funding could not be counted on.

In addition, states have seen their public health efforts undermined repeatedly by social media and disinformation campaigns, by political influences on federal governmental health agencies, and by the ever-present risk that a president and his or her administration might effectively sabotage public health messages by failing to be effective role models of desired behaviors or by making statements that hamper public health efforts. Again and again, they encountered barriers of poorly structured and inadequately equipped public health infrastructures at the state level, the result of decades of underfunding.

As we fight to bring this pandemic under control, it will be wise for states to begin their planning for the next pandemic, while all of the mistakes and misjudgments remain fresh. First, state leaders and all state agencies need to review the state's performance during the pandemic and identify what lessons were learned. The sections of state emergency operations plans that deal with pandemics, epidemics, and other public health emergencies must be updated to reflect these lessons learned.

Recommendation #58

Update State Emergency Operations Plans

States should update the section of their emergency operations plans that deals with pandemics, epidemics, and other public health emergencies to reflect the lessons learned from the COVID-19 pandemic.

Public Health Structure

An intensive review of the state's public health structure is called for. These public health infrastructures may have been put in place decades ago, long before lawmakers were prompted to contemplate pandemics. Some states have a very decentralized public health structure; this will need to be reconsidered. The challenges that we experienced during this pandemic were a patchwork of widely varying public health measures from city to city, county to county, and public health district to public health district. This, of course, led to people in one location who did not like the restrictions of their city, county, or district to merely relocate their party, sporting event, wedding, or bar hopping to the very next city, county, or district.

Recommendation #59

Reevaluate the Public Health Structure

As appropriate, states should reconsider whether they were well served by a decentralized public health system if that structure led to a patchwork of inconsistent public health measures, conflicting messages, different degrees of control of disease transmission, and people moving their activities to avail themselves of weaker restrictions.

As state and local public health departments or agencies review their plans, it would be prudent to establish a decision-making framework that reviews the range of public health issues that confront them and determine which should be subject to evidence-based standards that should be set by the state and adopted throughout the state, and which require varied approaches that are unique to each locale that should be left to the individual health districts or local public health departments to decide. Further, guidelines should be developed, perhaps based upon the extent of involvement of a public health threat throughout the state, or in a part of the state that overlaps multiple health districts or public health agencies, as to which level of government will set the public health guidance and orders, so as to eliminate irrational variation across the state in response to the same public health threat.

Plans should also include how resources can be shifted from one public health district to another during a public health threat.

Qualifications

It is also important for states to review the makeup and experience of their public health boards and authorities. In Idaho, most members of public health boards have no medical or public health training and, in some cases, do not embrace fundamental public health principles and practices. This becomes an issue during a pandemic because these non-health care board members may follow political pressures rather than science.

In Idaho, one public health board was especially egregious. While there was room for debate on some issues early in the pandemic, by November 2020, many of these issues had been settled by clinical trials and the resulting medical evidence. Yet this particular board was meeting in person, with very few people wearing masks. They were inviting testimony from a physician who was touting widely debunked or unsupported notions that modifying one's diet could improve immunity and gut health, which in turn could prevent a coronavirus infection. This was a physician who asserted that hydroxychloroquine could be used to effectively treat COVID-19 (a claim made by the president, but largely disproven by clinical trials and refuted widely by public health and medical experts) and declared that people of color were disproportionately impacted by the pandemic because of vitamin D deficiency.[1]

That same board invited a non-physician naturopath to testify, who downplayed the severity of the pandemic and then made the outrageous claim that there was no medical evidence that masks and face coverings could slow the spread of SARS-CoV-2.[2] We have emphasized that while not everyone on a public health board needs to be a health care professional or expert in public health, it does not make sense to place people on these boards who reject basic public health tenets and principles, since it is these boards that are charged with protecting the health and safety of the public.

Recommendation #60
Public Health Board Composition

States should review the composition of their boards or decision-making bodies to determine whether these boards are comprised of people who can, without conflicts of interest, put the public's health and safety at the forefront of their decision-making process. States should seek out board members that have well-suited backgrounds, experience, and knowledge to serve in roles where they will be making public health guidance or policy for the public.

Unfortunately, in some states such as Idaho, in a backlash to perceived infringements on personal liberties, the legislatures have prohibited or encumbered the ability of governors or public health agencies to declare states of emergency, issue mask mandates or stay-at-home orders, order the closure of schools or businesses, or limit the sizes of gatherings. These actions are shortsighted because these measures are often the only ones that can quickly stem the spread of a contagious disease and protect the public before therapeutics and vaccines can be developed. Setting aside the circumstances of this pandemic, there is no reason that the next pandemic couldn't be caused by an organism with a much higher mortality rate, one that does not largely spare our children from severe illness and death and causes our health care infrastructure to be overwhelmed.

If public health agencies do have their hands tied and cannot implement orders to protect the public, it will be even more important that these agencies present frequent, clear, and consistent guidance so that citizens who must act on their own to protect themselves are equipped with the knowledge to do so.

Communications

States should review their communications plans, as well as their capabilities. During normal times, the demands on communication for public health are generally quite manageable. However, during a pandemic, it can be challenging to stay ahead with messaging, responding to all the press and media requests while still retaining enough time to develop effective messaging campaigns.

In Idaho—and in many or even most other states, we are certain, particularly at the beginning of the pandemic—the press and media were running stories with various angles due to the public thirst for information, and inevitably they were calling hospitals and overwhelming their media relations' capabilities to instantaneously respond, or at least to respond in a timely way. At the same time, reporters were contacting the state and local public health districts, who were similarly overwhelmed and often also not able to quickly respond. This only further induced reporters to repeatedly and aggressively probe all these various information sources for the same story, hoping that at least one would return their call and allow them to meet an unforgiving story deadline.

Often, amid all the critical work a hospital, public health agency, or state is doing to deal with a crisis—in this case, a pandemic—press and media requests can seem like a nuisance and inconvenient intrusion. However, we encourage all of these parties to devise a plan to handle this burden in a timely manner—preferably with people who are not working on the front lines at the same time, directly dealing with the crisis—to ensure that we get our intended messages and reliable information out to the public. If not, the press and media will surely go looking for information in places, or from sources, that will not make or reinforce the messages that we desire or perhaps support.

It can be immensely frustrating and nearly impossible to keep up with, let alone be proactive on, social media channels, and yet this is where so many seek their news and information. Social media is also the venue that often clusters people who are neither expert nor mainstream together, providing them with a rich opportunity to amplify their misinformation messages to much larger audiences than would have ever been possible before. It must therefore be realized that even though social media attracts the least attention and resources from states and public health organizations, these platforms likely do the most to promote false or misleading information.

It follows that states and public health organizations need to have communication "surge plans," much as hospitals do. One way to surge is to temporarily hire or contract with professional communications experts or firms who can expand communications capabilities on short notice, but who also can be released when the immediate need recedes.

State and local public health departments must explore how they can improve the usefulness of their websites (while keeping in mind that these must serve two distinct stakeholders—the public and health care professionals) and how they can increase their social media presence and responsiveness. As we address elsewhere in this book, misinformation and disinformation thrives in a vacuum of reliable and authoritative information. We spend so much time on the back-end refuting misinformation and disinformation that for future pandemics, we must anticipate the most common misunderstandings and the common disinformation strategies, and get information out quickly to the public that is easily understandable. Thus, we won't allow misinformation to get so much traction.

We recommend that state health departments leverage their messaging by reinforcing (through retweets, likes, sharing, and so on) the messaging of other state health departments and other national and world health agencies, as well as medical professional associations, that have put out clear and effective messages. Likewise, we recommend that local public health agencies reinforce messages from those organizations, as well as other local public health districts in their state. Additionally, state and local health departments should identify social media influencers in their state who can amplify these messages, as well as regularly send messages to hospitals and state associations that can then send those messages out on their own social media platforms.

Much of the work should not wait for the next pandemic. Communications staff should identify the most common questions from the public and the media and begin drafting model answers that can be ready to go on short notice with the next epidemic or pandemic, after making any necessary tweaks to the answers based on the particular facts of the next pandemic. Similarly, the most common misinformation and misunderstandings from this pandemic should be catalogued. Communications staff should work with science communications experts and multimedia experts to create condensed educational material that can be easily revised to the particular circumstances of the next pandemic and rapidly deployed.

Recommendation #61

States' Public Health Communications Plans

State and local public health agencies should review their communications plans. They should review their current capabilities, and particularly address social media capabilities. They also need a "surge" plan to help expand communications capabilities during the next pandemic or public health emergency.

Data Sharing

The pandemic caused a significant need for data sharing and reporting. Every state has had to develop their coronavirus website quickly, as well as continue to revise and refine it as the pandemic progressed. Additionally, each state has needed to work with health care providers to ensure useful reporting of various pandemic impact data. There have been many challenges in sharing data, and it is important for states and public health departments to take note of their learnings from this pandemic to speed up data collection in future pandemics and avoid unnecessarily repeating the same errors. It is important to guarantee that what we have learned gets incorporated into an ongoing pandemic plan update.

Recommendation #62
Optimize State Data Reporting Systems

State and local public health agencies should identify the learnings from receiving, compiling, and reporting data so that these systems are in place and ready to go in the event of an epidemic, pandemic, or other public health emergency.

One of the challenges faced with data reporting was trying to get all hospitals to report data in a reasonable time frame, including obtaining reports on weekends and holidays. Another challenge in seeking better data reporting techniques was attempting to ease the burden of reporting on hospitals. Beyond that, data from urgent care providers and large medical groups would also have been helpful.

Recommendation #63
Automated Data Reporting

State and local public health agencies should work with hospitals to determine what options exist to automate reporting, so that data continues to flow to the state on weekends and holidays and the reporting burden on hospitals is lessened.

Recommendation #64
Expand Data Reporting Sources

To produce a more complete picture of disease activity, state and local public health agencies should explore options for urgent care and large medical group practices to report data during an epidemic, pandemic, or other public health emergency.

State and local public health departments, as well as hospitals, medical groups, and schools, should also try to define all of their data elements and post that information clearly on the website. For example, when rates are reported, it would be very helpful to post the formula for that calculation on the website as well as definitions of the terms used in that calculation. Further, when there are exclusions from a data set, that information would be helpful; for example, if a report excludes children under the age of 18, that should be made clear.

State Stockpile

Due to the federal government's undependable performance in adequately stocking supplies and Congress' failure in adequately funding the supplies and equipment needed, as sadly demonstrated during this current health crisis, states should make a key decision. Do they believe this will continue to be the case in the future, or do they believe that this was an aberrant event? If the former, states need to consider establishing their own stockpiles.

While establishing and maintaining a stockpile is an expensive undertaking, there are ways for a state to decrease these costs. One way is to partner with a distributor or health system within the state that already operates a warehouse and distribution system. In doing this, the state would need to determine whether the state should lease space within the warehouse or whether there is an option to build onto the existing warehouse. Such a strategy would preclude the need for the state to acquire land and build its own warehouse. In fact, the state may want to replicate this tactic in several parts of the state to ensure quicker access to needed medical supplies and equipment in the event of a natural disaster or if the pandemic resulted in a reduction in available truck drivers.

Another problem to tackle is the cost of the inventory, especially if goods otherwise languish for years without being used, forcing them to be disposed of and replaced to avoid reaching their expiration dates. Instead, the state can purchase the initial inventory but then partner with hospitals, health systems, and large medical groups to have them use and pay for existing inventory as they need new supplies, allowing the state to periodically purchase replacement inventory with those funds, thereby keeping its inventory fresh and ready to use. The state can also save money by contracting with the distributor or health system, delegating to them the operation and management of the stockpile.

Recommendation #65

State Medical Supply Stockpile

States should consider whether they should operate their own stockpile and, if so, whether cost savings are available by partnering with a distributor or health system in the state.

CHAPTER 9

Preparing Future Doctors, Nurses, and Public Health Workers for the Next Pandemic

The practice of medicine is an art, not a trade; a calling, not a business; a calling in which your heart will be exercised equally with your head.

SIR WILLIAM OSLER

The COVID-19 pandemic exposed many weaknesses in our health care workforce. It revealed that we did not have enough physicians or nurses in primary care, in emergency rooms, or in the critical care units of our hospitals. It also established that we do not have the right geographic distribution of physicians and nurses to respond to the demands of a nationwide public health emergency. In short, the pandemic overwhelmed—or threatened to overwhelm—our health care system in many parts of the country.

In addition to uncovering health care workforce shortages and distribution problems, the intensity and duration of the pandemic also exposed how vulnerable health care workers were to stress and infection. The pandemic imposed a heavy individual toll, weighing down health care providers with the sheer volume of very ill or dying patients. Excessive workloads, failed leadership, a lack of appreciation, inadequate staffing, and the emotional toll of the pandemic have caused an estimated 20 to 30 percent of front-line health care workers to contemplate a change in profession or early retirement, according to some studies and surveys.[1] Similarly, there are reports that many public health workers and experts have already left the profession or are planning to do so, given the stress of the pandemic and the lack of respect for and compliance with public health guidance. This is especially alarming because with the loss of their expertise, we are also losing experience—on-the-job training that cannot be taught in the classroom.

It should be pointed out that while there was volume overload in parts of the health care system, there was likewise a volume reduction in many of the outpatient and subspecialty clinical areas of the system. The need for face-to-face appointments as part of traditional patient care was soon reevaluated for the potential of conducting visits over the telephone or by video chat. This turn toward the virtual also revealed how many of these visits were actually unnecessary. Non-face-to-face health care, such as that provided by telehealth, became an essential piece of caring for people during the COVID-19 pandemic and arguably will result in the greater use of telehealth down the road. Telehealth became the lifeline when patients were afraid to leave their homes to visit hospitals and clinics, and quite likely it prevented more infections in health care workers.

So how do we prepare for the next pandemic? Preparing the next generation of doctors and nurses will require that we grapple with the following issues:

1. The number of physicians and nurses needed
2. The geographic distribution of physicians and nurses needed
3. The education and curriculum necessary for future physicians and nurses
4. The resilience and well-being of physicians and nurses in the next pandemic work environment
5. The development and evolution of new technologies and tools to be used by physicians and nurses in the next pandemic
6. The imperative to deal with the associated pandemic of intolerance
7. The need to understand and address the social determinants of health prior to the next pandemic

Let us take a deeper look at all of these issues.

The Number of Physicians and Nurses Needed for the Next Pandemic

The United States has just over 1 million professionally active physicians, with 54 percent being specialists and 46 percent being primary care physicians,[2] and there are about 3 million registered nurses.[3] This puts the United States in the 35th position in the world for physicians,[4] and the number of nurses per capita positions the country 19th.[5] As can be inferred from these numbers, the United States does not have a sufficient physician and nursing workforce to deal with the large number of people that can be seen in a health care crisis like the COVID-19 pandemic. This is especially true for particularly underserved areas of our population: inner city urban areas and rural and frontier locations.

This mismatch is magnified by the racial disparities among physicians and nurses in the United States. Although 17 percent of the US population is Hispanic and 13 percent is Black, only 6 percent of the physician workforce in the United States is Hispanic and 5 percent is Black.[6] On the nursing side of the equation, 6 percent of the workforce in the United States is Hispanic and 10 percent is Black.[7] This ethnic and racial disparity in terms of physicians and nurses, unsurprisingly, often translates into less physicians and nurses working in our inner cities and in our rural and frontier areas.

The nation needs to be able to rapidly mobilize large numbers of physicians and nurses and other health care workers to attend to areas where the patient demand is highest, be that in our cities or in our rural and frontier areas. Similarly, pairing resources by race and ethnicity should be performed in a way that would be culturally sensitive to areas that need these professionals most. At the time of the next public health emergency of this magnitude, we need to develop a rapid expansion of the physician and nursing workforce. In essence, we need to greatly expand our Medical Reserve Corps. These physicians and nurses could be retired from active practice but still desire, in a time of crisis and emergency, to lend a helping hand, or they could be actively practicing physicians and nurses from areas of the country that are not hard hit by the public health emergency.

We need to have credentialing processes in place that make the integration of these physicians and nurses into the workforce and their placements simple and efficient. There needs to be relaxation at the federal and state level for licensure at times of crisis that would allow physicians and nurses to temporarily practice in a different state when the need is high. Finally, we also need liability protection, such as Good Samaritan laws, that would be applied to these physicians and nurses in the delivery of appropriate medical and nursing care to patients in need.

Recommendation #66

Health Care Workforce Development

Health care workforce policies and incentives need to be developed that will promote an increase in the numbers of physicians and nurses in both ambulatory and hospital settings. The plan should be especially directed at medically underserved areas and health professional shortage areas to address their needs for primary care and specialty care, including mental health. Further, the plan should be directed at increasing the diversity of the health care workforce to better match the communities they serve.

The Geographic Distribution of Physicians and Nurses Needed

Twenty percent of the United States population lives in rural and frontier areas. However, only 9 percent of the physician workforce serves these areas.[8] The nursing distribution is somewhat better balanced, with 16 percent of registered nurses and 24 percent of licensed practical nurses living in rural areas.[9] There are 13 physicians per 10,000 people in rural areas, but nearly 2.5 times as many (31 physicians per 10,000 people) in urban areas.[10] Without a doubt, the United States has a problem with poor distribution of physicians and nurses by region.

And, as was noted above, not only is there a poor match in geographic distribution, there is a similarly poor distribution of physicians and nurses by race and ethnicity as well. To correct this problem, we need to seek out greater diversity and inclusiveness in the training of tomorrow's physicians and nurses to ensure that they more closely correspond to the diversity of our varied communities and that these new health care providers are incentivized to practice in such communities.

Shortages of physicians and nurses in disadvantaged and rural communities and communities of color lead to a reduction in timely access to health care and worse outcomes for these at-risk populations. We see this even more clearly during a public health emergency, such as an epidemic or pandemic.

Recommendation #67

Health Care Professional Geographic Shortages

A federal strategic plan must be developed for the geographic disparities and shortages in physician and nursing workforces across this country.

A group that can be instrumental in advising on and developing this plan is the Council on Graduate Medical Education. It is the federal advisory council to Congress and the secretary of health and human services. This council resides within the Health Resources and Services Administration and has the expertise needed to help formulate a plan.

An Education and Curriculum for Future Physicians and Nurses

What we have painfully learned from this pandemic is that we must improve basic instruction about public health principles and the science of epidemiology in our medical and nursing schools. Basic public health measures to combat an emerging epidemic or pandemic must be both planned for in advance and then implemented quickly in times of public health emergencies. So that all physicians and nurses can help educate and inform the community immediately at the time of the next health care crisis, they must be well-informed about science that demonstrates the effectiveness of face-mask wearing, social distancing measures, strategically limiting gathering sizes, handwashing, not going to work sick, and surface contact cleaning, depending on the transmission routes of the involved pathogen.

Recommendation #68

Medical and Nursing Education

Medical and nursing school curricula need to address training and preparation for public health emergencies, such as epidemics and pandemics. Education and training must also promote inter-professional teamwork and communication, professionalism, respect, and trust. Physicians must also be trained on medical informatics, data analytics, and how to critically evaluate clinical studies as our understanding of a novel pathogen during an epidemic or pandemic evolves.

Physicians and nurses must be trained in both medical and nursing schools on the importance of interprofessional teamwork and communication. These teams need to work together if they are to be successful in educating the public in a clear, measured manner to lessen their confusion and anxiety in the time of an emergency. Training should promote professionalism, trust, and respect between physicians, nurses, and public health agencies. Medical training should include informatics, data analytics, and preparation to receive and correctly interpret large amounts of data and emerging medical studies.

We also will need to prepare physician, nursing, and hospital administrative leaders how to develop evidence-based visitation policies for those admitted to the hospital or a long-term care facility. We saw widely varying policies throughout the country, and even in the same city, that often did not make sense from an infection control and patient safety standpoint and often had inexplicable internal inconsistencies, such as allowing a spouse or significant other to stay with a laboring mother, but not allowing a spouse or family member to stay overnight with a post-surgical patient. We saw one policy that allowed family members to stay with bone marrow transplant patients, but not with patients who were sedated and being given potent pain medications following surgery. Such policies did not align well with what we knew about the transmission risks of SARS-CoV-2.

While visitor policies do need to protect patients and staff, many policies included restrictions that were overly harsh and not supported by the evidence, and indeed may have compromised patient safety. Visitation policies should allow a designated family member or members to stay with a patient who is admitted to a non-critical care area of a hospital. There needs to be a balancing of the harms and benefits of having someone stay with a patient, especially those patients who might be prone to confusion or slightly impaired due to medications. A family member is often critical to reducing patient falls and medication errors and improving understanding of and compliance with post-discharge instructions.

Obviously, visitation must be drastically curtailed at the beginning of a pandemic when little is known about the biologic behavior of a pandemic virus. However, once we are aware of the transmission characteristics, we know how to effectively mitigate the risks of disease transmission in the hospital and can take the appropriate steps to protect patients, staff, and visitors. Overly restrictive visitor policies during the pandemic often meant increased risk of iatrogenic harm to patients, mental and emotional harm to patients resulting from loneliness and isolation, and psychological harm to family members who suffered increased anxiety associated with the hospitalization of their loved one and experienced unresolved grief in instances in which the family member died. These overly restrictive policies also created more stress for staff members who had to enforce these unpopular policies.

Recommendation #69
Evidence-Based Visitation Policies

Hospitals should review their visitation policies in light of what we have learned from this pandemic in preparation for the next. Visitor policies should be evidence-based and internally consistent.

Recommendation #70
Expand the Medical Reserve Corps

A greater effort should be made to inform physicians, nurses, and other health care professionals about the Medical Reserve Corps and to encourage their enlistment. The current focus on local health initiatives should be expanded to preparation for deployment anywhere in the country in the event of a public health emergency. Congress needs to make a greater commitment to sufficiently fund this effort and to ensure that, in the event of an emergency, proper laws are enacted to allow the practice of medicine, nursing, and other health professions in a state in which the professionals are not licensed, as well as providing the appropriate liability protections for these volunteers.

The Resilience and Well-Being of Physicians and Nurses

The stress, anxiety, and burnout observed in the physician and nursing workforce due to COVID-19 cannot be overestimated. Proactive education through medical school, nursing school, and graduate medical education training programs must emphasize techniques and strategies that will emphasize stress reduction, mindfulness, relaxation, resilience, and critical debriefing. Effective debriefing of physician-nurse work teams will be essential for both continued learning and performance improvement, as well as providing stress reduction for these professionals.

Ongoing continued medical education and continued nursing education must focus on interpersonal teamwork, communication, professionalism, and respect, along with mindfulness and stress reduction. Ensuring that physicians and nurses get adequate amounts of sleep during intense and prolonged crisis periods will be important.

Additionally, dealing with post-traumatic stress disorder, anxiety, and depression will be paramount not only for patients that have gone through a pandemic experience, but also for physicians, nurses, medical assistants, nursing aides, medical and nursing students, and other members of the health care workforce that have gone through this upheaval as well—who may have become ill themselves or been impacted by illness or death in their own family. The proactive application of cognitive behavioral therapy, counseling, and debriefing will help deal with many of these issues in a healthy, forward-looking way for the next generation of physicians and nurses meeting these challenges.

Recommendation #71

Education, Training, and Services to Support Health Care Workers

Education, training, and continuing education programs should address stress reduction, mindfulness, resilience, behavioral therapy, and incident debriefing to help prevent or address anxiety, depression, burnout, and post-traumatic stress disorder. During a time of increased and prolonged stress, leaders must be proactive in reaching out to their workforce and offering services to them.

The Development and Evolution of New Technologies and Tools

Telehealth became very important during this pandemic. Taking advantage of this experience, we need to continue to pursue strategies, policies, and appropriate payment methods for telehealth, using video platforms as well as patient telephone care, email care and text message care. All of these can be extremely helpful to patients, allowing them to safely communicate from a virtual environment—one in which the patient does not need to travel for excessive amounts of time or potentially expose themselves to environments where they might contract an infectious disease such as COVID-19. Our physicians and nurses need to be educated on the effective and compassionate use of these platforms.

Beyond this, what this pandemic has also revealed is the ever-increasing speed of information flow, both within the United States and around the world. We must help patients in need by responding to this torrent of information and work to incorporate lessons we have learned within the United States as well as other countries regarding how best to translate practices and therapies.

There is a role for hospitals to play in offering expert online continuing medical education, providing timely reviews of new developments with medical staff. Similarly, the Centers for Disease Control and Prevention (CDC) and other professional associations can offer weekly podcasts to review developments from clinical studies for busy clinicians who may be working long hours but can still listen to the podcasts on their way to and from the hospital. These organizations could maintain a library of the most important clinical studies on their websites and send out a weekly email summarizing updates from clinical trials.

In addition, medical and nursing students and residents need to be taught how to find reliable information and how to critically evaluate clinical studies. We saw many situations in which even seasoned physicians and public health experts did not critically evaluate study design or consider study limitations when reaching conclusions that they reported to the public. For example, in early studies examining the prevalence of long COVID, some experts failed to realize that if the inclusion criteria required a prior positive PCR test, this would eliminate many from participation in the study who had probable COVID based on the nature of their illness and a known close contact early on in the pandemic, at a time when there was lack of access to testing. Also, some researchers failed to appreciate that other studies looking at this same issue of long COVID and using the Veterans Affairs database to identify patients with long COVID would result in an underrepresentation of women, who appear to account for the greatest number of these cases, as well as young adults who are significantly impacted by long COVID. Trusted data sources that can be found online, especially with .gov, .edu and .org listings, will be helpful in times of emergency, not only to physicians and nurses but to patients as well.

Recommendation #72
Virtual Care Reimbursement

As long as health care reimbursement systems in the United States remain largely fee for service, we need those systems to cover and properly reimburse providers for their time and effort to manage the health of their patients without an in-person visit, such as telehealth, telephone, email, and text communications. To encourage providers to offer telehealth services for the safety and convenience of patients, these virtual visits should be reimbursed at parity with in-person visits.

Helping Prepare Future Physicians and Nurses for the Pandemic of Intolerance

As has been mentioned previously, we saw three ongoing pandemics at the same time. We saw the first, most obvious pandemic of COVID-19 rapidly spread across the world. We also saw how the second pandemic of the human response to this virus both helped and harmed our efforts to control COVID-19. Much of the book has been spent talking about the relationship between these two pandemics. The third pandemic, which we will now examine, is the pandemic of intolerance.

We have seen how the COVID-19 pandemic brought out the best in some people, but it also brought out the worst in others. A glaring item in the worst category was intolerant and prejudiced behavior. Dissecting this a bit, there are at the very least six different issues that were revealed during the epidemic. These items were discussed by Dr. Thomas J. Nasca, the CEO of the Accreditation Council for Graduate Medical Education. To help prevent future pandemics, an analysis of these categories must be part of what physicians and nurses are trained to recognize and inspired to overcome.[11]

Recommendation #73

Keep Clinicians Updated

To keep clinicians updated in the face of rapidly developing information about a new health threat, the CDC and professional associations should provide libraries of important articles on their websites, offer weekly podcasts to summarize and explain the latest developments, and send out weekly email summaries of important information and updates.

Inequity

Health care inequality was mentioned earlier in the book. We must proactively educate physicians and nurses on how to tackle the root causes of these health care disparities and inequities in a strong effort to ameliorate them. It is not acceptable to have greater numbers of cases, hospitalizations, and deaths for minorities and the socioeconomically disadvantaged. Awareness of these disparities must be taught to physicians, nurses, and all other health care workers so that we can confront these issues before the next pandemic.

Incivility

We also witnessed many examples of incivility in how people treated other people who didn't think or believe as they did. In a time of national crisis and emergency, we must all be more tolerant and realize that people will react differently to these crises. That said, we must center on what scientific data and evidence demonstrate, understanding that this is the most effective way to keep each other healthy and safe during a pandemic. We should refrain from being uncivil to our fellow community members for following those guidelines.

Incoherence

There was a lot of confusion and mixed messaging from the White House and the CDC in the early days of the pandemic. This inconsistent and incoherent communication must be eliminated in the future. It is important not only that we should be prepared for the next pandemic, but also that clear communication and guidance must be readied in advance so that we do not divide, polarize, and confuse the public. Most importantly, we must not deny or downplay the seriousness of the situation.

Inhumanity

There were many examples of inhumanity in the reaction of some individuals to the pandemic. Workers at meatpacking plants and transportation workers on buses were not provided with basic protections. There was open hostility and protests toward public health officials, physicians, nurses, community leaders, and others that were working hard on behalf of the public. Those who were trying to do the right things for the health of the community should be afforded respect and appreciation. We must all recognize that at a basic human level, every one of us is important and we must sacrifice some of our basic civil liberties in order for the population to stay as healthy as possible and thrive as much as we can in a pandemic situation.

Ignorance

We must strive to keep our minds open and receptive to new information. We must be careful not to get information from a single source without questioning the truthfulness and reliability of that information. We must all be open-minded, but also critical in our evaluation of what we are reading and being told. By being discerning and basing our beliefs on evidence, we can do a better job at rejecting misinformation and disinformation. We all must take responsibility and accountability for being informed and embracing the best science available.

Intolerance

We must all be able to perform at our best and elevate our thinking in times of an emergency. We must be tolerant of the fear, anxiety, and anger that we see in others. We must strive to be our best selves, our truly authentic selves to help calm and comfort people in times of stress. We must all serve as role models. If doctors and nurses cannot do this, then who can?

Physicians and nurses are ideally placed to ensure that the six I's of inequity, incivility, incoherence, inhumanity, ignorance, and intolerance are all handled in a professional and mature way. The one antidote that will help with this pandemic of intolerance is an abundance of compassion and empathy. If we can always strive to try to understand how others are feeling, as if we have walked in their shoes, and be compassionate for their situation and their fear, worry, and anxiety, we will be a better and more fulfilled society.

Recommendation #74

Combat Bad Behaviors

It is up to elected leaders, public health officials and board members, the medical and nursing communities, professional associations, licensing boards and other health care workers, and each of us to combat the inequity, incivility, incoherence, inhumanity, and ignorance that emerged during the COVID-19 pandemic and that will likely recur in future pandemics. All must speak truth, model desired behaviors, and speak out to correct misinformation and disinformation. Health care professionals must help disseminate the best evidence, facts, and data to better inform the public and advise decision makers.

Helping Prepare Future Physicians and Nurses to Address the Social Determinants of Health

Medical and nursing schools must make education about the issues that lead to inequities and disparities in health care, and the related challenges that can lead to worse outcomes in times of emergencies such as the COVID-19 pandemic, a curricular priority. Medical and nursing education at all levels, including graduate medical education, must train all physicians and nurses to address these social determinants of health. Issues such as housing, transportation, education, poor financial resources, domestic violence, adverse childhood experiences, food insecurity, and many others must be part of what physicians and nurses are trained to look for and to help improve in their communities.

We cannot remain a reactive health care system, responding only to people's illnesses and chronic conditions when they develop. We must all collectively move upstream to mitigate these problems before they result in bad health and disease outcomes. The negative impact of social determinants of health has been clearly demonstrated during this COVID-19 pandemic, as we have seen minorities and those who are socioeconomically disadvantaged bear the brunt of the disease. It is not only part of our social responsibility to remedy these inequities and disparities, but our moral responsibility as well.[12]

Efforts to address these social determinants can include better testing and better vaccination strategies in rural and underserved inner city and urban locations. We need better primary care access in these locations as well. We need better laws that protect workers, so that they can be quarantined and isolated without losing their income or their jobs. More physicians and nurses of Native American, Black and Hispanic backgrounds need to be trained, so that they can serve these communities and bring greater diversity and inclusivity to public health. Only by truly owning up to the social determinants of health care can we truly prepare the next generation to appropriately respond to and prevent a huge number of illnesses, hospitalizations, and deaths in the next pandemic.

Recommendation #75

Social Determinants of Health

It is imperative that we educate health care professionals in all phases of their education, training, and continuing education about the social determinants of health and strategies to address them. Students and trainees should be involved in community projects or initiatives to address and mitigate health care disparities.

Developing the Public Health Workforce

We have been extremely impressed with the hard-working, dedicated public health professionals that serve our public health districts and our state. These professionals were varied in their roles—contact tracers, epidemiologists, data analysts, website designers, media relations personnel, public health nurses, school liaison staff, microbiologists and other laboratory scientists, vaccine program managers, and more. Most were faceless and nameless to much of the public, but their work was critical to the deployment of accurate data and information to the public, health care providers, journalists and reporters, schools, businesses, and political leaders. They played critical roles in educating the public and decision-makers. They also played important roles in acquiring and distributing PPE, antiviral medications, and vaccines to hospitals and health care providers.

In 2020, while the president and his administration were largely undermining the efforts of these experts, promoting false information and failing to reinforce or model public health guidance, many of the experts were also thwarted in their efforts by governors, legislatures, local leaders, school boards, and even members of public health boards, shockingly enough, who at times embraced misinformation and conspiracy theories or deferred to health care professionals promoting interventions that were unproven or disproved over the expertise of their own public health experts.

In our experience, we have found that public health care professionals are extremely dedicated to and passionate about promoting and improving the health of their communities and state and protecting the public. Most could get higher-paying jobs in the private sector, but they are more driven by passion to help people and make a difference than they are by money, visibility, or recognition. In our state, Idaho, our director for the Department of Health and Welfare, Dave Jeppesen, is a cabinet official appointed by our governor. He was a high-ranking executive for the largest commercial health insurance company in Idaho before taking on this role. Many of us considered him a likely potential successor to the CEO of that company upon her retirement. Nevertheless, he turned away both the opportunity and undoubtedly a significantly higher salary in order to enter public service and lead the department through this unprecedented pandemic, in a way that neither of us can imagine anyone else could have managed, and performed his duties with such grace, patience, and commitment to doing the right thing.

Similarly, Dr. Christine Hahn, our Division of Public Health medical director and state epidemiologist for nearly 25 years, has brought a calm, guiding hand and common-sense solutions to our state while no doubt forgoing more lucrative private practice opportunities in her field of infectious diseases. Dr. Hahn received national recognition when she received the highly coveted Pumphandle Award from the Council of State and Territorial Epidemiologists in 2021 for outstanding achievement in the field of applied epidemiology.

Many public health experts worked an excessive number of days in a row during the pandemic, and far greater hours per day than during more normal times. They, too, risked burnout, as we have seen among front-line health care workers. These public servants received little recognition or appreciation for all their efforts; in fact, they often saw their hard work lead to guidance that in many cases was ignored or disregarded.

While there was a good deal of discussion about the mental health challenges faced by the public and by students due to the pandemic and the measures enacted to prevent the spread of the disease, there was little discussion about the mental health implications for health care workers and these public health experts.

A study of public health workers was conducted during the months of March and April in 2021 to assess the psychological effects and impacts on these professionals. The study's authors summarized their findings as follows: "Among 26,174 respondents, 53.0% reported symptoms of at least one mental health condition in the preceding 2 weeks, including depression (32.0%), anxiety (30.3%), PTSD (36.8%), or suicidal ideation (8.4%). The highest prevalence of symptoms of a mental health condition was among respondents aged ≤29 years (range = 13.6%–47.4%) and transgender or nonbinary persons (i.e., those who identified as neither male nor female) of all ages (range = 30.4%–65.5%)." For those "public health workers who reported being unable to take time off from work," they "were more likely to report adverse mental health symptoms. Severity of symptoms increased with increasing weekly work hours and percentage of work time dedicated to COVID-19 response activities."[13]

In preparing the future public health workforce to face future public health emergencies, we believe that the most important step is preserving and maintaining the current workforce with its accumulated experience and expertise. We call on the president of the United States, Congress, governors, state legislatures, and local elected officials to declare a day of public recognition of and appreciation for our health care and public health workers. We encourage the use of proclamations, publication of the proclamations in local newspapers, flying of flags over the United States and state capitols, and public service announcements by leaders at all levels of government to recognize the efforts, contributions, and sacrifices of all these unsung heroes. We need to express our appreciation, but also reinforce to all these workers that their actions made a difference, saved lives, and helped our country, states, and local communities to navigate through this pandemic.

We also call on the president and Congress to renew our country's commitment to science and, much like we did back in the 1960s, invest in strategies and programs to stimulate the interest of children in careers in STEM fields: that is, science, technology, engineering, and mathematics. We will have trouble convincing young people to pursue education and training in public health if we send the simultaneous message, inadvertently or purposefully, that we do not value science or expertise or respect the work that these professionals do. We must also educate students about careers in public health and the exciting and meaningful contributions they can make in these roles.

Physician, Nursing, and Community Collaboration

An organization that one of the authors, Dr. Epperly, is a member of was approached by the city of Boise, Idaho, in concert with three of the community's homeless shelters, to request help from them in providing medical care for those living at the shelters, as well as caring for them at a local hotel if they became ill. The response was the idea of one of the family medicine residents, Dr. Julie Duncan, and her faculty advisor, Dr. Abby Davids, working in conjunction with our chief medical officer, Dr. Penny Beach.

Starting March 30, 2020, we offered COVID-19 testing six nights a week at all three shelters using our mobile van. The testing was done by a medical assistant and a physician/resident physician, physician assistant, or nurse practitioner using the van as an outreach site. We also did multiple rounds of mass testing at the shelters, recruiting for medical provider volunteers and asking medical assistants to work overtime.

The second part of this project was supporting the local COVID-19 isolation hotel for patients experiencing homelessness. The City of Boise rented out an entire hotel to isolate COVID-19-positive patients living on the streets who were not sick enough to be admitted to inpatient facilities at local hospitals. At a minimum, our providers saw these patients on the date of their admission and at the end of their isolation period in order to assess their medical status. Anyone teetering on hospital admission was seen daily.

To date, we have run over 1,000 tests. Unfortunately, we observed a high test positivity rate, driven by the fact that one of the shelters did not require masks. We have taken care of over 200 patients experiencing homelessness in the COVID-19 isolation hotel, and we are now vaccinating shelter patrons against COVID-19.

In the last year, we have had one person living on the streets die of COVID-19—a patient that was transferred to the hospital directly from the shelter without staying in the hotel. We have admitted two patients from the hotel to the hospital, and both survived. Everyone else has done well.

During the height of the pandemic, we were able to reduce the burden on our local hospitals by taking discharged patients into the hotel who otherwise might have needed to stay in the hospital a few days longer. We were also able to admit patients to the hotel from the local emergency rooms, alleviating the pressure on hospitals to admit patients who did not have homes to isolate in.

Collaborative partnerships with caring community members, physicians, resident physicians, physician assistants, nurses, and nurse practitioners were the key to the success of this project. Our collaboration with three homeless shelters and the City of Boise to provide testing, medical care, and vaccinations to over 1,000 patients experiencing homelessness in Ada County was critical to successfully managing a very high-risk population. Our goal was to keep our patrons free of COVID-19 and keep those who did get infected from transmitting the disease, being hospitalized, or dying.

This story speaks to caring, empathetic community partners who strongly desired to help other people. Our faculty and resident physicians, along with our nursing staff, medical assistants, physician assistants, and nurse practitioners, went above and beyond to make this community collaboration successful. In fact, it was one of our young resident family medicine physicians who, along with her faculty advisor, helped create and operate the program. The modeling of this caring and empathy goes a long way toward preparing the next generation of physicians, nurses, and other health care professionals to identify community needs and gaps and help be part of the solution—not only now, but in the future.

CHAPTER 10

Preparing Public Health Departments for the Next Pandemic

> Public health is something that has really nothing to do with politics . . . This is the worst outbreak . . . of a respiratory-borne illness that we've had in 102 years. You can't run away from the data.
>
> DR. ANTHONY FAUCI

The COVID-19 pandemic revealed critical fissures, cracks, and fractures in our public health system. Public health departments' typical business is primarily focused on restaurant and food inspection, on septic system approvals, on water and air quality, and on limited infectious disease outbreaks such as those related to fecal sources in swimming pools. They also track small foodborne disease and tuberculosis outbreaks, where traditional contact tracing, isolation, and quarantines can be effective. They are not designed to handle huge, full-scale, ongoing epidemics and pandemics. Public health departments do mass disaster planning in collaboration with area hospitals, fire, police, and other community agencies, but their charters typically did not appreciate the scale or persistence of a public health emergency such as occurred with the COVID-19 pandemic. Simply put, the public health departments were not prepared for this infectious disaster.

An analysis of public health departments across the nation reveals anywhere from a 16 to 18 percent decrease in funding since 2010.[1] In the United States, three quarters of the states fund their public health departments with less than $100 per person per year.[2] This compares with the nearly $11,000 per person per year that is on average spent on health care costs. That is a 110-fold difference between the amount of money that is spent on health care and the amount of money made available for public health. Because of health department funding decreases, 40,000 jobs at the state and local public health agencies have been lost since the recession of 2008.[3]

In Idaho, there are seven public health districts. These districts were enacted by state law and went into effect in 1970. The objective was to provide all 44 counties with reasonable access to all public health services. The districts were structured around geographical units consisting of rural counties augmented by an adjacent urban center—seven urban cities and seven health districts. The boards of these seven public health districts are made up of one physician and either county commissioners from each of the counties in the district or a person designated by the county commissioners. Idaho's public health system was designed this way primarily to equitably distribute infrastructure resources (such as environmental health specialists, women-infant-children coordinators, health education and disease coordinators, and so forth) between the more highly populated counties and the rural counties that could not afford this expense without a considerable tax burden. Funding for these public health resources is generated from county taxes assessed to the citizens of a county, as well as from the state and federal government, along with fees for certain services. This is an efficient and effective way to help rural counties secure public health services and recruit expertise, resources they would otherwise be unlikely to be able to obtain on their own.

This model works relatively well under normal conditions, but during the worldwide pandemic and the resulting national emergency, public health departments were suddenly placed fully in the spotlight and were ill prepared for it. Public health districts, whose funding had been stripped away since 2008, had little extra infrastructure, funding, or resources to handle a crisis of this magnitude. The public health boards were inevitably exposed as lacking the knowledge, expertise, capability, or preparedness to tackle the depth and complexity of this crisis.

As the COVID-19 pandemic continued to gain ground in the United States, politics, ideology, and the economy started to overpower public health measures. In fact, this has gotten so bad in our state of Idaho that the state legislature passed a bill that requires public health departments' countywide or districtwide orders to be reviewed by the county board of commissioners for the counties affected by the order within seven days of being issued. The county's elected officials have the authority to overturn the order with no recourse by the public health department. This bill was signed by the governor and is now a law in Idaho, and it is a formula for disaster. It prioritizes politics and ideology over science and public health. It places medical and public health decision-making into the hands of political county commissioners with no medical knowledge needed to make informed public health decisions.

Several other laws have been enacted or proposed in our state to no longer allow health boards to close schools, along with laws that interfere with colleges and universities dealing with pandemics. Additional constraints target the governor's authority during a public health emergency. The proposed restrictions on the governor's authority range widely, from reducing the ability to order closures to restraining vaccine requirements, limits on the size of gatherings and the ability to order a mask mandate. In the entire current legislative session, not one bill was passed to ensure that Idaho is better prepared for the next pandemic.

Useful legislation could have been considered, such as creating and maintaining a stockpile of face masks, respiratory protection for health care workers, and sufficient personal protective equipment (PPE). An effort could have been made to improve county and statewide communication plans and provide more effective testing. Better coordination among public health districts and vaccination preparedness could have been championed. Instead, the Idaho legislature took steps to prohibit many of the most effective public health measures available to us in a time of a major public health threat.

So, what can we do to develop a better public health department for the next pandemic?

Increase the Visibility of Public Health

Public health in the United States clearly suffers from an identity and an invisibility problem.[4] Public health departments are not well known in their communities. There is little understanding of their roles and functions. Average citizens do not know what the public health departments do in normal times, let alone how they operate during a crisis such as the COVID-19 pandemic. There must be increased messaging and communication about the importance of public health, with an emphasis on understanding the function of public health departments in all communities. This should focus on emphasizing the importance of their day-to-day activities, as well as explaining their essential role in the face of an emergency. That emergency can be local and man-made or a natural disaster, such as earthquakes, fires, and floods, or it can be an event at a national or even worldwide scale, such as the COVID-19 pandemic. The ability to form lasting, trusted, collaborative relationships in communities between the leadership of the community, the hospitals, the health care providers, and the public health department must be enhanced.

Recommendation #76

Inform the Public about the Role of Public Health

There should be organized and targeted messaging and a communication plan that educates the public, health care providers, and social organizations about the many roles and functions of public health departments under normal conditions, as well as during times of emergency.

Increase Public Funding for Public Health

As mentioned above, spending for public health agencies has dropped by 16 to 18 percent over the last decade. Federal support for public health, emergency preparedness, and hospital preparedness has dropped by 30 percent since 2006.[5] As an example of this sort of funding mismatch, one of the authors, Dr. Epperly—as a member of Idaho's largest public health district's board of directors—has seen firsthand how there is always strong tension between the Idaho legislature's portion of public health funding and the local county commissioners' own assessment of their necessary public health district funding requirements. Most elected officials think they are spending too much of the taxpayer's money and need to reduce their expenditures. Public health departments, on the other hand, do not understand why the county commissioners and the state legislature do not understand that their functions are important for the well-being and safety of the community, and that the amount of public spending per person needs to increase. They point out that preventing illness or poor health will save money in the long run.

But after all this wrangling, in the end, there must be an increased prioritization of funding to public health departments. It is important that this imbalance between mission and funding be tackled in order to nurture this vital community function. Public health funding needs to be enhanced at the federal, state, and county level. Our goal should be to increase the level of support from the current $100 per person per year expenditure to closer to $300 per person per year.

Recommendation #77

Increase Funding for Public Health

Appropriate levels of funding of the public health infrastructure should be established by the federal government and each state, as well as locally by county, driven by the creation of national benchmarks. This funding should be sufficient to allow for all the functions of public health, but also with a sufficient investment for planning and preparation for future public health emergencies. A practical benchmark would be to move this funding from $100 per person per year to $300 per person per year.

The Structure of Public Health Departments

All too often, the structure of public health departments lacks much to be desired in terms of the board membership chosen to oversee these departments and their functions. Form follows function. Since the function of public health departments is to oversee and monitor the public's health, there must be people that have appropriate knowledge placed on the public health boards. At a minimum, board members must be knowledgeable about the principles and science of public health, social determinants of health, and infection control principles. When the board is largely made up of elected officials, it is not surprising that decisions become political and the public health departments become lightning rods in their communities if something big flares up.

In Idaho, this is exactly what occurred. Even though public health districts had talented executive directors and staff, their boards were unable to reliably stick to evidence-based data and science. This resulted in inconsistent decision-making and conflicting rulings by neighboring public health districts, and this disarray undermined the credibility of the districts. It led to decisions spurred primarily by the lobbying of board members by the public or by special interest groups, rather than those founded on applied science. It was more common to hear "This is what my hundreds of emails say" than "This is what the science and data say." Boards were acting vigorously on behalf of their constituents' interests as they perceived them, filtered through their own political agendas and beliefs. They were more interested in ensuring that the economy stayed open and that people's personal liberties and individual rights were being honored than ensuring the public's health and preventing the spread of the pandemic. We stopped focusing on what a public health district's actual charter is, which is to evaluate and monitor data so that the best informed, evidence-based, scientific answers can be applied to the community in the interest of the entire public's best health.

Recommendation #78
Appointments to Public Health Boards

The boards of public health departments in the future should be made up largely of physicians, nurses, social workers, educators, people who work to provide shelter for the homeless, and those who run food banks. We must have people who are serving the health and social well-being of the citizens of the counties that will use evidence, data, and deference to expertise in their decision making.

Recommendation #79

Qualifications of Public Health Board Members

Public health boards should not be primarily comprised of elected officials. Like other fiduciary boards, board members should not have conflicts of interest—political, ideological, or financial—that conflict with the mission and essential function of the public health board. Members of these boards should embrace foundational public health and infection control principles.

The Function and Education of Public Health Department Board Members

Many public health departments across the nation were ill prepared for their function in the pandemic. As noted above, to mitigate against this in the future, there needs to be membership on the board that brings knowledge of and familiarity with public health principles. All new public health department board members must be provided with a standard orientation and curriculum upon arrival to the board. This curriculum should educate them in moderate detail about what the public health department's functions, goals, principles, and values are, as well as instructing them on infection control principles, along with an understanding of the social determinants of health. They need to be educated on what emergency, epidemic, and pandemic preparedness and implementation look like. They need to be taught how the funding works, and then they need to be advocates for the public health departments to help secure that funding while meeting the mission of the departments. The emphasis must be on the public's health, and not on politics.

Recommendation #80

Education of Public Health Board Members

Public health department board members should undergo an extensive orientation and complete a curriculum and training in public health principles, infection control, social determinants of health, and public health emergencies.

One function of public health departments is to issue public health orders. These have the same effects and consequences as laws, and they should only be issued when absolutely necessary. But public health orders without enforcement are nothing more than suggestions. As the pandemic raged on, this became ever more apparent. People complied with the governor's stay-at-home order at the start of the pandemic out of uncertainty and fear. After we gained more experience and observed that people were not dying in massive numbers, voluntary compliance faded.

People's interest in voluntary compliance resurged in November and December 2020, driven by the reality that most everyone now knew someone close to them who had become ill or died. Other countries like South Korea and Australia did a great job with compliance in their communities through consistent messaging, and had enviably low infection numbers and positive outcomes as a result. Instead, back in the United States—and particularly in Idaho—we had sheriffs proclaiming on the news that they would not enforce mandates and county commissioners unilaterally passing resolutions to make state orders null and void in their county. While—to use an extreme example—we are not China, with its nearly unfettered ability to impose top-down restrictions, we can nevertheless do better. All future board of public health department members must understand the difference between public health recommendations, advisories, and orders. If a public health order is given, there must be cooperation from the city mayors, police, and sheriff's departments to enforce the orders. If not, the orders will have considerably less that the desired effect.

Recommendation #81

Range of Interventions by Public Health Boards

All public health board of directors must be educated about the differences between and implications of public health recommendations, advisories, and orders. If a public health order is issued, it is essential that mayors, police officers, and sheriffs are willing and committed to enforcing the order, or the order is unlikely to be effective.

Public Health Districts

The concept of public health districts themselves may need to be tweaked and realigned for maximum performance. For example, in cases such as Idaho, with its many rural and frontier counties currently coupled with adjacent large population centers to take advantage of economies of scale, health district partitions may need to be redrawn so that they now contain a combined metropolitan area, such as Ada and Canyon Counties. We previously mentioned the conundrum caused by these two adjoining health districts with large populations taking very different approaches to the pandemic, even though their citizens intermix for work, shopping, athletic events, concerts, and other social events. These different approaches undermined the acceptance of public health messages, and in many cases shattered compliance with them by eroding the public's trust.

This dilemma was most noticeable within the four counties comprising Central District Health, which contains Ada County, the county with the largest population in the state and home to the state capital, Boise. This meant that the state's largest city was conjoined with three smaller, much more rural counties. This led inexorably to an uneven application of public health policy that tangled up the concerns of the most densely populated county in our state with very different worries that other commissioners had gleaned from their small, rural, and frontier counties. This misalignment generated strongly heated disagreements over public health mandates regarding face masking, group sizes, and social distancing.

The smaller, more rural counties wanted to be excluded from policies that would mandate masking, whereas masking clearly needed to be done in Ada County. Over to our west in Canyon County, another large urban area was paired with five much more rural and frontier counties to form Southwest District Health. There, a similar urban/rural mismatch occurred. Because most of the county commissioners in Southwest District Health were from the smaller rural and frontier areas, Canyon County did not adopt a face mask ordinance despite their physician board member imploring them to do so. This left a very uneven application of face masking across the Treasure Valley, which is the valley that contains both Ada and Canyon Counties. It was a bit like a single car with both an American and a British steering wheel installed, manned by two drivers at the same time, all the while strongly disagreeing on which side of the road to drive.

All of this led to not only intra-health district disagreements, but also an inter-health district lack of cooperation. In essence, the tail was wagging the dog. Rural and frontier counties, in order to meet their local requirements, were blocking the larger urban counties' ability to implement appropriate public health initiatives. There needs to be a thoughtful reconsideration of how these public health districts and counties can share resources in good times and work more harmoniously in times of emergency and disagreement.

Recommendation #82

Realignment of Public Health Districts

Functional and geographical alignment of counties into health districts by size, population density, and resource distribution will better ensure that similar issues that nevertheless impact populations differently are more effectively addressed with the goal of achieving consistency of effort and outcome.

The Role of the Governor and State Health Department

In many of our country's states, the pandemic started out being managed by the governors in conjunction with their state health departments. The states that managed this best stayed with this model. This approach led to consistent efforts and clearer messaging, while the states that did not follow this formula had inconsistent efforts and confused messaging.

Idaho started out with a governor-led model. This made sense and worked well initially. Disease transmission was brought under control quickly. However, in the early part of the pandemic, the impact of COVID-19 varied throughout the state, with some counties having very little, if any, disease identified. Increasingly, the governor therefore shifted the management of the public health response to the public health districts, which are created by the legislature to manage local public health issues.

However, with public health boards largely made up of elected officials and not health experts, with some board members rejecting science and embracing debunked theories, and with aggressive protests and significant lobbying of board members on whether or not to implement public health measures, we encountered inconsistent public health approaches, inconsistent public health messages, and inconsistent results in controlling the spread of the coronavirus. The fragmentation and confusion led to disbelief, anger, and frustration on all sides of the issues. It has become evident that while the public health model established by the legislature may work well under normal circumstances or with localized outbreaks, this model is not effective for managing a statewide health emergency. In the example we've provided in Idaho, we would recommend that in the event of a statewide health crisis, the legislature place the public health response in the hands of the governor and the Idaho Department of Health and Welfare. By extension, it is recommended that an equivalent approach be strongly encouraged across the nation.

Recommendation #83
Coordinated, Unified Approach to a Statewide Public Health Emergency

While local public health districts or agencies can function well during normal times and times of localized outbreaks of disease, in a time of an epidemic, pandemic, or other statewide public health emergency, state legislators should authorize the governor and state health department by law to lead the public health efforts in a coordinated manner across the state.

A New Workforce and New Policies of Tracing

During the COVID-19 pandemic, contact tracing was quickly overwhelmed in all health districts across the United States. It very quickly became apparent that as the case numbers mounted, we did not have a sufficient number of public health workers to track or trace people who had potentially been in contact with a person known to be infected with COVID-19. This is important because an identified infected case needs to be isolated for a period of up to 10 days, and the people they come into contact with need to be quarantined for up to 14 days. However, because of the lack of adequate tracking resources, the system was rapidly overwhelmed and because of this, we lost control over the spread of the pandemic.

We need the ability to immediately enlarge the contact tracing workforce during a pandemic. Because this workforce is not needed in large volumes during normal times, there must be a mechanism in place to cross-train individuals so that they can do other jobs within public health departments (or elsewhere in the community) during regular times, but then be rapidly redeployed into these emergency roles when needed. Perhaps something like a public health National Guard is needed, where workers can do their regular jobs to stay gainfully employed but be activated at a moment's notice to serve the public health districts if needed. Another possibility would be to use community health workers as potential contact tracing personnel. They know the communities in which they live and work and could help appropriately isolate, quarantine, and track people who are positive or have been contacts of those who are infected.

Recommendation #84
Contact Tracing Surge Staffing

Public health departments need the flexibility to rapidly ramp up and ramp down the number of trained persons available for contact tracing. Considerations should be given to cross-training public health workers who have different responsibilities under normal conditions, so that they can rapidly be redeployed. It would also be useful to create a volunteer corps of individuals who can be called on from their regular jobs or retirement to help when needed, along with a focus on cross-training community health workers who can be redirected to contact tracing efforts in a time of need.

Additionally, there needs to be proactive policy development at the local, state, and federal levels to assist people who have been identified as infected or who are contacts of someone who is infected. Some workers may resist isolation or quarantine due to concerns that they might lose their job or that they will not be paid during that time. We need protections in place for these workers so that their jobs are protected and they have access to some financial assistance during this period when they cannot go to work. During this current pandemic, many people with housing insecurity feared eviction and homelessness if isolation requirements or quarantine threatened loss of their pay and a resultant inability to pay rent. Therefore, a federal or state law must be enacted which helps protect people from financial ruin, loss of employment, and eviction if they need to quarantine or isolate. If we are not able to protect people's jobs and finances, then there will be an ongoing underreporting of cases and incentives for people to go to work when potentially ill, allowing pandemics to continue to surge.

Recommendation #85
Protect Low-Wage Earners
It is critical for lawmakers to understand the financial impacts that may cause people to resist complying with critical public health procedures aimed at isolating those who are sick and quarantining those who are close contacts. To control the spread of a pandemic disease, it is critical that those who are asked to isolate or quarantine do not have to fear loss of employment, income, or housing.

Improved Data Systems

The ability to get rapid, accurate, and meaningful data in the early days of the COVID-19 pandemic was highly constrained. As the caseload grew exponentially, it not only overwhelmed the capacity of the system to contact trace, isolate, and quarantine, but also led to incomplete and lagging data. Soon, public health departments were working blind. We must invest in data systems and bring public health departments up to speed with electronic databases that can work closely with the state and federal governments to unearth information concerning the numbers of cases, hospitalizations, deaths, and test positivity. We have become so siloed in our health care system that health care entities such as hospitals, health care systems, and clinics often will have such data well before public health departments and state departments of health have it. Hospitals and health systems must be willing to share timely and accurate data—including personal protective equipment inventories, bed availability, confirmed cases and cases under investigation, test positivity rates, deaths, and more—and we need a way for physician offices and clinics, including urgent care, to report what they are seeing on the ground. We need to put systems in place that share data simultaneously so that the best decisions can be made for the public's health, driven by the goal of controlling the infection as quickly as possible.

Recommendation #86

Improved and Automated Reporting

Federal, state, and local governments should pursue an integrated and interconnected public health data system that allows for data to be shared instantaneously. This data needs to be aggregated, reported, and examined with analytic tools to give governments, public health agencies, and health care providers real-time information and data as to the emergence and control of transmissible diseases.

Recommendation #87

Public Health Organizations Must Revise and Update Their Pandemic Plans

The very first action for public health organizations as they prepare for the future is to learn from the past. They must review the entire course of the current pandemic and reflect on what went well and what did not. As they review and update their public health emergency history, they must capture the lessons learned and incorporate these lessons into their future pandemic plans.

As can be seen above, there is much to be done to help prepare public health departments of the future for the next pandemic. A great deal of work must be undertaken to overhaul existing public health departments that have changed only minimally over the last 50 years.

Personal Story: "The Tail Wagging the Dog"

Dr. Epperly tells the following story.

In the darkness of December 2020, COVID-19 was ravaging the southwestern Idaho region represented by CDH. We were at the peak of the most recent surge at that time, with case rates over 90 cases per 100,000 people per day and a test positivity rate of nearly 30 percent.

CDH is the largest public health district in Idaho and the health district for four adjacent counties—Ada, the largest of them with a population of 482,000, and three rural and frontier counties: Elmore County with 28,000, Valley County with 11,000, and Boise County with 8,000 people. On the evening of December 15, CDH was poised to have one of its most important votes: whether to mandate compliance with public health guidance to slow the spread of the virus.

Our hospitals were at capacity and we were fearful that with the added infections anticipated during the upcoming holidays, individual hospitals might be overwhelmed, requiring them to go on divert or be bypassed until hospital capacity had improved. Worse yet, there was a lingering dread that hospitals would be so inundated that the state might have to declare crisis standards of care. Such a declaration would provide for rationing of care and resources based upon the likelihood of therapeutic benefit.

On the table at the CDH meeting was a motion that would mandate the wearing of face coverings in public, physical distancing, and group size restrictions for all four counties. Such a mandate was already in place for Ada County due to the prior action of CDH. Board members had to decide between individualism or collectivism in our public health crisis.

The three board members representing Ada County all voted yes: public health supersedes individual rights. The three other board members, one from each of the rural/frontier counties, all voted no: personal rights and freedoms must not be infringed. The board chair, a nurse by background and a representative of one of the rural counties, abstained. A tie vote meant that the motion failed.

The outcome is illustrative of the dysfunction of public health boards whose members are political appointees. Politics and ideologies overruled science and public health. The county with more than ten times the population of its surrounding counties was blocked from acting in accord with what the science and data was telling us needed to be done.

The citizens of all four counties are, metaphorically speaking, in a public swimming pool together. What one does in the pool affects every other swimmer. People commute between these counties for work, play, shopping, and health care, and the virus respects no borders and no political ideology. This is a classic story of the tail wagging the dog.

CHAPTER 11

The Rejection of Science

You know it's true . . . Every disaster movie begins with a scientist being ignored.

NEIL DEGRASSE TYSON

It is overly simplistic to conclude that many people rejected science during the COVID-19 pandemic, when the truth was far more nuanced.

We say this for several reasons. We did not see people rejecting *all* science; we did not have a rash of people jumping off of buildings or cliffs, believing that the laws of gravity were no longer valid. Some of the legislators, public health board members, and school board members who rejected public health guidance and the science it was based on availed themselves of testing—often additional testing that was not available to the general public—and were among the first in line to receive COVID-19 vaccines created by the new messenger RNA, or mRNA, technologies that had been developed by scientists over the years. They did this eagerly, even though these were the first vaccines of their kind to be authorized for use.

It was also common for those who rejected the consensus of the mainstream scientific community then to endorse the few physicians who advocated for positions inconsistent with the results of scientific studies, such as promoting the use of hydroxychloroquine and ivermectin for the prevention and treatment of COVID-19 or asserting that masks are not useful in preventing the transmission of the SARS-CoV-2 virus. Consequently, there was not so much a wholesale rejection of science but more of a selective dismissal of science by some when it did not support their beliefs or desired outcomes.

We also saw some members of the lay public reference solid scientific papers but then cherry-pick isolated facts that they believed proved their position when the conclusions they came to, in many cases, were not justified by the study's design or findings or, in other cases, were not supported by adequate sample size or statistical power. As we said above, it seemed that the problem was less a complete rejection of science than it was a rejection of science that did not support their positions and an embrace of pseudoscience that supported their preconceived notions or desired outcomes.

While undoubtedly it is too simplistic to sort those who failed to embrace scientifically sound public health advice into a scheme of categories—especially because categories overlap—it did seem that many who challenged us fell into one or more of the following groups:

1. People with an unwavering, unquestioning devotion to a tribalistic or a hyper-partisan view of the pandemic. For convenience, we refer to members of this group as the hyper-partisans.
2. Those who were medically and scientifically uninformed, who failed to understand science and the scientific method, who lacked an understanding of how to evaluate new information critically, and who often failed to distinguish trustworthy sources of information from those that were not. For convenience, we refer to members of this group as the scientifically undiscerning.
3. Those who embraced conspiracy theories. The members of this group probably met all the criteria for the scientifically undiscerning group, but they went beyond just being unaware or misled. Instead, they embraced conspiracy theories that often had no basis in fact and would be deemed too far-fetched or incredible by members of the scientifically undiscerning group. For convenience, we refer to members of this group as the conspiracy theorists.

There were certainly many who blindly followed the president, accepting everything he said, no matter how outrageous. After the president made a comment to his medical advisors during a press conference, suggesting that perhaps there was a way to inject or otherwise get disinfectants inside the body to fight the SARS-CoV-2 virus, there was a rise in calls to poison control centers all over the country, with callers inquiring about the president's suggestion or seeking help for someone who had ingested disinfectants.[1] Concern by public health officials led the State of Washington to issue the tweet in figure 11.1.

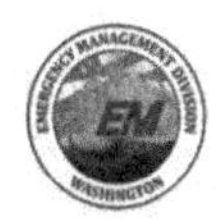

WA Emergency Management
@waEMD

Please don't eat tide pods or inject yourself with any kind of disinfectant.

If you do need help with #COVID19 issues, we have lots of resources at coronavirus.wa.gov

Just don't make a bad situation worse.

5:57 PM · 4/23/20 · Twitter Web App

1,365 Retweets **542** Quote Tweets **3,625** Likes

Figure 11.1. A tweet from the Washington Emergency Management Division pleading with people not to eat laundry detergent or inject themselves with disinfectant to combat COVID-19. *Source*: Washington Emergency Management Division, "Please don't eat tide pods or inject yourself with any kind of disinfectant," April 23, 2020, 5:57 p.m., https://twitter.com/waEMD/status/1253473167017865216

The Hyper-partisans

For some, this devotion to the president or groups like QAnon was cult-like. Even when confronted with evidence of the president's bad behavior, many excused it or justified it. When presented with evidence of the president's lies, such as Bob Woodward's tape recordings of his conversations with the president, in which the president admitted to knowing early on that the novel coronavirus was severe and intentionally downplaying the threat to the American people, it seemed that few Republicans believed the president had done anything wrong or were willing to call him out for this behavior.[2]

Even though we do not think that the response to any emergency, including a public health emergency, should be partisan, it inevitably is. We have seen elected leaders praised for their response to a disaster, such as former mayor Rudy Giuliani for the rescue-and-recovery efforts in response to the September 11 terrorist attack,[3] and we have seen elected leaders pay a heavy political price for a failed or inadequate response to a disaster, such as former president George W. Bush's response to Hurricane Katrina.[4]

The public's perception that the pandemic was mishandled would certainly make for bad politics. Given the intense criticism of the federal response to the COVID-19 pandemic leading up to the 2020 presidential election, perhaps it is not surprising that many Republicans took up the defense of President Trump, his words, and his actions. Although the pandemic was at the forefront of voters' minds, President Trump hoped to run on a strong and vigorous economy. Therefore, the president's comments were often far rosier than reality in an effort to keep the stock market up. Republican supporters strongly opposed restrictive public health measures that might negatively impact the economy.

Of course, holding the president accountable proved extremely difficult. One of the coauthors, Dr. Pate, interviewed an award-winning investigative reporter with the Idaho Statesman—Audrey Dutton, currently the senior investigative reporter for the Idaho Capital Sun—for additional background and perspective on this issue.

In many ways, the president set himself up to be the sole source of truth by labeling reporting that was unfavorable to him as "fake news." Many in the public seemed to be quite receptive to embracing this notion of fake news. Ms. Dutton was asked whether this notion of "fake news" began with President Trump. She indicated that in large part, it did. However, there certainly have long been both left-leaning and right-leaning news sources, which could help perpetuate the idea that the press and media are biased.

Ms. Dutton was asked whether this stirring up of public mistrust in the press and media has hurt the ability of reporters to hold leaders accountable. Her response was that in some cases it has, because of the willingness of many in the public to dismiss legitimate criticisms of leaders as merely the result of political bias from the opposition. In other cases, it is in large part due to the reluctance of those within the same party to be interviewed on these issues due to fears of political retribution.

Ms. Dutton explained that the key to maintaining her credibility in this environment is to research the issues she is reporting on thoroughly, get many perspectives, present the issues in a balanced matter, and make sure that she and her newspaper are holding leaders of both parties accountable.

The use of fear and retribution has been a major tool of President Trump and the Republican Party. Because of the loyalty of the president's supporters, legislators—who, under constitutional principles, are supposed to hold the executive branch accountable—came to fear the damage to their political standing that could come from a single tweet from the president. Such a tweet could be magnified millions of times through retweets and the cable news eruption that often followed. The president was also not hesitant to suggest a primary challenger or to campaign for one if he perceived a lack of loyalty from a member of Congress.

President Trump also used intimidation and retaliation to discourage members of the press or media from asking him questions that were critical of him or his handling of various matters. "In some cases, the president has gone so far as to call reporters 'terrible,' 'fake,' and 'nasty,' and telling some that they're 'never going to make it.'"[5] If a newspaper consistently wrote articles unfavorable to him or his administration, it was not uncommon for him to assert that the particular company was "failing."

In another unprecedented move, the White House revoked a CNN reporter's press credentials after he asked President Trump questions about his immigration policy and persisted in his efforts after the president refused to answer his questions.[6]

When Ms. Dutton was questioned about the impact of such intimidation tactics deployed against journalists who did not provide favorable stories about the president and his administration, she pointed out examples of behaviors that others are now displaying in response to this change of norms perpetuated by the former president. She called attention to the increased number of personal attacks on journalists on social media that are "unlike anything I've experienced in (more than) 15 years." Obviously, this runs counter to our long-held cultural belief that America promotes the free and open exchange of ideas and debate of issues. At her newspaper, some of the attacks have been threatening and necessitated the filing of police reports, the development of safety plans, and reports of abuse to the social media platforms. She told us that reporters would spend hours listening to grieving families and traumatized health care workers and then find abusive emails in their inboxes, including some alleging that the reporters were merely making all the COVID-19 news up to sell newspapers. She also noted that there have long been challenges in getting people to go on the record to state their opinions or positions on topics of the day, but this is much more difficult today, as people fear retaliation from their employers and personal attacks and bullying on social media in response.

We now have a new president, one who has committed to bringing the country together and helping us heal. When Ms. Dutton was asked if this provided her with a sense of renewed optimism, she replied, "The president can set the tone for a country, but the horse is out of the barn, especially with people radicalized."

We will go much further into this in a later chapter on leadership; however, for now, several recommendations can be made.

While ideally the management of a public health emergency should not be influenced by politics, often there are political consequences stemming from what the public perceives to be good or bad handling of the emergency.

Recommendation #88

Leaders Must Inform the Public Truthfully and Factually

Leaders are more likely to be politically successful if they tell the American public the truth. They need to communicate clearly and often with the public, embracing science and allowing scientists and public health officials to stand before the people at press conferences to provide guidance and answer questions. Leaders need to develop a strategy for dealing with the emergency and then effectively communicate that strategy to the public.

Clear and truthful communication is the best way to engage Americans in public health measures that will bring an end to a pandemic sooner and avoid the loss of life, the added health care costs, and the negative impact to the economy. Reporters are an asset to help disseminate the information that the American public needs to know.

Recommendation #89

Combat Disinformation with Proactive Communication

Speaking clearly, openly, truthfully, and often to the public helps to decrease anxiety and fill the information gaps so that others do not plug those gaps with misinformation, disinformation, and conspiracy theories.

The Scientifically Undiscerning

This group of people do not intentionally reject science, but they tend to be science skeptics. They are uncritical when judging information sources that claim to know what "science" tells us about the SARS-CoV-2 virus and COVID-19. They often are not discerning about the education, training, or reputation of those in the information outlets they embrace, nor are they aware of the biases or conflicts of interest within the organizations they work or speak for.

As a result, they were quick to send us selected data, statistics, articles, and studies which they believed supported their point of view. Most often, this was an effort to try to make the case that face coverings do not work, COVID-19 is no worse than the flu, or that the mortality rate is infinitesimally small. Often it became clear that the scientifically undiscerning did not appreciate the scientific method and the need to assess the limitations and accuracy of data, nor were they knowledgeable about the definitions of terms and the sources of data. We would also see instances where people pulled a fact out of a well-designed clinical study to support their position, but unfortunately not select a fact that actually answered the question they were trying to answer. This biased sorting of information was accomplished without the necessary skills needed to analyze clinical data and interpret its statistical significance.

The scientifically undiscerning did not approach science as something to be tested, an endeavor requiring large numbers of repeatable observations. Instead, they were often willing to accept as proof nothing more than anecdotal reports, if those reports supported their point of view. In other words, this group was characterized by confirmation bias—the tendency to search for and embrace any information or data that seems to support preconceived notions. Those with an understanding of the scientific method understand that we may start with a hypothesis, but we need to accept that the hypothesis may be proved or disproved.

This group had another interesting trait. Physicians and scientists become skeptical when there are clinical studies with different results. We look carefully at the studies to determine differences in the quality of the study designs, in the study participants, in the study protocols, or in the study measurements and outcomes, to see if we can reconcile the results or conclude which study is stronger in the evidence it provides. In our experience, the scientifically undiscerning were not disturbed by the fact that the article or study they enthusiastically touted, upon further investigation, conflicted with peer-reviewed studies appearing in prestigious journals or was contrary to positions supported by leading scientists or public health experts. Again, unrecognized confirmation bias allowed them to accept an isolated article or study as proof in support of their position, even though it was not peer-reviewed, not accepted by the public health and scientific community, and inconsistent with findings by well-designed studies.

Social media played a huge role in allowing the scientifically undiscerning to regurgitate bits and pieces of information that would further contribute to confirmation bias within their own circles. Much of the misinformation and disinformation circulated on social media increased the risk of harm to people who were earnestly looking for answers but not skilled at discerning between good and bad sources. In one case, one of us was informed by a friend of a substance this friend's sister was taking because of reports she saw that this substance would prevent her from getting COVID-19. Unfortunately, this substance—colloidal silver—was already known to be quite toxic to a number of organ systems in the body, and there was absolutely no evidence to support its use or effectiveness in preventing COVID-19. The friend was urgently advised to plead with her sister to stop ingesting this substance immediately.

Returning to Ms. Dutton's view on how we should react to social media's tendency to spread dangerous misinformation and disinformation, she observed that "Social media platforms created a forum for millions of people to be independent publishers. We (The Idaho Statesman) use social media, and we regularly monitor comments. Social media platforms need to figure this out."

She also noted that a side effect of the evolving and changing guidance offered as we learned more about the virus seemed to sow more distrust in some members of the public. She made a great point: "Truth has context to it. It can change as we learn more."

Recommendation #90
Schools Must Teach Students How to Assess the Credibility of Sources

We need to reevaluate our educational curriculums to ensure that we are teaching children and young adults the critical thinking skills they need in an age of social media. We must teach students how discern the truth, how to evaluate the veracity and reliability of sites they may go to for information, and how to evaluate the credentials of those they are looking to for information. They need to be educated in the importance of peer review in medical and scientific literature, in the role political bias and financial conflicts of interest can play in shaping someone's opinions, and in the importance of looking at multiple sources for confirmation.

Recommendation #91
Promote Science Literacy

We must promote science literacy among students. All students should have a working knowledge of the scientific method and how to judge the strength or weakness of scientific studies, as well as the limitations of such studies.

The Conspiracy Theorists

Conspiracy theories are not new. Probably the best examples of conspiracy theories that received the most time and attention devoted to them, the greatest notoriety, and the widest embrace by the American people in our lifetimes are those associated with President John F. Kennedy's assassination.

President Trump even rehashed old conspiracy theories concerning President Kennedy's assassination involving the father of one of his Republican primary challengers, Senator Ted Cruz. Trump picked up on a sensational story run in the *National Enquirer* connecting the senator's father, Rafael Cruz, with assassin Lee Harvey Oswald. President Trump exclaimed, "I mean, what was he doing—what was he doing with Lee Harvey Oswald shortly before the death? Before the shooting? . . . It's horrible!"[7]

One may wonder why people believe some of the most far-fetched conspiracy theories out there. But when people are shaken by the unexpected—the assassination of a president, or the onset of a deadly pandemic—many question how something of this magnitude can just happen out of the blue. Surely there was some reason that was hidden and unknown to us. The assassination must have involved a secret Mafia hit; the pandemic must have been a purposeful or accidental release of a virus from a laboratory in China. As humans, we feel the need to rationalize that which we do not understand.

Today, these conspiracy theories can easily be spread and reinforced through social media, giving such theories greater than justifiable credibility to the undiscerning. This often leads to the circular argument that since so many other people have come to the same conclusion, it must be true.

Many people, as the conspiracies become more and more reinforced, tend to seek out and read those sources that build further on their beliefs, through confirmation bias, rejecting sources that attempt to disprove or reject the theories. The reinforcement is all the more significant if the president of the United States, who obviously has access to our country's greatest secrets, gives these conspiracy theories credence.

The psychological concept of rationalism, a concept that can lead a person to embrace conspiracy theories to explain something that would otherwise be unexplainable to them, should not be confused with the idea of denial. Denial is a psychological defense against anxiety. It is usually not considered a productive or positive psychological defense mechanism, but it can, at least temporarily, relieve significant and distressing anxiety.

Anxious over reports of a novel virus, its spread and its toll, the most productive psychological response would be to devise a plan that incorporates the best available guidance from public health officials. But, of course, that response acknowledges the threat, and that may mean some continuing anxiety.

Thus, the alternative to devising a plan is to deny that the pandemic exists. Another variation is to acknowledge the pandemic, but deny that it is any worse than the flu, searching for others who also believe this or data that will support and reinforce that position. We heard both denials repeatedly during the pandemic. Of course, what starts as denial can then incorporate conspiracy theories to help justify why that person denies it, even though the pandemic is on television and in the newspapers every day. So, instead of just denying it, it becomes an active hoax, and then a hoax created by the liberal media or the opposing political party to undermine the president. Doctors and the media are just trying to scare people. As was mentioned earlier in the book, President Trump even started another conspiracy theory that would be picked up and further perpetuated: that doctors and hospitals were falsely reporting the numbers of COVID-19 cases and deaths because they were financially benefiting through increased federal reimbursements for their COVID-19 patients.

Of course, denial as a psychological defense mechanism is much more successful when you have not been personally confronted with what you are denying. Early in the pandemic, this psychological defense could be reinforced by confirmation bias. If the person in denial had not been infected themselves (as was the case for most), had not known anyone who had been infected, or had any family members who were infected, it was all the easier to deny. But denial was a harsh partner and placed people at risk because of their failure to follow public health guidance. This increased the chances that they or someone they knew who participated with them in ill-advised activities would become infected. We saw less and less denial over time and more of a shift to acceptance as the disease spread, with now more than an estimated quarter of all Americans having been infected. With this amount of disease transmission, it has become far less likely that any given individual has not been personally affected by the pandemic. Awareness was more clearly focused for a growing number of people based on their own infection or the infection of someone they cared about, and perhaps even severe outcomes. In some cases, there were deathbed conversions.

Though denial and rationalization are common, if not the most effective defense mechanisms, it is another thing altogether to embrace conspiracy theories. When something significant and shocking occurs, it is natural that we all seek to make sense of what happened, and many of us often toy with conspiracy theories that emerge that might seem to make sense of it all. Having an explanation helps decrease anxiety and helps us maintain a sense of control. However, most of us will consider new developments and information and displace conspiracy theories with evidence.

However, during the pandemic, we saw many people persist in their belief in conspiracy theories—and particularly in some that were so far-fetched that they were not even temporarily entertained by most people, or quickly dismissed when confronted with repeated evidence of their falsity. A recent movement that embraces and profligately promotes conspiracy theories is called QAnon, or "Q." Lia Eustachewich wrote a story for the *New York Post* that provides the background and history of this movement. According to Eustachewich, an anonymous user of a "seedy" message board called 4chan, later appearing on another message board called 8kun, began posting conspiracy theories under the name of "Q Clearance Patriot." The anonymous "Q" claimed to have insider knowledge of the Trump administration and put forward the outrageous claim that President Trump was waging a secret war against a "global cabal of pedophile elites that includes an array of Hollywood actors and Democratic politicians who allegedly worship Satan."

As preposterous as it sounds, many people embraced this conspiracy theory and believed that President Trump was sending them coded messages in his public comments. Taking a comment made by the president while standing alongside military generals—when he said, "Maybe it's the calm before the storm"—members of QAnon believed the president's message was really that "The Storm" is coming. This would bring "a day of reckoning . . . when Trump uncovers the cabal, leading to the arrest of thousands—and a so-called 'Great Awakening' will bring salvation."[8]

In analyzing this bizarre mix of denial, rationalization, and conspiracy theory, Eustachewich points out that members of the QAnon community believe that COVID-19 is a hoax. It thus follows that members of Q promoted a further theory to reconcile the denial of COVID-19 with the president's COVID diagnosis and admission to the hospital: a claim that the president was not really ill but rather was pretending to be in a design to arrest Hillary Clinton.

One would think that when the many predictions made by QAnon, including the arrest of Hillary Clinton, the overturn of the election on January 6, and the disruption of the hypothesized global cabal, failed to materialize, the movement would dissolve and its supporters would disperse. Certainly, some former members have denounced QAnon after suffering great disappointment over these unfulfilled predictions. But there is little evidence that QAnon has been significantly harmed by all this; in fact, a new member of Congress who embraced many of the QAnon conspiracy theories, Marjorie Taylor Greene, the Republican representative of Georgia's Fourteenth District, was elected in 2021.

What is different about these people who will embrace the most outrageous of conspiracy theories? According to a study out of Emory University, as reported by VOA News, "The people most likely to embrace conspiracy theories are less inquisitive and often exhibit narcissistic tendencies, such as an inflated sense of self-importance, a deep need for attention and admiration, troubled relationships, a lack of empathy for others and fragile self-esteem."[9]

So, what are we to learn from all of this? There are many lessons:

1. Leaders must be forthcoming with the American public. We should not promote panic, but we must be truthful, and we must inform the public of what we know, what we don't know, and what they can do to protect themselves.
2. Although public health officials and physicians will be very busy during a pandemic, we must make time to hold press conferences, respond to questions from the public, sit for interviews with reporters, and engage in social media so that we get facts out to the public. We must fill the voids with facts, or it will be filled with denial, rationalization, and conspiracy theories.
3. We all must call out false or misleading information.
4. We must be clear that we are learning as we go and some things that we think we know today may be different when we get more information. However, we promise to tell the public what we think we know as we know it.
5. We must admit when we were wrong. Maintaining trust is critical.
6. When we debate issues or refute misinformation, we must attack the facts and not the people. We must keep people engaged in the dialogue.

Recommendation #92

Preempt Unhealthy Psychological Responses with Clear and Frequent Communication

Fear, anxiety, and the need for humans to make sense of serious, unexpected events can lead to several unhealthy psychological responses, including denial, rationalization, and conspiracy theories. Governments, public health agencies, and physicians with expertise in the area must make the effort and devote the time to communicate openly and frequently about what we know so as not to leave gaps that can be filled with misinformation and disinformation. Experts must refute the misinformation and disinformation clearly and strongly.

Probably the most concerning aspects of the pandemic to us, especially while we were working to refute misinformation and disinformation being circulated by the general public, were reports of physicians and other health care professionals not embracing and utilizing public health guidance in their own practices, and some who were publicly giving support to false information.

Physicians are certainly entitled to have different opinions. After all, that is where our concept of second opinions came from. But in the modern age, physicians have not been entitled to any arbitrary opinion or demonstrably false facts they want when it comes to patient care and risk to the public.

Since the early 1900s, states have had licensing boards and medical practice acts that regulate who can be licensed and the obligations of those who are licensed. The single most important role of a state medical board is to protect the public.

Since medical science is not always clear, physicians can, and often do, have different opinions about treatments for various conditions, especially given the wide range of people that we treat who may also have other diseases that may be material factors in the treatment decisions. Because of this, physicians are given broad latitude—but that latitude is not indefinite. There still must be a medical or scientific basis for the treatment. When there is no such basis, or when science has disproved a treatment, then physicians can face discipline by state licensing boards and liability for harms under our malpractice laws. As an example, if a physician were to take to the airwaves or social media and advise the public that they should not undergo colon cancer screening and that colon cancer is a hoax, I would suspect that that physician would soon be held to account by the medical boards for the states in which that physician holds a license. This is for a good reason: physicians are privileged to be highly regarded and trusted by the public, and health information that they promote is likely to be more readily accepted by the public. If people were to take this physician's guidance, we could certainly anticipate harm to the public.

We have heard from individuals whose health care providers, in the first six months of the pandemic, did not wear masks in their offices and did not require their patients to do so, allegedly replying to their patients' questions about this that they were trying to achieve herd immunity. This behavior would seem to squarely fit under the purview of the state board that regulates these providers to discipline them. First, it was inconsistent with the public health advice of the Centers for Disease Control and Prevention (CDC) and every public health agency in the United States. Second, that policy would place the providers' patients at risk. Keep in mind that the individuals seeing a provider during a pandemic are often those who are at high risk for severe COVID-19. Finally, by sending the message to people that getting infected is desirable and that they should not wear masks, these providers were not only endangering their patients, but everyone whom these patients lived with or associated with. We will not dwell on how absurd the theory that exposing patients in health care practices would help us get to herd immunity is—a practice that should be grounds for discipline—because we address this fallacy in chapters 1 and 12.

The Oregon Medical Board took emergency action to suspend the license of a physician who was, according to the board's findings of fact, not only violating the orders of the board but also engaging in extremely reckless behavior, endangering his staff (by not wearing masks in the office while seeing patients) and his patients (by urging individuals who were wearing masks to remove them) and providing dangerous instructions to his patients. According to the order, a patient was told that asymptomatic persons should not be tested and that wearing masks does not prevent transmission of COVID-19. Another patient was directed not to self-isolate because being around other people would provide the patient with immunity to COVID-19. The order additionally stated that "Licensee regularly advises, particularly for his elderly and pediatric patients, that it is 'very dangerous' to wear masks because masks exacerbate COPD and asthma and cause or contribute to multiple serious health conditions, including but not limited to heart attacks, strokes, collapsed lungs, MRSA, pneumonia, and hypertension. Licensee asserts masks are likely to harm patients by increasing the body's carbon dioxide content through rebreathing of gas trapped behind a mask."[10] If the facts are substantiated, as alleged, this case would clearly qualify for discipline because so many of them are counter to official public health guidance and contrary to the scientific evidence, and these are not matters for which there is legitimate debate among medical experts and associations.

It is important to remember that with a pandemic involving a novel organism and thousands of articles coming out each week, it is impossible for any health care professional to be aware of every new development right away while also working long hours to try to help people in need. Discipline is not appropriate for not knowing every nuance or being unable to answer every question about this new organism and the disease it causes. However, there is an expectation that health care practitioners will be familiar with a certain amount of basic knowledge about how to prevent the disease, how to recognize the disease, how to test for it, and when to refer their patient to a specialist.

What we are really talking about here are two points. First, health care providers should not be acting in a manner that is inconsistent with the main public health measures and guidance that are in place at the time. Second, if you are not well-versed in the science of the organism and disease, then you should not be stepping forward into public venues while espousing beliefs that are contrary to established medical and public health guidance, incorrectly characterizing yourself as a health care professional with expertise on the subject.

We applaud some state boards that have been active in this area, but we see a need for all boards to take an active role to ensure that their licensees are not placing their patients at risk or endangering the public. We are not suggesting that all these cases merit license revocation. In many cases, an investigation, fine, or requirement for continuing medical education will be sufficient.

Recommendation #93

State Boards Must Be More Active

State boards of health care professionals need to play a more active role in ensuring that their licensees are following the CDC and their state's public health guidance, and that providers who are promoting disinformation in the press, on media outlets, or on social media are disciplined. Unfortunately, these health care professionals, though few in number, have played into the public's distrust and the denial, rationalization, and conspiracy theories of some of the public.

Teaching the Public How to Recognize Disinformation

During this pandemic, those of us dedicating significant amounts of time to educate the public found that we still couldn't keep up with all the false information. In this case, we are referring to addressing *disinformation*, the spread of incorrect information with the intent to harm, confuse, mislead, or otherwise affect people's hearts and minds to accept lies or support the position of those who are spreading the false information. This is opposed to *misinformation*, which is incorrect information that the person spreading it did not realize was incorrect (or incorrect at the time). Whether it be misinformation or disinformation, the other thing we found is that combating it was like playing a game of whack-a-mole; every time we successfully countered incorrect information, new misinformation or disinformation popped up to replace it. Because of this, we cannot successfully win this battle for the truth on our own. We must educate the public about how to recognize suspicious information. Fortunately, we had so many examples of people spreading disinformation that certain patterns emerged.

Disinformation comes from many sources, including foreign countries. The motives of those who spread disinformation can be diverse. For a foreign country, it often is the intent to sow distrust in the United States government and discontent among the populace. For homegrown purveyors of disinformation, perhaps they stand to financially benefit from their actions; sometimes there are political aspirations or motivations, and sometimes these sowers of disinformation like the public attention and adoration they receive from those who want to believe the lies. There may be other reasons as well. But a common thread found in all of the incidences was narcissism and lack of empathy. These individuals do not care if they harm others, so long as they gain whatever benefit it is they are seeking for themselves.

What are the patterns that can alert the public to be suspicious of the information being conveyed?

Misuse of Credentials to Gain Undeserved Credibility

We often saw that physicians and other health professionals who were promoting misinformation and disinformation were not in specialties that generally treat patients with COVID-19 or have expertise in treating acute infections, respiratory disorders, or hospitalized patients. Some examples were pathologists, neuroradiologists, ophthalmologists, and chiropractors. Of course that does not mean that the physician may not have very specialized knowledge about COVID-19, but this should be a red flag when that advice is contrary to physicians who are specialists in those areas of practice, in much the same way that a dermatologist offering advice about prenatal care that is inconsistent with information put out by the American College of Obstetricians and Gynecologists should be suspect.

Use of Grandiose or Inflammatory Language

Reputable physicians and scientists generally try to maintain objectivity and professionalism. It would be greatly out of character for these experts to use inflammatory or offensive language in explaining science or public health recommendations to the public. On the other hand, one physician who was spreading disinformation repeatedly referred to the COVID-19 vaccines as "needle rape."[11] To compare vaccination to one of the most psychologically and physically traumatizing events that can happen to a person is beyond the pale and offensive in its trivialization of what victims of sexual assault have suffered. The language is obviously intended to inflame the hearts and passions of those they are spreading disinformation to rather than to stimulate the mind. We also heard many of those spreading disinformation about the vaccines using language to conjure up images of Nazi Germany, making reference to the Nuremburg Code, and often using variations of the phrase "crimes against humanity," all of which were intended to create a false equivalency between vaccinations and various historical atrocities. When you hear or read this kind of language, a red flag should be raised to suggest that an attempt is being made to emotionally manipulate you and that the information is likely unreliable.

Use of Emphatic and Absolute Statements

There are very few things that we can say are absolutes in medicine—things that always happen or never happen. That is because diseases can manifest themselves and behave differently between children and adults, between young adults and the elderly, between men and women, between the immunocompromised and the healthy, and even in individuals of the same age and gender. Thus, another warning sign is when sources make statements that are absolutes. Physicians and scientists will often qualify their statements and advice with phrases such as "based upon what we know today" (understanding that new data may come along in the future that could change our understanding of the disease or its treatment) or "based on a recent study" (leaving open the possibility that more studies or larger studies might change our understanding), or "based on the limited data we have available" (acknowledging that we have some data, but it may not apply to people that are different than those who were study participants, or to people with additional medical conditions than those studied). An example of an absolute statement that should raise a red flag that we heard during this pandemic was "Masks do nothing." Now, we can debate the effectiveness of different kinds of masks, their effectiveness under different conditions, or their effectiveness when it comes to different variants, but if someone tells you that masks provide absolutely no protection or that masks provide complete protection, this should be reason enough to look for another source.

Another very helpful indicator as to whether you can trust a source is that reputable physicians and scientists will often answer questions when there is a new development with some variation of "we don't know" or "we need more information before we can answer that," whereas those spreading disinformation rarely answer questions by admitting that the science is evolving or that it is too early to answer the question with any certainty.

Use of Anecdotes as Evidence

We often heard those promoting misinformation making comments such as "I treated [fill in the number] patients with ivermectin and they all did great." That is an anecdote; that is not science. Were all of their patients young, healthy, low-risk, and expected to have good outcomes even without treatment? Did all of the patients have confirmed infections? How do they know none of the patients deteriorated and didn't go straight to the hospital without notifying them, especially since a number of physicians making this claim did not treat patients in hospitals?

Internal Inconsistencies in Their Arguments

Think about a person in an interrogation room at a police station. A skilled detective can tell when the person is being truthful, because truth has an internal consistency to it. The various pieces fit together, and it makes sense that they would occur in the manner and order the witness describes. On the other hand, when you can get a person to talk for an extended period of time and that person starts out with a lie, it is incredibly difficult to maintain the lie because things eventually don't make sense and cannot be connected in a logical way. In the same way, if you give someone spreading disinformation enough time to talk, you will generally see them get tripped up.

Let's look at an example. A very common internal inconsistency arose when some doctors made the argument that people should not take the COVID-19 vaccine because it was only authorized for emergency use and not yet fully approved by the United States Food and Drug Administration (FDA). That certainly could be a reasonable concern for some people, and was a point worthy of discussion. However, what they suggested as the alternative—and what patients seemed more than willing to do—was to take various medications that were neither authorized or approved by the FDA for the prevention or treatment of COVID-19. In fact, the FDA even warned the public not to take one of the recommended medications. The inconsistency was using FDA approval as the criteria for the prevention of COVID-19 and using it to argue against one measure, but then disregarding it in recommending another.

Misuse of Data

One common tactic used by purveyors of disinformation to generate fear of vaccination was to point to the thousands of deaths reported to VAERS (the Vaccine Adverse Event Reporting System) as being due to the vaccines. This would make sense to the majority of Americans who are not familiar with VAERS, but can tell from the name that this is a system that reports vaccine-related adverse events. But this was an intentional deception by the physicians who were suggesting causality, when in fact the site is for reporting by the public so that the CDC and FDA can be alerted if the frequency of an adverse reaction exceeds the background rate of those symptoms or conditions. Prior to the pandemic, more than 8,000 persons in the United States died each day on average. To keep the math simple, if you consider that about half of the United States population was vaccinated this year, you would expect roughly 4,000 deaths each day unrelated to COVID-19 among the vaccinated—in fact, even higher than 4,000, because those being targeted for vaccination were the elderly and those with underlying medical conditions. Those perpetuating fears of vaccination attributed all of the deaths in VAERS that would be expected under pre-COVID conditions and unrelated to COVID-19 or the vaccines to the COVID-19 vaccines. Even just using common sense, if the FDA temporarily stopped vaccinations with the Janssen (Johnson & Johnson) COVID-19 vaccine when only three cases of thrombosis with thrombocytopenia syndrome were identified through the VAERS reporting, it should cause everyone to question that the CDC and FDA could then believe that there were thousands of deaths caused by the vaccine, yet take no action or even issue a warning.

Failure to Cite Studies and Identify Any Limitations to Those Studies

It is common for purveyors of disinformation to proclaim that studies show support for their position, but then not produce those studies when asked. Further, we have never heard these disseminators of falsehoods ever describe any limitations to the studies they are referring to. Reputable physicians and scientists are always willing to provide the evidence for their statements or opinions, and they are quick to point out the limitations of these studies, such as patient selection or study design. They will usually provide caveats that they cannot be certain that the findings will apply to patients that are different than those who made up the study participants or who are treated under different conditions than those used in the study.

Health professionals can certainly have differing opinions about the best treatment for a particular patient. These differences can arise because clinical trials have not yet provided us with evidence of the best treatment or because the particular circumstances of the patient are different than those who have been enrolled in clinical trials. These professional differences of opinion are appropriate.

Our objection is to health professionals who offer the public and their patients advice that is clearly and demonstrably erroneous, contrary to the guidance of the CDC, FDA, professional associations, and their own peers, and has great potential to harm patients. As physicians, we always have a duty to act in the best interests of our patients, and we have an obligation to inform our patients and tell them the truth, as best we understand it. Lying to and deceiving patients should be abhorrent to physicians.

We are starting to see physicians being held accountable for purposeful and repeated dissemination of disinformation, and we believe that appropriate actions can include discipline by state medical boards, loss of hospital privileges, and revocation of board certification. However, the disciplinary process is a lengthy one because of the need for investigations and hearings. In the meantime, it is essential for the public to be aware of the red flags of disinformation that we have listed above in order to protect themselves until the system can, because in an internet and social media age, disinformation spreads faster than the virus.

A Proponent of the "Scamdemic" Faces His Own Mortality

Reproduced with permission, the excerpt below comes from a guest column written by Tony Green for the *Dallas Voice*, titled "A Harsh Lesson in the Reality of COVID-19" and published on July 24, 2020.[12] We follow it with our own reflections.

Tony is a Texas Republican, a conservative gay man, and someone who voted for Trump in 2016. He now admits that he fell hard for conspiracy theories and dug in to protect his "God-given rights." He believed that SARS-CoV-2 and COVID-19 were a hoax. "I believed the mainstream media and the Democrats were using it to create panic, crash the economy and destroy Trump's chances at reelection."

In defiance of public health guidance, Tony and his partner hosted a party on a Saturday in June 2020 for members of their families. On Sunday, Tony was sick. On Monday, Tony's partner and parents were all sick as well. Over the next few days, six more family members became ill, some of whom had attended the party while others were infected by subsequent contact with those who had been at the party. Later, five more family members would test positive.

Tony, his father-in-law, and his father-in-law's mother all required admission to a hospital. Tony reports that the virus attacked his central nervous system, and the hospital staff stopped him from having a stroke. Tony and his father-in-law eventually recovered, but his father-in-law's mother died in the room next to her son, alone.

> You cannot imagine the guilt I feel, knowing that I hosted the gathering that led to so much suffering. You cannot imagine my guilt at having been a denier, carelessly shuffling through this pandemic, making fun of those wearing masks and social distancing. You cannot imagine my guilt at knowing that my actions convinced both our families it was safe when it wasn't. [. . .]
>
> The next time you're put out because your favorite spots are closed or because they won't let you enter without wearing a mask, and you decide to defy them rather than comply because you're defending your rights and freedoms from being trampled, just remember: Your family and friends may be next. [. . .]
>
> Now imagine one more thing: That pool party, the mixer or family reunion you're pushing for resulting in you being cold and alone in a hospital bed, fighting for your life. Imagine the only human contact you feel is a stranger's rubber glove giving you medication, checking your vitals and changing your diaper.
>
> That is exactly what has happened to our family.

This is a variation on a story that we heard far too often during the pandemic. It highlights how easy it seemed for well-educated, intelligent people to fall swiftly and hard for misinformation and conspiracy theories, and how effortlessly people could be persuaded by the influence of the president, even after evidence was presented in his own words that he had purposely misled the American public.

An observation we made above was that people who embraced misinformation and conspiracy theories often limited their sources of information to those that reinforced their beliefs. They did not seek out differing thoughts or expert judgments prior to forming their opinions, or question their beliefs once they were formed. Oftentimes in our discussions with people holding these beliefs, when we provided evidence that called into question their belief or proved it wrong, rather than reevaluating their belief structure, they merely shifted to a different piece of information or argument to support these strongly held viewpoints. It was quite surprising—and quite disappointing—to see the contrast and conflict play out in those who fiercely held onto their "God-given rights," at the expense of God-given commandments and teachings such as being kind and compassionate to one another, forgiving each other (Eph. 4:32) and looking out for each other's interests (Phil. 2:4).

This story also highlights the popular belief in the need to preserve the economy in order to preserve President Trump's reelection chances, when—as we have pointed out elsewhere in this book—that is a false dichotomy. The best way to preserve the economy is to contain the spread of disease and keep workers and the public safe. Furthermore, while we don't want to oversimplify or generalize voter motivations, it appears that the ineffective management of the pandemic was in large part to blame for the failure of President Trump to be reelected. Thus, it appears likely that competent and effective management of a public health emergency is good for both the economy and one's political future.

Another point raised by this story was the belief among many that convening one's family would be a low-risk activity. There was a lack of understanding that family members from other states might bring infection and potentially variants from that state with them, or acquire infection during their travels. Moreover, the risks posed by family members related in large part to the risks they incurred in the weeks preceding the visit. Grandma, for example, who stayed at home, avoided gatherings, and wore a mask when she went to the grocery store, would have a relatively low risk of infecting others; daughter Susan, however, who worked in a congregate living facility, and grandson James, who attended college, lived in a dorm, and frequented bars and parties at school, would have a much higher risk of doing so.

CHAPTER 12

Dangerous and Erroneous Approaches

For the most part we do not first see, and then define, we define first and then see.

WALTER LIPPMANN

In this chapter, we discuss two theoretical approaches to end the pandemic that were embraced by many but, when tried, utterly failed. The first approach was to sequester those at high risk of infection, allowing everyone else to get back to normal quickly; the second approach was to promote opportunities for the young and healthy to get infected, as a means of achieving herd immunity.

Approach 1: Sequester Those at High Risk of Infection

At the beginning of the pandemic, as infections first spread and then surged across the United States, many states imposed restrictions that ranged from simply closing selected businesses thought to be at high risk for transmission all the way to issuing broad stay-at-home orders for all citizens, with exceptions granted only for essential workers.

Recommendation #94

Essential Workers

For future public health emergencies, avoid the phrase "essential workers." In reaction to such a designation, some workers not falling into the state's definition of "essential" will take offense, incorrectly assuming that "essential" means important and, by extension, "non-essential" means not important. Furthermore, politicians and protestors who opposed restrictions will be tempted to take up the rallying cry that *all* jobs are essential. This can prove to be a huge distraction. While there is unlikely to be any categorization that completely escapes criticism, perhaps a designation such as "critical infrastructure" or "critical public infrastructure" might be less prone to attack.

At first, with little known about the virus, how it was transmitted, what the mortality rate was, and what could be done to prevent or treat an infection, there was a fair degree of willingness by the public to comply with these restrictions. However, that did not last long.

A common early suggestion was that the elderly, who were at higher risk of death if infected, should remain sequestered in their homes. Meanwhile, younger people should be allowed to return to their normal lives because their risk was so much lower. In fact, it might be desirable, so the argument went, for young and middle-aged adults to get infected to achieve "herd immunity," and providing support for both approaches. Let us now address these flawed approaches.

The first problem with this suggestion of sequestering only those at high risk of infection was in the underlying meaning of the phrase "high risk." Health care and public health officials tried to educate the public as to who was at particularly high risk for severe illness and potentially death—namely, the elderly and those with certain chronic medical conditions such as diabetes, obesity, cancer, chronic kidney disease, chronic obstructive pulmonary disease, and various heart conditions. It also included patients with underlying immune disorders and those who were immunocompromised by medications, as well as those with sickle cell disease.[1]

When evaluating these categories, many people not in these groups—specifically, young and middle-aged adults who were otherwise healthy—

concluded that they were clearly not at significant risk of getting ill or being hospitalized with COVID-19, and certainly there was some truth to this. But while young and healthy people, if infected, often had only a mild or undetected illness, for reasons that still elude us at present, there have been young adults infected with COVID-19 who have experienced severe illness, hospitalization, and the need for intensive care and, in some cases, mechanical ventilation. In some cases, they have died.

Furthermore, people often thought that those at highest risk of contracting COVID would be restricted to a nursing home or at the end of their life. We would repeatedly hear the very insensitive comment: "Well, they have to die of something." There was a lack of understanding that many who are at high risk by virtue of their age may still be working; may be retired, but still very active in and engaged with their communities; most likely have families and friends who cherish them; and may have years or even decades of remaining life if it is not cut short by the coronavirus.

In thinking of COVID-19 as an old person's disease, many people missed the fact that there are several medical conditions that can place young and middle-aged adults in the high-risk category. They can have illnesses such as diabetes or cancers being treated with chemotherapy. They can be on immunosuppressive therapy for an autoimmune disease, or they may have undergone an organ transplant. These were often adults who needed to work to support their families and maintain their health insurance, and could not, in all cases, work from home.

We also struggled to bring home the message that while it did become clear over time that certain age groups and underlying medical conditions placed people at higher risk of severe disease, hospitalization, and even death, there were still others who did not fit neatly into any of these categories and developed very severe symptoms and, in many cases, died. Worse, we often had no way of identifying them ahead of time.

Similarly, we never seemed to succeed in explaining to people that death was not the only outcome to be avoided. Even though in many cases we were able to identify age groups and underlying medical conditions that significantly increased the risk for severe disease, hospitalization, and death, we could not accurately predict who in their 20s,

30s or 40s would suffer major strokes, heart attacks, myocarditis (heart inflammation, which in some cases ended in sudden death), loss of limbs due to the need for amputation, or the so-called long COVID—post-acute sequelae of COVID-19, or PASC—that we described in chapter 1.

In other words, even if we had accepted a reasonable theory of age-related and pre-existing medical condition vulnerabilities and then had thoughtlessly implemented it, there were still those who were at high risk who we could not identify before they developed severe symptoms or an even more terrible outcome. If we were to do this, we would miss many who would then be returning to their normal lives, thereby increasing their risk for exposure by taking a path that would place them in even greater danger than if we all embraced the public health precautions.

The second major flaw in this sequestering approach was that throughout the pandemic, we have seen how challenging it is to keep the elderly and those with multiple chronic illnesses in a "bubble"—the term used to describe the isolation of a specifically selected group of people for the purpose of avoiding contact with others who might expose them to the SARS-CoV-2 virus. Time and time again, we saw that those in communal settings such as long-term care facilities, prisons, and so on were exposed to the virus and became ill not from contact with a new resident or a new prisoner being introduced to the facility, but rather from the young people who served as staff in these facilities. Such staff would acquire the infection through activities outside of work, but then expose the residents or prisoners when they came to work. These staff members would often be contagious, but not yet symptomatic. They could also be infected and "pauci-symptomatic," meaning that the symptoms were mild and perhaps overlooked. It was not uncommonly, but incorrectly, thought that the staff member had just overdone things or not gotten enough rest, or that their symptoms could be ascribed to something else, such as allergies. Oftentimes, and discouragingly, it appeared that many young people failed to understand their role as intermediaries in the transmission of this disease to those who were far more vulnerable.

Even outside of communal settings, the elderly or individuals with multiple chronic illnesses often felt the need to go to the grocery store or their dentist's or doctor's office. If all those young and healthy adults who worked at or sought services from these establishments simply returned happily to their lives as if times were normal, the jeopardy to high-risk individuals would be even higher than if everyone complied with public health recommendations. This is because while the highest-risk age groups were the elderly, the age groups with the greatest role in the transmission of the virus were generally 20 to 40 years old.

Furthermore, during the pandemic, in what has been described as an epidemic of isolation, loneliness, and mental health issues, elderly grandparents longed for opportunities to visit with their families and their grandchildren. In some cases, appropriate precautions were exercised; in other situations, either through misunderstanding of what precautions were needed or a common misconception that family members would be unlikely sources of the virus, many seniors were infected even though they believed they were employing precautionary measures. Beyond this, while many felt that it might perhaps be manageable if isolation were needed for only a few weeks or months, significant resistance was created when the majority of public health experts predicted that the pandemic would last well over a year.

It was especially difficult for families to remain separated during the holidays. Repeatedly throughout the course of the pandemic, we would see surges in the numbers of cases, followed by increases in the number of hospitalizations, and then, finally, an increase in the numbers of deaths. This was especially the case following holidays where it is traditional for friends and family to come together, and many continued to do so through the pandemic, despite pleas from public health officials not to do so.

Recommendation #95

Public Health Measures

As happened with COVID-19, it is likely that the elderly will have the highest risk for severe illness and death in a future pandemic with another pathogen. We must remember that when there are not yet effective therapies and vaccines, and when the strategy to preserve life and minimize the impact on hospitals is to sequester the elderly, young adults must abide by public health mitigation measures because the elderly will inevitably come into contact with them. Young people can pose a significant threat to the elderly, especially when they belong to an age group with a high rate of infection.

Approach 2: Reaching Herd Immunity through Infection

Many suggested, including at least one of President Trump's advisors, which achieving herd immunity through natural infection would be a desirable way to bring the pandemic to an end. Herd immunity in a group is the level of immunity to a contagious organism (whether acquired through natural infection or vaccination) that results in such inefficient transmission of that infectious agent that the infection fails to spread to others in the population who are still susceptible to the infection. For example, infants are not generally vaccinated against most infectious diseases in the first six months of life. However, if a large percentage of the population is immune to an infectious agent, which resulting herd immunity is enough to prevent the infection from circulating among the population, eventually finding its way to that infant.

There were many problems with this hypothesis. First, in the modern era of vaccines, the proponents of this idea were unsuccessful in finding an example of another viral disease for which herd immunity had been achieved through natural infection. Second, no one knows the level of population immunity required for herd immunity against this novel virus. It is thought that at the very beginning of the outbreak, when no one had preexisting immunity and no one had applied any proactive mitigation measures, that the reproduction number (R-naught, or R_0) was 2.2–2.7 (and there are some that believe the true number could be almost double this due to instances of so-called super spreaders). This means that a person infected with SARS-CoV-2 would on average have been expected to infect 2.2 to 2.7 additional people. An accepted epidemiological model would then predict that herd immunity would require that roughly 60 percent of the population be immune to safeguard vulnerable individuals within the herd from infection.

To make matters even more problematic, these data points were based upon the original SARS-CoV-2 virus circulating at that time. SARS-CoV-2 is an RNA virus, and all such viruses mutate fairly frequently. SARS-CoV-2 seemed to mutate less frequently than many other RNA viruses, but because of the large number of worldwide infections (more than 113 million as we write this),[2] variants of concern have arisen. The development of variants is one of the strongest arguments against the strategy of creating herd immunity through natural infection. It clearly argues against either encouraging people to seek out opportunities to be intentionally exposed (including so-called COVID parties) or unwisely, intentionally avoiding precautions meant to protect against unintended exposures.

While most variants are of no significance or concern, some may be problematic for any or all of the following reasons. First, mutations may result in increased transmissibility (contagiousness).* Second, mutations may produce a more severe disease (increased virulence); or the mutations may confer some degree of immune evasion. Immune evasion or escape means that a change in the virus's structure will make it less susceptible to the immune defenses developed previously during a natural infection with a prior variant or, alternatively, from an immunization. Because of this biological advantage, some variants with enhanced transmissibility have become the dominant forms of the virus in many parts of the world. At the time of this writing, the United States has several COVID-19 variants of concern circulating in low numbers. Of particular concern, the 20I/501Y.V1/B.1.1.7 (Kent) variant, also designated by the WHO as Alpha but commonly known as the UK

* Authors' note: While we use *transmissible* and *contagious* interchangeably in this book, these terms are not synonyms for medical scientists. The contagiousness of an infected individual is certainly one factor in determining the transmissibility of an infection, but other factors contribute to the transmissibility of a virus as well, such as the infectivity of the pathogen, the susceptibility of those who are exposed to the infected person, and environmental factors. For example, a variant may be more transmissible by virtue of mutations that promote immune evasion or escape, even though the variant is not inherently more contagious than the wild-type virus.

variant, has been estimated to be anywhere between 30 to 70 percent more contagious than our prior variant. The CDC has projected that this variant will become the dominant variant in the United States sometime in March of 2021.[3]

An increase in contagiousness or transmissibility means that the reproductive number has increased. It is now estimated that herd immunity may require up to 85 percent of the population to be immune. Unfortunately, with the current estimates of those who refuse to get vaccinated, along with those who have a contraindication to vaccination, those who remain vaccine-hesitant, and all those children under the age of 12, for whom there is no currently authorized or approved vaccine at the time we are writing, there is no way to get to this level of immunity in the near future. This would be true even if the CDC estimates are correct that roughly 25 percent of the American public have had COVID-19, even if we assume that immunity is durable in each of those individuals, and even if we assume that immunity from natural infection with prior variants is protective against the emerging variants of concern.

Though New York City became an epicenter of COVID-19 activity in March 2020, with overwhelmed hospitals, inundated health care workers, and an excessive mortality rate compared to many other countries, including China, a seroprevalence study conducted in New York City at the end of that month indicated that only 22.7 percent of the population had antibodies to the SARS-CoV-2 spike protein.[4] If the mathematical projections were anywhere near correct in estimating the level of population immunity required for herd immunity, New York City was far from it. Therefore, those who advocated for this strategy risked overwhelming the country's health care system and causing large numbers of deaths, not to mention the health care costs that would be associated with such resource-intensive hospital care. As further evidence of the lack of herd immunity in New York and the consequences of uncontrolled spread, at this time a new variant, B.1.526 (or Iota), has just been identified in patients in New York and has mutations that might result in increased transmissibility and some degree of immune evasion. Undoubtedly, by the time you are reading this, many other variants of concern will have come and gone.

A third problem was that touting the idea of natural herd immunity—some of the promotion emerging from the White House—became even more outrageous and irresponsible as we entered into clinical trials for vaccines. In record time, two mRNA vaccines were shown to be safe and effective in phase 3 trials, ultimately receiving emergency use authorizations from the US Food and Drug Administration (FDA) before the end of 2020. On February 27, 2021, the FDA gave emergency use authorization to a third COVID-19 vaccine that uses an adenovirus vector for persons at least 18 years of age. With these advances in mind, giving preference to chaotic natural herd immunity strategies over concentrated and focused vaccine efforts seemed all the more foolish.

The fourth problem with arguments in favor of achieving herd immunity through natural infection was a huge difficulty contained within the very foundation of herd immunity—that of individual immunity. In 2020, we simply did not know whether people who recovered from a SARS-CoV-2 infection were immune; if so, whether everyone or just some of those who recovered were immune, including those with asymptomatic or mild infections; and if they were in fact immune, for how long. As of February of 2021, we still do not know the answers to these questions. We certainly could detect antibodies to the spike protein in most people following infection, but communicating to the public that the presence of antibodies does not necessarily mean immunity has been achieved has been a challenging concept to convey, since it is contrary to commonly held beliefs.

Explaining to the public that not all antibodies are created equal and that the body produces a wide array of antibodies in response to an infection, not all of which may be protective against subsequent infection, was very difficult. It was further confused by the fact that others were promoting antibody tests as a way to determine whether a prior illness was a common cold or COVID-19, whether they were now protected, and whether they should be cleared to return to work. A further complication was that due to numerous challenges in having adequate testing available, the FDA allowed several of these tests to enter the market without their approval. Many tests were available with widely varying sensitivity and specificity levels established by the manufacturer of the test, which could not always be substantiated when tested by third parties.

Early studies showed that while most (but not all) persons mounted an IgG antibody response to infection, few people made high levels of neutralizing antibodies and most people made some, but at comparatively low levels. Furthermore, antibody levels tended to decline significantly over two to three months, with some people becoming seronegative (their blood testing negative for the presence of antibodies). While these data were generally discouraging, we still did not clearly know the indicators of immunity for this disease until the vaccine trials were well advanced. Therefore, while we suspected that any immunity gained from natural infection might be short-lived—on the order of three to six months, perhaps, as is typical for other more common coronaviruses—declining levels of IgG antibodies would not necessarily imply a loss of immunity, especially given that we had little data on the cellular immune response to this disease.

Though it has been difficult to document cases of reinfection because testing was generally done by nucleic acid amplification methods (polymerase chain reaction, or PCR), which did not preserve a sample of the virus for future genetic sequencing, there have been, as of the time of this writing, 57 documented cases of reinfection, with two resulting in death, and 11,765 suspected cases of reinfection, with 32 resulting in death. Supporting our impressions that immunity from the SARS-CoV-2 virus infection may be short-lived, the average time interval between infection and reinfection for the confirmed cases was 95 days.[5] While with other infections, we often see that a reinfection is milder than the initial infection, that was not true in every case with COVID-19; there were instances where the reinfection was serious enough to require hospitalization, and the two previously mentioned cases of documented reinfection in which the patients died as a consequence of the reinfection.

And finally, in a case of "last but not least," a fifth herd immunity problem soon emerged: while many of those who advocated for a rush to herd immunity through natural infection considered the initial United States case fatality rate of 1.77 percent to be low and acceptable, they typically took little consideration (if any) of the emerging evidence of morbidity associated with COVID-19.

The Sweden Experiment

If you ask those who advocate for achieving herd immunity through natural infection to present a COVID-19 case study, they will most often point to Sweden. Swedish officials deny that their goal was to achieve herd immunity, asserting that it was to focus on encouraging voluntary measures among its population rather than issuing edicts to close businesses, schools, and its borders and imposing so-called lockdowns, which—as they correctly pointed out—were difficult to sustain.

With this approach of voluntary compliance with public health measures, Sweden was an outlier among European countries in its region. Though in the spring of 2020, many Americans pointed to Sweden as the example for the United States to follow, "in late June, Sweden announced a commission to evaluate its pandemic response, reacting to criticism over a death toll far exceeding that of its neighbors. At the time, more than 5,300 Swedes had died compared to around 250 in Norway, 600 in Denmark and 325 in Finland, all of which have populations around half the size."[6]

The Swedish Corona Commission (Coronakommissionen) has issued the first of its two anticipated reports. This first report was focused on Sweden's handling of the pandemic with respect to the elderly population as of December 2020.[7]

The report cited more than 7,000 deaths due to COVID-19 at that time, with those aged 70 years and older accounting for almost 90 percent of the deaths. Half of these deaths occurred in long-term residential settings. One conclusion of the commission was: "We find it most likely that the single most important factor behind the major outbreaks and the high number of deaths in residential care is the overall spread of the virus in the society." This is further evidence of the failure of Approach 1, which we reviewed at the beginning of this chapter. In fact, the commission sums it up by stating: "The strategy of protecting the elderly has failed."

Nevertheless, after the surge in cases in April through July 2020 dissipated, Swedish health officials pointedly questioned other nations' decisions to lock down and indicated that they believed the worst was now behind the Swedes and that there would be no more surges. They could not have been more mistaken. The epidemiological curve (epi curve) for what unfolded in Sweden is shown in figure 12.1.

As you can see, a new and far greater surge began in November and peaked on December 25, 2020, with a seven-day moving average of 70.7 daily cases per 100,000 population. The Swedish health care system became stressed, and Stockholm's ICU capacity was strained at 99 percent. There were reports of more and more health care workers

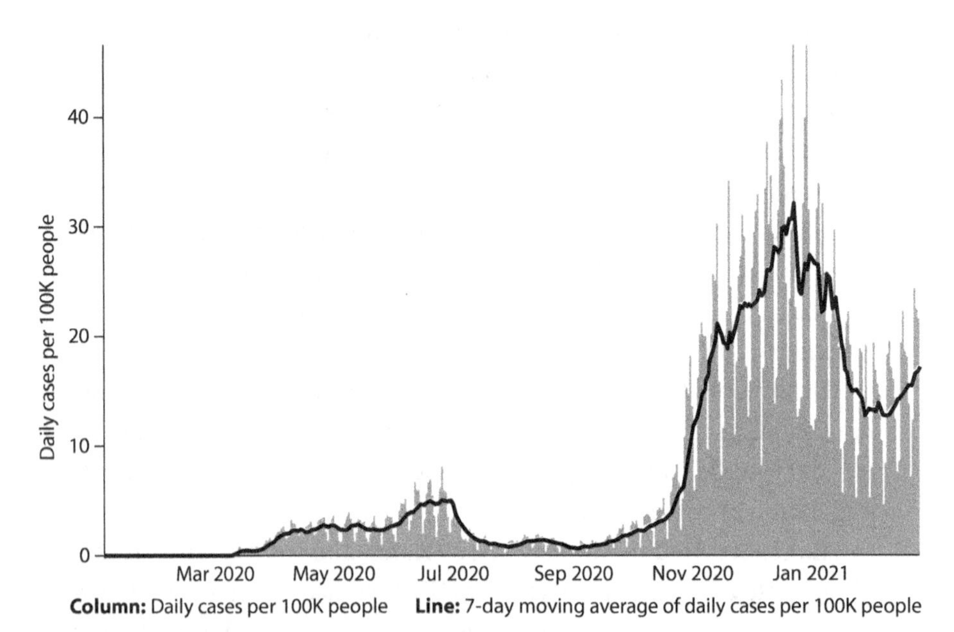

Figure 12.1. The epidemiologic curve for Sweden during the COVID-19 pandemic from March 2020 through January 2021. The columns indicate daily cases per 100,000 people, while the line is the seven-day moving average of daily cases per 100,000 people. *Source*: Brown University's School of Public Health

resigning because they were overwhelmed. Finland and Norway closed their borders to Sweden to prevent spillover into their countries.

This surge prompted Swedish government officials to reverse their prior policies and to ban gatherings of eight or more people, close certain entertainment venues (cinemas and theaters), prohibit bars and restaurants from serving alcohol after 10 p.m., and shift all high schools to remote learning in early December.

Sweden's neighboring nations had taken the more common approaches to managing the pandemic with restrictions from the beginning. The most recent comparative statistics from the Johns Hopkins Coronavirus Resource Center are presented in table 12.1.

From this analysis, we can conclude that both Approach 1 (sequester only those at highest risk) and Approach 2 (attempt to achieve herd immunity from natural infection) are flawed and dangerous. However, we now address one final, often-used argument to support Approach 2: avoiding lockdowns, restrictions, and closures of businesses averts damage to the country's economy. While the final word is not yet out on this, it does not appear to be the case. Because Sweden reversed its course in the fall of 2020, we tried to find an economic analysis from the summer to see if the data supported that contention. We found an analysis by Dhaval Joshi, chief European investment strategist at BCA Research. Joshi compared Sweden, with its lack of restrictions, to Denmark, a country with similar culture and demographics, but one that imposed one of the strictest lockdowns found worldwide.

He found that both countries had a rise in unemployment of two percentage points at that time. Both suffered similar drops in consumer

Table 12.1. COVID statistics for Sweden and its Nordic neighbors

Country	Case fatality rate	Deaths per 100,000 population
Sweden	2.0%	125.31
Norway	0.9%	11.67
Denmark	1.1%	40.57
Finland	1.3%	13.41

Source: Johns Hopkins University of Medicine Coronavirus Resource Center, "Maps & Trends: Mortality Analyses," accessed February 28, 2021, https://coronavirus.jhu.edu/data/mortality

confidence, though Denmark's appeared to be recovering more quickly by July. Other news reports suggest that Sweden gained no economic advantage from its lack of restrictions. Here is Joshi's explanation: "The simple answer is that in a pandemic, most people will change their behavior to avoid catching the virus. The cautious behavior is voluntary, irrespective of whether there is no lockdown, as in Sweden, or there is a lockdown, as in Denmark."[8]

These findings support our positions. We have long said that those who say we must either fight the pandemic or save the economy were offering a false dichotomy. In fact, the way to save the economy is to aggressively fight the pandemic. When consumers are fearful of the risks of infection, they will restrict their activities and avoid events and certain businesses. If governments and public health authorities do not take action to control the spread of disease, businesses without subsidization will reduce hours, lay off or furlough employees, or close down, driving increasing unemployment—and unemployment further reduces consumer spending.

Recommendation #96

Controlling the Pandemic Is Key to Protecting the Economy

The best way to preserve the economy is to control the spread of infection; to make people, particularly those who feel at greatest risk, feel safe; and clearly communicate the successes in preventing infection through the adoption of public health guidance. Inevitably, if efforts to control spread are not successful, consumer confidence will suffer; governments are then invariably left with few options other than restrictions and closures, and employee productivity will decline, along with a surge in employer health costs.

CHAPTER 13

Vaccines and Variants

A Race against Time

Misinformation or distrust of vaccines can be like a contagion that can spread as fast as the measles.

THERESA TAM, CHIEF PUBLIC HEALTH OFFICER OF CANADA

Vaccines

It soon became clear that the SARS-CoV-2 global pandemic was not going to be contained in the same way as the original SARS coronavirus was back in 2003, and we have already discussed in chapters 1 and 12 why we never believed we would achieve herd immunity through natural infection. No, for us to get back to any sense of normalcy, it was increasingly clear that our only way out of this pandemic was the development of one or more safe, effective vaccines and the vaccination of a high percentage of the population.

It was certainly an intimidating thought, depending on a vaccine to end this pandemic. "An average vaccine takes about 10–12 years to be developed," wrote Jens-Peter Gregersen for the science blog *Eureka*,[1] and there are a number of viruses for which we have not yet been able to develop an effective vaccine, despite intensive efforts and to our great frustration. Even if a SARS-CoV-2 vaccine were developed and then approved, how long would it take to manufacture, distribute, and administer enough doses to vaccinate the world's population of about 7.8 billion people?

The United States launched an innovative approach to encourage the development and manufacture of potential vaccines on a fast track. The White House announced Operation Warp Speed on May 15, 2020. This initiative was conducted through the US Department of Defense in partnership with private vaccine developers and manufacturers. The mission was to "deliver 300 million doses of safe and effective vaccine by January 1, 2021."[2] While the operation fell quite short of achieving the targeted doses on the designated timeline, we nevertheless applaud the Trump administration for setting out a moonshot initiative with a stretch target.

Vaccine development is a lengthy, costly, and financially risky undertaking, especially when dealing with a novel virus. We did not yet know the indicators of immunity, nor the potential for durability of the immune response. Despite such deterrents to vaccine development, there were stronger incentives for creating a SARS-CoV-2 vaccine than is typical for most other contagions. A SARS-CoV-2 vaccine would serve a market consisting of everyone on the planet (as opposed to other vaccines that target certain at-risk populations) and would assist many who were desperate to be vaccinated.

It is typical procedure for a vaccine developer and manufacturer to wait for the results of clinical trials of their vaccine and the subsequent approval by the US Food and Drug Administration (FDA) before they begin producing and storing large quantities of vaccine. A brilliant part of the Operation Warp Speed program was funding up to six of the leading vaccine developers whose phase 3 clinical trials showed promising results (figure 13.1). These developers could then produce and store vaccine in advance of an authorization from the FDA so that doses could be shipped out to states immediately upon federal authorization.

As you can see in figure 13.1, there was a systematic plan to accelerate the vaccine development and review process. The first step was to take three months off of the typical determination of vaccine candidates by using vaccine platforms that had already been tested and proven successful for other diseases and by creating vaccine candidates immediately after the viral genomic sequence was known. Researchers had already sequenced the virus's genome early in January 2020.

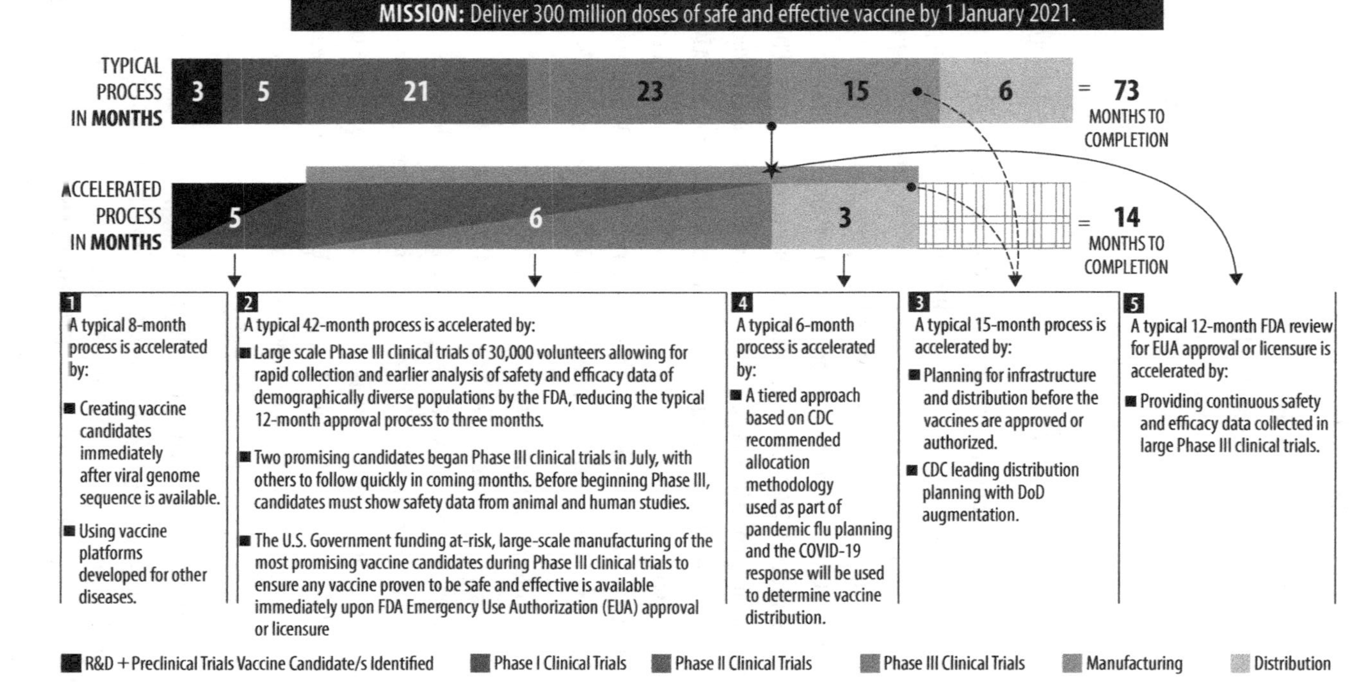

Figure 13.1. A timeline for Operation Warp Speed's accelerated vaccine development.

In fact, many companies had already begun to develop vaccine candidates before Operation Warp Speed was implemented.

Recommendation #97

Public-Private Partnership for Vaccine Development

In future pandemics, as was done in the current one, the United States should consider providing advance funding to the leading vaccine candidate manufacturers that get their vaccines to phase 3 clinical trials so that they can ramp up production and supply of vaccine in anticipation of FDA authorization and so begin shipping as soon as that authorization is given.

A notable success of this manifold approach was that it led to the development of a variety of vaccine types—mRNA, viral vector, protein subunit, and so on. Thus, we were not repeating the mistake we pointed out in chapter 1 where the United States put all its eggs in the basket of a single COVID-19 test developed by the Centers for Disease Control and Prevention (CDC) that then turned out to have flaws. The advantage of developing multiple types of vaccines was that it increased the odds that at least one of them might turn out to be safe and effective. At the time we are writing, the FDA has authorized two mRNA vaccines as safe and effective—Pfizer-BioNTech's Comirnaty and Moderna's Spikevax—along with one viral vector vaccine: Johnson & Johnson's Janssen.

Recommendation #98

Develop Multiple Types of Vaccines Concurrently

The United States should encourage the simultaneous development of different vaccine types when faced with the next pandemic with a novel contagion, so as to increase the chances that at least one of the vaccines will be safe and effective. The goal should be to have at least several manufacturers' vaccines authorized to allow for greater vaccine production and distribution on a rapid basis.

Another advantage of developing multiple vaccines is addressing the problem of a huge demand for vaccine that cannot be met on a reasonable timeline by a single manufacturer. To the extent that there were two, three, or more manufacturers with an authorized vaccine, the production and distribution of vaccine would be much greater and faster.

The next step was the attempt to reduce a typical 42-month process of clinical trials to six months by working with the FDA to create large-scale (30,000+ study participants) phase 3 clinical trials to determine the safety and efficacy of the vaccines.

mRNA technology had been studied for many years as a potential vaccine candidate for a number of viruses. No mRNA vaccine had ever been previously approved for use by the FDA, but fortunately, vaccine scientists at Pfizer and BioNTech and Moderna started to work on developing vaccine candidates for SARS-CoV-2 soon after the genome of the virus was published in January. One beauty of the mRNA technology is that you do not need an actual sample of the virus, nor is it necessary to grow the virus in cell cultures to design the vaccine; all you need is the genetic sequence. Thus, mRNA-based developers were able to get a head start and begin animal trials as soon as possible, followed by early human trials. By July, vaccine candidates from both companies were ready to begin phase 3 clinical trials.

In the end, vaccines were developed and authorized well under the target of 14 months; however, only 1 percent of the distribution target was met by January 1, 2021. Nevertheless, this was an amazing scientific achievement, the likes of which has never been seen before, and frankly, few thought it would be possible.

Despite this major accomplishment, the handoff to and coordination with the states raised several hurdles that obstructed the goal of efficiently vaccinating Americans:

1. As we pointed out earlier in this book, public health infrastructures within the states have been downsized and inadequately funded for the past half-century. Given the resulting limitations to the public health agencies' capacity to conduct mass vaccinations, states have had to largely rely on private health care providers and pharmacies to vaccinate their citizens. Furthermore, the first available COVID-19 vaccine was the Pfizer-BioNTech mRNA vaccine, which required an ultra-cold supply chain and subsequently special freezers that few providers had. This challenging storage and handling requirement, in turn,

limited the number of providers who were willing to sign up to administer the Pfizer-BioNTech vaccine.

2. States were ill prepared to urgently administer mass vaccinations, and many were already financially strained by the unanticipated needs of the first nine months of the pandemic, leaving them disadvantaged in their efforts to become prepared. States thus needed funds from the federal government to assist them in their vaccination efforts. Congress did not approve these funds until well after the states began receiving vaccines.
3. In the first months of vaccine distribution, the state allocation of vaccine was frequently changed, and states generally did not learn how much vaccine they would receive until a few days before the shipment would arrive. The short notice and unpredictable supply made it very difficult for providers to know how much vaccine would be available to them and how many appointments they could offer. This led to huge frustration aimed at health care providers from the public due to the difficulty in scheduling a vaccine appointment. The public's frustration was even greater when providers had to cancel appointments because they'd received less vaccine than they were expecting.
4. Neither the federal government nor most states had created a website, or a call center for those without computer and internet service, where people could express their interest in being vaccinated. Thus, many lacked an easy way to communicate the days and times they would be available to be vaccinated, the distance they were willing to travel, and the pertinent personal health information that would allow them to be placed in a priority group so that the computer or call center could determine a date, time, and place for them to go to be vaccinated. Instead, people were left to their own devices. This created significant frustration, especially for our seniors. Many were unclear as to when it was their turn to be vaccinated, even though priority groups were posted on public health websites and communicated in the press and media. When new priority

groups or vaccine appointment options opened, people had to choose a provider, go to that provider's website, and attempt to grab one of the available appointments. Oftentimes, early on, this was preceded by an announcement that these new appointments would be available starting on a particular day at a particular time. Unsurprisingly, many providers' websites crashed due to the tremendously high volume of people all trying to access the system at the same moment, reminiscent of how concert tickets for a hugely popular show go on sale.

For people who were initially unsuccessful in obtaining an appointment, the advice was to keep returning to the site in the hope that a new appointment might open. This frustrated many people, as they would spend hours every day checking repeatedly for an appointment. They wondered why they could not simply be added to a waiting list and have the provider contact them once an appointment became available, and many providers did ultimately change their processes to do just that. However, when they did, large numbers of people then signed up with multiple providers to increase their chances to receive the vaccine earlier. Quite often they did not go back and cancel the other appointments that had become available; effectively, people became chaotic gamblers, pulling the levers of several slot machines simultaneously and hoping for a payout. This produced problems for providers who were attempting to use up all the vaccine doses they had for the day so that none had to be discarded. A centralized appointment scheduler that also maintained a backup list of people willing to come in for vaccination at a moment's notice in the event of a cancellation would have helped streamline operations and reduce disenchantment with the system.

5. Due to demand greatly exceeding supply, states had to create priority groups to restrict who could show up for vaccination and to ensure that those with the most urgent need received the vaccine first. This itself proved to be incredibly difficult and complex.

It seems to us that there were three possible approaches to determining vaccine priority, which would, in general, make a big difference in who would get vaccinated first. One approach would be to minimize deaths and the burdens on hospital capacity. This would select those over 60 years of age to be vaccinated first. A second approach would be to minimize transmission of the virus as much as possible, in which case you would likely prioritize those ages 20 to 40. A third approach would be to protect essential services and infrastructure—for example, health care workers, firefighters, police officers, paramedics, utility workers, and so forth.

There were merits to each strategy, and problems with each. With respect to vaccinating high-risk individuals based on age, there were many high-risk individuals who were under age 60 and had underlying medical conditions, and thus also highly vulnerable to COVID-19 complications—not to mention that based on the amount of vaccine some states were receiving, it could take months just to vaccinate all the seniors who wanted to be vaccinated.

Most states established their vaccine priority groups using various combinations of the first and third options above. We are not aware of any state that went for the second option—trying to disrupt the transmission of the disease by vaccinating those age groups most likely to be transmitting it. The reason why is likely because trying to explain to seniors, whose lives were at risk, why vaccinating young adults, who rarely die, would reduce their risk and bring the pandemic to an end sooner would be a tough sell, difficult to explain, and a huge political risk.

One might think that the third approach would make sense and be easy to implement. It was anything but. There was little, if any, resistance to the notion that we should vaccinate health care workers. But which health care workers should be vaccinated before their age group otherwise comes up? In a hospital, should all environmental services workers be vaccinated in the first tier, or just those who worked on COVID-19 units? Should chiropractors and podiatrists be included in this first tier? What about a massage therapist?

At one hospital that ended up with an extra dose of vaccine at the end of the day, staff contacted their media relations person to see if she wanted to come in for immunization so the vaccine would not go to waste. Since she was in her thirties to forties, this opportunity would likely be four or five months earlier than when she would be eligible for vaccine based on her age risk group. She jumped at the chance but then later had to defend her organization's decision by stating that there were occasions where she had to go to the COVID-19 units to film stories she was working on. We certainly have no problem with this, but exasperation mounted among the elderly who continued to watch people half their age get vaccinated before they could. And why didn't this hospital have a waiting list of elderly patients who were willing to come in at a moment's notice if there was a cancellation or extra dose at the end of the day?

Recommendation #99
Computer-Assisted Vaccine Scheduling

For future pandemics, when people must be assigned to priority groups due to limited vaccine, the federal government should create a website for each state's use that will allow people in that state to indicate that they wish to receive the vaccine, how far they are willing to drive for the vaccine, what days and times they are available for a vaccine appointment, the demographic and clinical information that will allow them to be prioritized, and whether they wish to be placed on a waiting list if a provider has vaccine left over at the end of the day. The system should not allow the double-booking of appointments and should automatically cancel an existing appointment if the person is on a waiting list and has called in prior to their appointment.

Those over age 12 are currently being vaccinated. Clinical trials are under way to determine the safety of vaccinating those under the age of 12. By the time you are reading this book, we expect that everyone from age six months and up will be eligible for vaccination. It is also likely that booster shots will be available to deal with waning immunity. We certainly expect to see additional types of vaccines (such as inactivated whole virus vaccines, protein subunit vaccines, and perhaps intranasal vaccines) become available, and likely there will be new versions of the existing vaccines to deal with future variants of this virus.

As one might imagine, with high demand and short supply at the beginning of 2021, there were allegations of wealthy people line-jumping. The US House Select Subcommittee on the Coronavirus Crisis launched an investigation into a health care company, One Medical, based upon reports that the company diverted "vital vaccine doses away from vulnerable populations to benefit wealthy concierge clients and friends and family members of [the] company's executives who are not eligible under state and local guidelines." One Medical has denied these allegations.[3]

Florida's agriculture commissioner called for a congressional investigation of the Florida governor's vaccine rollout. According to her allegations, pop-up vaccination sites were set up in wealthy communities to benefit political donors.[4] As yet, no investigation has been completed, nor have these allegations been proven.

Of course, there are bigger concerns than whether some people of privilege in the United States are getting vaccinated ahead of others that are of higher priority. One such concern is that wealthy countries are getting vaccine far in advance of poor countries. There are some estimates that it may take two years to get vaccines out to all countries. We must remember that as long as we have large populations of people who are not immune to the SARS-CoV-2 virus, we will continue to see spread within that country and to other countries when there is international travel. Furthermore, the continued spread can be expected to produce new variants, and potentially one that can evade the immunity generated by natural infection and our current vaccines.

Another big concern is vaccine hesitancy. One survey of 13,426 people in 19 countries, while COVID-19 vaccines were still in clinical trials and not yet approved, showed that 71.5 percent of participants reported that they would "be very or somewhat likely to take a COVID-19 vaccine, and 48.1 percent reported that they would accept their employer's recommendation to do so. Differences in acceptance rates ranged from almost 90 percent (in China) to less than 55 percent (in Russia). Respondents reporting higher levels of trust in information from government sources were more likely to accept a vaccine and take their employer's advice to do so."[5]

Trust in the government and trust in the information provided to people about a new vaccine is critical to decreasing vaccine hesitancy. Elected leaders must use government agencies, public health leaders, doctors, and scientists to regularly educate and update the public about vaccines that are being developed and why vaccination is so important. Because of mistrust and lack of access to health care among minority groups, it is important to ask doctors, scientists, and influential leaders of color to make and reinforce these messages through media sources that are more likely to target these populations and to offer vaccines in their communities by trusted providers. Messages need to be put out in the native languages of those for whom English is not their primary language.

Recommendation #100

Promote Vaccines within Disadvantaged Communities

When vaccines become available, public health departments must make vaccines available to socioeconomically disadvantaged communities and communities with barriers to accessing care, including low English fluency, low levels of health insurance, and employers that do not provide time off from work for vaccination, using individuals fluent in the languages spoken in that community and who live in the community. Efforts to leverage people much trusted in those communities to help bring folks out for vaccination—trusted people such as teachers, coaches, clergy, doctors, nurses, community health workers, social workers, and pharmacists—should be made to the greatest extent possible.

In the United States, the Pew Research Center published a study showing an increase in willingness to receive the COVID-19 vaccine as the vaccines were undergoing authorization by the FDA, in contrast to when they were still in clinical trials. In the two months between

September and November 2020, the percentage of those surveyed who indicated that they would definitely get the vaccine increased from 21 to 29 percent, while the percentage of those who indicated that they definitely would not decreased from 24 to 18 percent. The percentage of those that we refer to as "vaccine hesitant"—those who either "probably would" or "probably would not" get the vaccine, with an emphasis on the word "probably"—changed little over those two months: 55 percent in September and 52 percent in November. But even among those who indicated that they probably or definitely would not get the vaccine, 46 percent did indicate that they might get the vaccine after others did and they received more information about the vaccines.[6]

Given the tremendous improvement in the times from development of the vaccine to clinical trials to authorization of the vaccines, many Americans worried that the process was rushed and that necessary steps might have been cut from the process. Of course, in retrospect, the title "Operation Warp Speed" may have contributed to these concerns. There were also understandable worries that politics may have interfered with the scientific process because President Trump was touting the vaccines as an important reason for his reelection, and we had previously seen instances where it appeared that the White House had pressured the FDA and CDC to alter their positions during the pandemic.

Some states have resorted to incentives in order to try to get more of their population vaccinated—for example, an entry for lottery drawings and cash prizes upon vaccination. Some businesses have offered incentives, such as a "shot for a shot," in which a person over the legal drinking age is given a free alcoholic drink in exchange for receiving their vaccination. It is not clear whether these programs have been effective at this time. The hope is that it may be just enough of a nudge for those who were on the fence about getting vaccinated, but no one seriously believed this would influence those who are strongly opposed to the vaccine.

As of the time of this writing, the country with the highest percentage of fully vaccinated residents is the Seychelles at 69.32 percent. Despite relatively high levels of vaccination, the Seychelles has recently had some of the highest disease transmission rates. The same has been true for some other countries with relatively high vaccination rates, and this has often been attributed to a new, widely circulating variant with greatly increased transmissibility, the Delta variant, moving through populations and largely infecting those who are not vaccinated. It seems to support the notion that "herd immunity," if even attainable, is likely to require significantly higher levels of immune protection in the population, and perhaps our estimates on the order of 85 percent are realistic. Despite our early access to the vaccine, and because of vaccine hesitancy or resistance, the United States is only the 13th highest ranked country by percent of population vaccinated and stands at 47.6 percent.[7]

Aggravating the United States' efforts to get Americans vaccinated were unprecedented levels of misinformation and disinformation, the likes of which we have never seen before. Much of the disinformation was promoted on social media and certain cable news networks. While there was a significant increase in activity from the well-established anti-vaccine groups, there were also new organizations such as America's Frontline Doctors and various "freedom foundations" that became very active—and, most concerningly, a seemingly much larger number of doctors and health-related professionals spreading disinformation.

It is also important to note that there are still many countries with few or none of their citizens vaccinated, particularly developing countries. We reiterate that, setting aside our moral obligation, it is in the world's best interests to get high vaccination rates in all countries, as unfettered transmission will continue to generate new variants—perhaps even one that will significantly threaten the efficacy of our current vaccines and threaten the rest of the world.

Americans may not feel the pressure to be vaccinated at present due to relatively low levels of disease transmission in the United States. However, the Delta variant is increasing in prevalence in the United States and it is expected that in a few months' time, it will be the predominant variant in the United States, displacing the Alpha variant that has been predominant since late March and early April. The expectation is that we will have enough people vaccinated to avoid the kinds of surges we saw in disease transmission last year and early this year, but also that we are likely to see outbreaks in those states and areas with relatively low vaccination rates, which currently are predominantly in the midwestern and southern United States. However, given the amount of vaccine hesitancy, aggressive disinformation campaigns, and emerging variants with increased transmissibility, many of us remain concerned as to whether we can get high enough vaccination levels to prevent significant outbreaks and even surges anytime soon.

A number of Republican governors and legislatures rushed to prohibit or limit the use of vaccine passports to limit services or admission of persons to state buildings—or, in some cases, businesses operating within their states—without evidence of vaccination. These prohibitions have generally not been extended to health care providers.

A number of hospitals and health systems have announced that their employees will be required to be vaccinated against COVID-19. Among the first to make this requirement was Houston Methodist, a large and well-respected health care system in Houston, Texas. A group of employees facing the loss of their jobs sued Houston Methodist, making a number of claims as to why it was illegal for their employer to require vaccination. That case has now been decided. Before we go through the court's analysis and decision, let's explore some of the issues.

The requirement for vaccinations is not new. Schools have long required certain immunizations for their students. Many readers of my age will remember getting our polio vaccine sugar cubes at school. Hospitals have long required new employees to show evidence of immunity to certain diseases such as hepatitis, measles, rubella, and mumps, or get vaccinated against these diseases. Most every hospital in the country requires their employees to receive an annual influenza vaccination. Of course, exceptions are made for those with medical contraindications or sincerely held religious beliefs that would prohibit them from receiving the vaccines.

Conflict arises when an employer has a legitimate interest in protecting its workforce and customers from health risks caused by a contagious disease and when individuals believe that the exercise of their personal freedom not to be vaccinated will mean the loss of their employment.

Hospitals face additional pressures to require vaccination than most businesses. First of all, those infected with the contagious disease (in this case, COVID-19) are more likely to seek services from a hospital than many other types of businesses. Whereas with other businesses, someone who is infected with the SARS-CoV-2 virus may be in and out of that business in minutes to hours, those requiring the services of a hospital are often hospitalized for days or weeks, posing a more protracted risk to the hospital's employees. In addition, unlike the services of most businesses, hospital services may require health care workers to be in very close contact with infected patients and, through the performance of certain medical procedures, cause a patient to cough or expel more virus than with normal breathing that would occur in most businesses.

Not only do infected persons create a special risk for health care workers, but health care workers can create special risks for certain patients. By the very nature of hospital services, patients often tend to be those that are at highest risk for infection and for worse outcomes from infection. This would include the elderly, those with multiple underlying medical conditions, and patients who are immunocompromised, including patients undergoing chemotherapy, patients preparing for or who have received bone marrow or solid organ transplants, and newborns and infants. In one recent poll, 62 percent of respondents indicated that they want health care workers to be vaccinated to ensure their own safety as potential future patients.[8]

Hospitals obviously have an interest in ensuring that they keep employees safe and maintaining sufficient staffing levels to care for patients. Many hospitals also offer their employees and their families self-funded health plan coverage and have an interest in keeping those health care costs down for everyone. It also is unclear at present what liability a hospital may have if a patient were infected by a staff member and suffered harm.

Now, let's turn to the interest of the plaintiff employees and their claims and examine how the court addressed those claims. The lawsuit brought against Houston Methodist was decided by Judge Lynn Hughes in the United States District Court for the Southern District of Texas; the judge entered his decision on June 12, 2021.

The first claim addressed by the court was that the plaintiffs were wrongfully terminated. It is important to note here that Texas is an "at will" employment state. The premise of the plaintiffs' claims of wrongful termination was that Houston Methodist was requiring employees to take an experimental vaccine that was dangerous, and because these plaintiffs would not do so, they either had been terminated or were facing termination. The judge concluded that both claims—that the vaccine was experimental and that the vaccine is dangerous—were false and that, in any case, whether those claims were true or not, they were legally irrelevant.

The judge pointed out in his decision that Texas law (even though the case was heard and decided in federal court, the court was required to apply Texas law in deciding the case) only protects employees from being terminated for refusing to commit an act that would potentially impose criminal penalties on the worker. The judge set out the case that the plaintiffs would have to prove in order to be protected under a claim of wrongful termination: (1) that the plaintiffs were required to commit an illegal act—one for which they could suffer criminal penalties, (2) the plaintiffs refused to commit the illegal acts, (3) the plaintiffs were terminated, and (4) the only reason for termination was their refusal to commit the illegal act. The judge quickly dismissed this cause of action, because receiving a COVID-19 vaccination is neither illegal nor exposes the plaintiffs to any criminal penalties.

Next, the judge addressed the plaintiffs' assertions that Houston Methodist's vaccination requirement violates public policy. The judge pointed out that Texas law does not recognize an exception to at-will employment for actions inconsistent with public policy, but went further to state that even if it did, this vaccination requirement would not be contrary to public policy. Judge Hughes referenced Supreme Court precedent stating that neither involuntary quarantine for contagious diseases nor state-imposed requirements for mandatory vaccination violate an individual's due process rights. Further, the Equal Employment Opportunity Commission issued guidance in May 2021 that employers can require employees to be vaccinated against COVID-19 subject to reasonable accommodations for employees with disabilities or sincerely held religious beliefs, and Houston Methodist complied with this guidance.

The plaintiffs also alleged that Houston Methodist's vaccination requirement violated federal law, in that employees cannot be required to take "unapproved" medications, and none of the COVID-19 vaccines had received full approval from the FDA. Judge Hughes pointed to federal law that does allow the US secretary of health and human services to introduce into commerce medical products intended for use during a public health emergency. Furthermore, the court pointed out that the federal law neither expands nor restricts the rights and responsibilities of private employers; in fact, the federal law in question does not apply to private employers. Moreover, the federal law does not provide for a private cause of action against either the government or private employers.

The plaintiffs likewise alleged that the vaccine requirement violated federal law that protected human subjects in clinical trials. They asserted that because the COVID-19 vaccines were not fully approved, their use was experimental, and thus, employees could not be coerced into receiving the vaccines. However, Judge Hughes held that the vaccines were not experimental, Houston Methodist was not conducting a clinical trial with its employees, and therefore, this provision of federal law also did not apply.

Another claim made by plaintiffs was quite shocking. They alleged that Houston Methodist's vaccination requirement violated the Nuremberg Code, comparing Houston Methodist's actions to those of forced medical experimentation on Jewish people during the Holocaust. Judge Hughes rightly chastised plaintiffs for making such a reprehensible analogy and pointed out that private businesses are not subject to the Nuremberg Code.

In his opinion, Judge Hughes repudiated the claims made in behalf of the lead plaintiff, Jennifer Bridges:

> Although her claims fail as a matter of law, it is also necessary to clarify that Bridges has not been coerced. Bridges says that she is being forced to be injected with a vaccine or be fired. This is not coercion. Methodist is trying to do their business of saving lives without giving them the COVID-19 virus. It is a choice made to keep staff, patients, and their families safer. Bridges can freely choose to accept or refuse a COVID-19 vaccine; however, if she refuses, she will simply need to work somewhere else.[9]

Where do things go from here? Bridges and the other plaintiffs in this case could file an appeal, but most of the holdings in Judge Hughes's opinion are well-settled law, and it would seem unlikely to us that this decision would be overturned on appeal. We think this case likely settles the matter—at least, for workers in Texas.

It is likely that there will be other lawsuits in other states, and their states' laws regarding wrongful termination may differ from Texas' law to an extent that would allow plaintiffs to prevail on this claim. However, many of us expect that the FDA will grant full approval to the currently available COVID-19 vaccines in the United States, in late 2021 or early 2022. If that happens during the process of these lawsuits, it will likely make some of the suits, or at least some of the causes of action, moot, in that the plaintiffs are likely to make similar arguments to those made in this Texas case: that the fact that the vaccines are not fully approved should be a rationale to prevent employers from requiring them. The result will be that many of these lawsuits will then be dismissed by the courts.

Variants

RNA viruses mutate frequently. Most viral mutations are inconsequential and have no appreciable impact on the transmission, severity, or control of the disease those viruses cause. However, when a virus has high levels of transmission across much of the world, the rate of mutations increases and the risk that consequential mutations will occur increases significantly.

Viruses with mutations that result in an increase in transmissibility (especially contagiousness), an increase in virulence (cause more severe disease), or the ability to evade the immune response are referred to as variants of concern.

Mutations arise as errors in transcribing the genetic code of the virus. When a virus invades a cell, it hijacks the cell's machinery, which is then used to replicate the virus and make its proteins based upon the instructions in that genetic code. Just as when you might make an occasional error when transcribing something with a pen and paper, so too an error can be made when the virus' RNA is being transcribed. The more you must transcribe with your pen, the more transcription errors you are likely to make. Similarly, when the SARS-CoV-2 virus is infecting millions of people and replicating at very high rates, more transcription errors will occur that will result in more mutations, which subsequently can result in more variants of concern.

One way that you could reduce your own transcription errors is to have someone proofread your work. Not all viruses have the ability to proofread the transcriptions of their genetic code, but the SARS-CoV-2 virus does have that ability. Proofreading certainly reduces the number of transcription errors, but it does not completely eliminate them. Thus, the SARS-CoV-2 developed mutations at a much slower rate than other RNA viruses without a proofreading function, but because of the huge levels of transmission, we did see the emergence of a SARS-CoV-2 variant of concern as early as the end of January/beginning of February 2020, but many more near the end of the year and into 2021, and no doubt we will see even more concerning variants in the future, until such time as we can significantly slow the transmission of this virus globally.

What is the impact of a variant of concern? It depends. First, we try to determine whether the variant is more transmissible, more virulent, or able to escape prior immunity acquired either due to infection with a previous version of the SARS-CoV-2 virus without the mutation or due to vaccination. Then, we look to see how the variant virus is behaving. An increase in transmissibility can give the variant an advantage over the original strain of the virus (wild-type) that may result in the variant displacing the wild-type virus. Sometimes this is referred to as a "fitness" advantage for the variant, or the variant may be described as being more "fit." In this case, as was the case for a variant that was first detected in the United Kingdom (B.1.1.7/501Y.V1/VOC202012/01, now referred to as "Alpha" under the WHO's naming convention), when virus samples are taken from those who are infected over time and genetically sequenced, we see a progressive increase in the percentage of infections that are caused by the variant compared to the wild type. In the United Kingdom, despite an intervening lockdown, this variant of concern became the predominant variant in just three months.

When we see a variant gain a fitness advantage, we also look to see whether it is causing more severe disease or even deaths. We must be careful in looking at mortality, because a variant that is more transmissible and infects more people will result in more deaths, just by virtue of the fact that it infected more people. Instead, what we look for are whether infections are now resulting in a higher percentage of people developing severe illness, requiring hospitalization, requiring ICU level care and mechanical ventilation, or deaths. Of course, when a variant causes more severe illness and deaths, that can actually be detrimental to its transmission if the time interval between becoming contagious and becoming more severely ill is truncated, because children with more severe symptoms are less likely to go to school or play with friends; adults with more severe illness are less likely to go to work or events; and if the person is in the hospital, they are likely to be in isolation.

For the apparently more transmissible variants of concern that we have seen thus far, it remains unclear as to why they have gained a fitness advantage and become more transmissible. It is commonly believed that a mutation involving the spike protein of the virus that results in the spike protein having a greater affinity for the ACE-2 receptor with which it binds or enables it to bind more tightly to it may contribute to increased infectiousness, but this hypothesis remains unproven. Further, transmissibility is itself a complicated concept that includes both biologic characteristics of the virus as well as factors intrinsic to the host (such as genetics) and extrinsic to the host (such as the environment) While the wild-type virus appeared to infect children less commonly and not be transmitted as effectively by children in comparison to the rate of transmission by infected adults, some of the new variants of concern that were more transmissible also infected children more often and allowed children to transmit the virus more effectively.

In variants that develop the capability for immune evasion or immune escape, one of the first signs we may see is a huge spike in cases after a region has already been through a big wave of infections, suggesting that people who were previously infected may be getting reinfected. We have seen this with the South African variant (B.1.351/501Y.V2/VOC202012/02, now referred to as "Beta") and, most recently, with the Brazilian variant (P.1/20J/B.1.1.248/501Y.V3, now referred to as "Gamma"). Brazil is having a huge surge in cases that is overwhelming their health care system, despite the fact that some had assumed that prior levels of infection in parts of Brazil had likely resulted in herd immunity due to a large wave of infections in 2020. It can be difficult to tell if these variants are also more transmissible. It may be that they merely take advantage of a population with a high degree of immunity to wild-type virus. Such a population could have, as a result, a reduced amount of circulating virus, allowing the new variant with immune evasion capabilities to spread without competition from the wild-type virus or other variants that may otherwise be more transmissible.

Fortunately, when a variant acquires the capability for immune evasion or escape, it is not always, or even usually, complete escape. In other words, it does not mean that prior immunity confers no protection. Immune evasion can render convalescent plasma or monoclonal antibodies less effective. Fortunately, one of our current monoclonal therapies is a combination of two monoclonal antibodies. While we have seen a variant with immune evasion capabilities render one of the monoclonal antibodies much less effective, it appears that the other monoclonal antibody remains effective. Similarly, we have seen evidence that our current vaccines continue to offer protection against severe disease and death, even though they appear to offer less neutralization of the South African variant (B.1.351/501Y.V2/VOC202012/02, or "Beta"), which could result in a higher rate of reinfection (infection with a new variant in a person who was previously infected) or breakthrough infection (infection in a person who has been vaccinated). This has been our experience thus far in that variants of concern with immune escape capabilities have effectively reduced the titers of neutralizing antibody, which may allow for more infections with the variant than would occur with variants without significant immune escape capabilities. But perhaps even the reduced levels of neutralizing antibody, together with SARS-CoV-2-specific T cells, are able to prevent most individuals from becoming severely ill and thus still offer a level of protection. As of the time of this writing, the variant with the greatest degree of immune escape or evasion is the so-called Delta variant that arose in India. While our vaccines remain highly protective, the efficacy of only one dose of the two-vaccine series is markedly reduced and the efficacy against symptomatic disease in fully vaccinated individuals is reduced in percentage from the mid-90s to the high 80s, and the protection against very severe disease, hospitalization, and death appears to be reduced in percentage from nearly 100 percent to the mid-90s.

Of great anxiety to us is the fact that we now have three or more variants of concern circulating in many states. The potential exists for two variants to infect the same person, and this concern may be even greater in a person who is immunocompromised, which may allow these viruses to replicate over a much more extended period of time, resulting in a new variant through mutations or a new variant through recombination (the combination of genetic material from one virus with that from another) that has the worst features of both variants. This appears to have already happened in the city of Bristol in England, where a new variant appears to have the increased transmissibility of the United Kingdom variant (B.1.1.7/501Y.V1/VOC202012/01, or "Alpha") and the E484K mutation that appears to confer immune evasion capabilities found in the South African variant (B.1.351/501Y.V2/VOC202012/02).

The spread of a virus through a population is dependent upon many factors. Those factors include the inherent transmissibility of the virus, the immune characteristics of that population, human behavior, and environmental factors. While viral mutations can certainly change the fitness of the virus, it would be overly simplistic to ascribe all attributes of transmission and spread to these mutations. In fact, countries that were willing and able to implement significant travel restrictions and non-pharmaceutical interventions were successful in blunting disease transmission even in the face of these more transmissible variants.

Yet another concern for accelerating mutations or recombinations involving SARS-CoV-2 is the ever-growing number of animals that have been identified as being able to be infected with this virus. We explained that COVID-19 is likely a zoonotic infection, meaning that the natural host for this virus is in an animal (in this case, we believe, bats) and that the virus has expanded into a number of animal reservoirs (perhaps pangolins, among others) and then spilled over into the human population, which is not a natural host for this virus. So, too, there can be reverse zoonotic infections. In other words, humans that are infected may transmit the virus to animals that are not normally the hosts for this viral infection. We have seen many cases of what we believe are reverse zoonotic infections, with wildlife and zoo animals becoming infected by the SARS-CoV-2 virus.

The viral replication process in animals can promote more and different mutations. One example of a reverse zoonotic infection is the infection of mink on a mink farm in Denmark, presumably from a mink farm worker who was infected. The virus was then transmitted widely among the mink, which were housed in close quarters. It appears that the mink then infected a farm worker with a new mutation that we had previously not seen with human-to-human transmission.

Animal reservoirs of infection are the reason that we continue to see episodic cases reported of MERS-CoV in humans, even though we successfully thwarted a potential MERS-CoV pandemic a decade ago. One reason that we were able to eradicate smallpox through a worldwide vaccination program was that there has never been an animal reservoir identified for the smallpox virus to circulate in and eventually reintroduce itself into humans. Unfortunately, we fear that the large, and growing, animal reservoir for the SARS-CoV-2 virus means that eradication is unlikely, though this categorically does not mean that the efforts to reduce the transmission of this virus cannot and should not be pursued.

There remains much that we do not understand about this virus. Two of the most perplexing unknowns are why SARS-Co-V-2 infections come in the surges or waves that we have seen, and what accounts for the regional distribution of these surges or waves. Specifically, what causes the acceleration of disease transmission and what accounts for the often-sudden decline in transmission that produces these surges, only for another surge or wave to occur months later? And why have we seen very high levels of disease transmission in some parts of the country, while other geographic areas are having much lower levels of transmission? To use one example, why did Oregon and Washington experience fourth surges in the months of March through May of 2021, while Idaho did not experience its fourth surge until the fall, even though Oregon and Washington had much higher vaccination rates than Idaho?

A final point: the development of variants of concern is one of the major reasons that the proposals by some to encourage young adults to get back to their normal lives and get infected to accelerate our progress toward herd immunity, as discussed in chapter 12, is so dangerous and ill advised.

Recommendation #101
Concern for the Development of Variants

In future pandemics, the public and its leaders must be better educated about the dangers and risks of variants that can result if every reasonable effort is not made to control the transmission of the infection, especially when dealing with an RNA virus. Efforts for lower-risk persons to get infected to obtain immunity or for a population to intentionally try to achieve herd immunity are dangerous and risk the promotion of the development of variants.

Personal Story: "Ready to Give Life a Shot Again"

Dr. Epperly recounts his experience with a patient.

I heard him coming before I saw him. *Kerflop . . . kerflop . . . kerflop . . .* The sound grew louder as a pale, gaunt man in a red Toyota pickup truck pulled into our clinic's lot. He parked in front of the window where I was seated. As the man shut off the ignition, I could not help but notice his truck's front left tire: it was totally destroyed, with rubber shards hanging off the rim. Today was the first day of our COVID-19 vaccination clinic for patients over the age of 65.

The man, visibly shaken, was ashen gray and panting for breath. "My name's Robert, and I'm here for my vaccine," he gasped. I helped him out of the truck and into a wheelchair, then wheeled him into our clinic.

"Robert, I'm amazed that you even attempted to get to us," I said.

"For a whole year, I haven't once left my home," he replied breathlessly. "But there is no way I was going to miss this. My pickup has had that flat for over a year, and I had to drive twelve miles on it to get here. It took more than an hour." Panting and distraught, he described the trek—how passing drivers had honked and cursed at him, pointing unhelpfully at his shredded tire as the truck crawled along. "I have emphysema," he said. "I had to leave my oxygen tank behind because the tubing is all worn out."

Hearing these words, I felt stunned. What an ordeal he'd endured to reach our clinic!

After the clinic staff took him to an exam room and gave him oxygen, he started to calm down. At that point, we were able to give him his first dose of the vaccine. As he rested, I asked him how he planned to return home, and he indicated the truck: the same way that he got here. I asked him if he had family or friends to call for a ride home, but he responded no and added, "Can't leave it." I then asked him if he would allow us to replace his ruined tire with his spare. He looked up at me with dark, deep-set eyes and replied, "Won't make any difference; it's flat too."

So I asked him if he would mind us fixing his tire for him. He slowly looked up into my eyes and responded, "Would you do that?" I said we most certainly would. He then reached slowly into his pocket, pulled out his keys, and said, "Your clinic has always been full of sweethearts."

My friend Tad, our chief operating officer, happened to be at the clinic. I loaded Robert's flat spare tire into Tad's truck and Tad took it to a local tire dealer, who brought over a new tire plus a mechanic to install it on Robert's truck. When he'd finished, I wheeled Robert outside to the truck. His eyes darted to the front left tire. He didn't say a word, but tears started to roll down his face and into his mask. He was clearly overcome.

Eyes wet, he thanked me profusely for our care. "Don't worry about it," I told him. "Consider this one covered by the clinic, since it matters to us how people navigate through life."

"Would it be all right if I just sit here in the wheelchair for a while with the oxygen tank before driving back home?" he asked.

"Sure, take your time," I said. We agreed that he would take the oxygen tubing for use with his tank back home. Five minutes later, I helped him into the truck, handed him the tubing, and watched him steel himself, turn on the ignition, and drive off.

Later on, reflecting on Robert, I was struck once more by his desperation. Leaving his house for the first time in a year to drive on a flat tire down a road that must have seemed endless, all the while feeling increasingly suffocated from a lack of oxygen, testifies to just how much this vaccine meant to him.

It is powerful proof of the value of the vaccine to people who lived sheltered lives for months on end, people who were now catching their first glimpse of hope in this long, dark pandemic. For me, Robert's new tire perfectly embodied a renewal of hope.

Four weeks later, I saw Robert again, when he returned for his second vaccine shot. "I'm doing much better," he told me. "I drove here in fifteen minutes, and I have my oxygen with me. Thanks to your clinic and this vaccine, I'm ready to give life a shot again."

"Wow, Robert looks a lot better than he did a month ago," a nurse said to me as he drove away. "And so does his truck!"

At times like these, may we all pull together and take every opportunity to look out for one another.

CHAPTER 14

Preparing Schools for the Next Pandemic

> We should not expect individuals to produce good, open-minded, truth-seeking reasoning, particularly when self-interest or reputational concerns are in play. But if you put individuals together in the right way, such that some individuals can use their reasoning powers to disconfirm the claims of others, and all individuals feel some common bond or shared fate that allows them to interact civilly, you can create a group that ends up producing good reasoning as an emergent property of the social system.
>
> JONATHAN HAIDT

In many cases, school administrators and school boards were ill prepared to manage a pandemic and quite understandably so. Few, if any, had any specialized knowledge of or expertise in public health or infection control. As it turned out, however, this was not the biggest problem. There was actually plenty of expert help available for the asking from physicians and local public health organizations.

As an example, one of us (Dr. Pate) worked extensively with many local schools, both private and public, and with the largest school district in Idaho. When problems occurred, it was generally because experts were not called in soon enough. Oftentimes there was inadequate communication with both teachers and parents and an inadequate operations plan. In almost every case, there was also poor governance.

Nonetheless, there are many lessons to be learned from those schools that operated successfully in comparison with those that did not.

Lessons for School Leaders

In March of 2020, under the governor's stay-at-home order, most Idaho schools either went fully remote or just ended the school year early. Even in those early months of the pandemic, the consensus of public health experts was that the pandemic would still be with us at the start of the new school year in the fall.

Over the summer, concern grew that no one in our network of local health care leaders was aware of any public school engaging physicians to help them with their planning for the fall. In response to this, one of our most respected and expert leaders, Dr. James Souza, went before local school boards to stress the importance of having a detailed operating plan to reduce the risk of in-school transmission of the virus, just as hospitals had done to protect their staff and patients. Soon thereafter, several private schools reached out to Dr. Pate, asking for an assessment of their plans.

Recommendation #102
Include Experts in Pandemic Planning Early
School administration and boards should engage a broad array of experts early to advise them on planning during an epidemic, pandemic, or other public health emergency.

Recommendation #103
A Robust Operating Plan Is Essential
A robust operating plan is essential to operating schools safely during an epidemic or pandemic. It is critical to have the input of physicians and public health experts in creating and reviewing the plan.

The plans tended to be very good efforts on the part of schools, but most were heavily focused on the risks in the classroom, and few offered sufficient details. Seldom did plans address risks that arose from children arriving at the school campus prior to class, including the risk of students congregating near each other without masks. Similarly, the plans seldom addressed physical distancing in the hallways when changing classrooms. Plans omitted precautions for the cafeteria when students would be eating without their masks on. Infection control measures were missing for physical education and extracurricular events, including choir rehearsals, band practices, cheerleading practices, and sports and clubs. Also absent was specific guidance for students and parents when students were leaving campus at the end of the day. They frequently did not address what measures should be taken in special education classes, which pose particularly high risks since some of the students in said classes cannot tolerate wearing a mask and require hands-on instruction from a teacher. For early elementary students and some special education students, as well as for students that were deaf or hard of hearing, teachers indicated that it was important that students be able to see the teacher's tongue and mouth movements as they learned to sound out letters and words—or, in the latter case, lip-read.

Recommendation #104

Operating Plans Need to Be Comprehensive

School pandemic operations plans should address all risks from the time students and staff arrive on campus until the time they depart, and not focus solely on traditional classroom risks. As examples, plans should address the cafeteria, physical education, sports, special education, and extracurricular activities. These plans should also contain mitigation strategies for all modes of transmission of the disease.

The plans reviewed contained mitigation measures for contact (hand sanitizers and cleaning of frequently touched surfaces) and respiratory droplet transmission (physical distancing and mask wearing), but no plans were in place to address the risk of airborne transmission or how to mitigate such risk (holding classes outside when weather permits, increasing air exchanges, opening windows and doors, air filtration, the use of ionization or ultraviolet light, avoiding placing students and teachers' desks directly under air returns, and so forth). Such counteractions were especially useful given that many school buildings were old and did not have high efficiency HVAC (heating, ventilation, and air conditioning) systems, and some classrooms did not have windows.

Fortunately, private schools did ask for help over the summer prior to the opening of schools, so we had time to strengthen their plans before the first day of classes. These schools tended to have fewer outbreaks once school resumed in the fall.

For the rest of this chapter, let's take a deeper dive into the question of how to plan for a response to a pandemic by recounting the personal experience of one of us coauthors, Dr. Pate.

My many years as a hospital and health system CEO taught me that you can have plans and policies, but you never know how well they are being implemented until you actually watch your employees put them into action. Therefore, I designed a process called "walk-throughs," where I go to the school and physically walk through it to determine what risks had been missed in the plan, how well staff understood the plan, how well the plan was being implemented, and what the barriers were to implementing the plans. My walk-through methodology can be used both before students are in session and while they are in school.

Recommendation #105

School Walk-throughs

School and public health officials should consider implementing walk-throughs of schools after developing the pandemic operations plan in order to assess staff knowledge of the plan, how effectively the plan is being implemented in the school, risks that might have been missed in creating the operations plan, and barriers to the implementation of the plan.

In conducting the walk-throughs, I ask that the school principal, one of the building maintenance personnel, a classroom teacher, a teacher from each of the extracurricular activities that were not planned to be held remotely, the school nurse, and a note-taker meet me outside of the school. After introductions, I then ask what areas they are most concerned about, what questions they have about the plan in specific or the virus in general, and how have they communicated the plan to teachers, staff, parents, and students. We also discuss incentives that might work against the success of the plan, such as: would teachers lose income if they stayed home sick? Are there enough substitute teachers available that teachers do not feel pressured to come to work sick or return to work before they are completely recovered? Is it required that students have a note from a doctor to return to school after an illness, which might discourage parents from keeping their sick child home in order to avoid the cost of the doctor's visit, to eliminate the difficulty of getting a doctor's appointment, or to circumvent the predicament of having to take time off from work to bring their child to the doctor? Do parents fear negative consequences for keeping their sick child home, such as encumbering them with a significant obstacle in making up missed schoolwork or penalizing them under the attendance policy?

Then, while we are still outside, I ask them to describe what happens when students arrive on campus if school is not yet in session. How early can students arrive? If students arrive long before the start of the school day, then we must be concerned about them clustering without masks, as at that time they likely are not under the direct supervision of teachers and staff. If it is a high school, I inquire whether students can carpool or gather in someone's car in the parking lot, either of which could create significant risks. To reemphasize this point, part of keeping the school safe is preventing students from becoming infected in the parking lot or the front schoolyard before they even walk in the school doors.

I also ask about how children arrive at school. For those who are dropped off by their parents, we discuss whether the school might want to screen students before they get out of their parent's car. If there are incentives for parents to bring students to school sick, this may be an important opportunity to identify a child with fever or symptoms and not let them out of their parent's car before sending them home. This can ease the difficulties for a school that would otherwise need to bring an infected student into the building, isolating them until a parent returns to pick the child up, potentially hours later.

Similarly, we discuss children arriving on buses. It is hard to do, but it can be helpful to require a parent to accompany the child to the bus stop, have someone screen the child before getting on the bus, and, if the child has fever or symptoms, return the child home with the parent, rather than having a potentially contagious child on the bus who does not get identified until they are at school. Buses are high-risk environments because it can be difficult to achieve physical distancing, it is difficult to supervise proper mask-wearing, and the air circulation is generally not good. When the weather is suitable, it is helpful to raise the windows of the bus.

Before staff, teachers, or students enter the school building, we want to ensure that they are correctly wearing a proper mask. We often see young children in adult-sized face masks that are loose around the sides of the face and slide down the child's face. I encouraged schools to have children-sized masks available for these situations. A common error in schools' operating plans were to allow face shields as an option in place of a face mask. Face shields are intended to serve as a barrier to secretions and body fluids landing on the face of health care workers, particularly when involved in medical procedures on a patient that may cause the patient to cough or vomit with the health care provider in close proximity to the patient. Face shields provide little to no protection with respect to the transmission of SARS-CoV-2 through respiratory droplets or aerosols. It is fine for a face shield to be worn in conjunction with a face mask, but in very few circumstances is it appropriate in lieu of a face mask.

At this point, we are ready to enter the school and conduct the walk-through. As we walk through the hallways, I observe the students. Are they congregating in the hallways? Are they wearing their masks properly? We often see face masks being worn below the nose, and these students need to be instructed to pull the masks up over their nose immediately. Occasionally, someone forgets to put their mask back on when leaving the cafeteria (where they had their mask off to eat) to go to the restroom, and they need reminding.

I also look for hand sanitizers outside classrooms and restrooms and test these to ensure they are keeping the containers full. Some schools have ATMs and vending machines, and I recommend that they place sanitizer next to these in case there is a line, and someone is going to be touching the buttons immediately following someone else.

We then go to a classroom. I again observe the occupants to ensure proper mask-wearing. As I mentioned above, it can be particularly challenging for teachers of young children, who need to see the teacher's mouth and tongue move as they learn the sounds of letters and words, and for teachers who teach the deaf and hard of hearing. I generally recommend one of several clear masks that provide a good fit to the teacher's face but have a clear window so that the teacher's mouth can be seen. In instances where distancing students makes it difficult for everyone to see the teacher's face, we have explored using the same technology the school uses for remote learning but using it for students spread out in a single classroom. This allows the teacher to use video while wearing a clear mask to allow the students to see more closely the mouth movements on their computer screens.

I then look at the physical distancing of students and the physical layout of the classrooms. I look for the air returns in the room and try to ensure that a student or teacher is not sitting directly under a return, as it often happens. If so, we look at the layout of the room to determine how to reposition desks, since the SARS-CoV-2 virus aerosols are carried on airstreams and will be directed right over the student or teacher sitting under a return, creating unjustifiable risk. I also draw an imaginary line from the air supply to the air return and we try to avoid a teacher or student sitting under that line.[1] Finally, I review which surfaces are frequently touched by students, such as countertops, sinks, tables, keyboards, and desks, and we discuss the need for regular cleaning of these surfaces between students. I should point out that while transmission through fomites (inanimate objects contaminated with the virus) was suspected to be a possible route of transmission early in this pandemic, there would be little evidence to support this over time. Nevertheless, this is a good infection control practice that may play a more important role in future outbreaks with other pathogens.

We then move on to nontraditional classroom settings. In physical education, I look to see if students can be distanced and wear masks consistently. I also review the types of activities the students will engage in, discouraging those activities where students will be passing balls or sharing equipment that is difficult to clean in between students. I also encourage the schools to hold physical education and other classes outside whenever the weather is conducive, as the resulting risks for airborne transmission are dramatically reduced, if not eliminated.

For choir, I have been amazed how well most students still can sing even with masks on. I discuss with the choir teacher whether there are instances when students sing without masks. If there are, I emphasize the need to double the physical distancing due to the risks of respiratory droplets being projected further with singing, but also warn that students will remain at risk from airborne transmission, since singing will generate aerosols that will travel on the ventilation airstreams. This is also generally the time I discuss ventilation with the building maintenance expert. I ensure that they are doing at least four air exchanges per hour and, if possible, in high-risk settings like the cafeteria and performance rooms, that they increase the air exchanges to six per hour.

For band and orchestra, we have two additional issues—the sharing of instruments and the use of spit valves. While many instruments are small enough to be transported back and forth to school and are used by a single student, there are other instruments that are quite large and generally kept at the school for students' use, such as percussion instruments and large string instruments such as cellos. I review the cleaning protocol with the band teacher for the large instruments between use by students.

Brass and woodwind instruments often have spit valves. This is because as the player blows into the instrument, spit often accumulates within the instrument. Though unpleasant, in normal times, players often empty their spit valves onto the floor in front of them by forcibly blowing through the instrument with the spit valve open. While I don't know of any studies on this subject, one must be concerned about a potential aerosolizing event given that if the player is infected, virus will be contained in the spit. Thus, we look at other options, such as providing small waste containers next to players with tissues that they can blow the spit into and then dispose of the tissue in the trash receptacle. I also encourage hand sanitizer to be at each of these player's seats so that they can sanitize their hands after handling the tissues.

We then go to the cafeteria. This is a high-risk environment because students must take their masks off to eat and drink. It also is often less supervised than classrooms, which may cause students to congregate closely to visit with each other. If students go through a lunch line, I check to see how physical distancing is maintained while in line. Many schools lay down marks on the floor where students are to stand while in line to ensure distancing is preserved. I also ensure that students keep their masks on until they are seated to eat, and then place their masks back on before getting up from the table to take their trays back.

A common mistake I see is that schools take great effort to physically distance students along each side of the table. Then they shift the alignment of students across the table so that they are not sitting directly across from one another, which is good, but they don't take into consideration that this still brings students too close across from each other without their masks on. Even if student seating is staggered, we still need to take into consideration the diagonal distance between students. Without a doubt, they will turn their heads towards each other to talk during lunch.

I then generally have a discussion with the school nurse about what he or she is finding on contact tracing, whether there is any evidence of in-school transmission, and whether the nurse has any concerns that we should discuss.

Finally, sports. Each sport must be examined specifically. Are the student athletes able to wear masks during practices and at games or tournaments? To what extent can students be distanced? Do the students have to travel to away games? Do they carpool or ride buses? Do they have to huddle or meet closely with the coaches without masks? Let me share a couple of examples to illustrate how I simply must observe the practice or game to determine the risks.

When I expressed concern about winter sports due to the high levels of community spread, a basketball coach told me about all the precautions they were taking—players and coaches wearing masks, each player having their own water bottle, keeping players distanced, and so on, which sounded very reassuring. And so, I went to observe a practice. As I entered the court with the principal, three players who had face masks under their noses immediately pulled the masks up. We must be particularly diligent about proper mask-wearing when students are exercising, because deep, rapid breathing can propel respiratory droplets further and with greater amounts of virus in the droplets. Though we transmit these droplets mostly though our mouths, we can transmit them from our noses, and more importantly, the nasal passages are lined with the ACE-2 receptor and thus completely exposed to infection from another player or coach when the mask is worn below the nose.

I then watched them perform a routine where they lined up to shoot baskets and then go off to the side of the court. After they made their shot, they moved off of the court, where they high-fived players already there. Obviously, we want to keep athletes distanced as much as possible and prevent them from coming into direct physical contact with each other. Just as we should not be shaking hands right now, so too should we not be high-fiving others.

I then observed a coach pull his mask down to yell out new instructions for the team. Again, when yelling, respiratory droplets are propelled a further distance and if the person is infected, the droplets will contain greater amounts of virus. Further, yelling also generates many more aerosols that can travel throughout the open space on air streams and increase the risk for airborne transmission. I recommended that the school get the coaches bullhorns to amplify their voices while allowing them to keep their masks on.

Here is one more example. I had a parent ask me whether it was safe for their child to participate on the swim team. Now, all things considered, from a COVID-19 standpoint, swimming should be one of the safer sports. I agreed with the parent that swimming itself, with swimmers in their own lanes and not coming into physical contact with one another, is pretty safe. But then I pointed out that this was not the end of the analysis. We must consider that some swim practices and meets will be indoors, and obviously swimmers cannot wear masks while swimming. If teammates were to congregate at the side of the pool without masks and then yell to cheer on their teammates, this could now transform a relatively safe sport into one presenting a much higher risk. We also must consider some of the same issues I raised for other sports—are there going to be team meetings with the coach in close contact without masks? Are there going to be carpooling or bus rides for away meets? Locker rooms pose an additional concern for both respiratory droplet and aerosol transmission, given the proximity of lockers and the inability to wear masks while showering.

So, in dealing early on in the summer with the private schools, there was plenty of time to review and improve their operating plans. By and large, those schools have done very well, with little in-school transmission and no need to shift to remote learning due to clusters or outbreaks.

In contrast, I was not asked for help by a large public school system until October 2020, when they were already in trouble. Parents and teachers were both unhappy, but for different reasons, on how the schools were being operated. Teachers were threatening a "sick-out," because they did not feel that they were being heard. Large numbers of teachers were on the verge of calling in sick for a couple of days, which would have closed the schools. Meanwhile, some parents were picketing and protesting outside the school district headquarters. Others were showing up angry at school board meetings. We had to work fast to restore the trust of these important stakeholders and improve the operational plans, because we were in the upswing of a new surge in cases in the community.

The first thing I did was review their operating plan. Unfortunately, it was poorly organized, way too lengthy to expect anyone to read and comprehend it. It contained ill-advised infection control measures and it did not cover the areas of risk that I discussed above in my discussion about walk-throughs. Thus, I asked whether I could just rewrite the plan, to which they promptly agreed. This gave me the opportunity, based on earlier experiences, to create a best-in-class operating plan.

What do I think was good about the plan? First, I reduced the former plan, which was heavily laden with more than 100 pages, to just 16 pages, something that we could reasonably expect everyone to read and comprehend. Secondly, because we desperately needed parents to be our partners in operating the schools safely, unlike any operating plan I had seen before, this plan was written for parents, not just for staff and teachers.

I started the plan with a high-level explanation about how SARS-CoV-2 is transmitted. We needed parents, staff, and teachers to all understand these modes of transmission so that they would understand why we were asking them to take the precautions we were asking of them.

I then included a section entitled "What are the most important things for me to know to protect myself, the staff and teachers at my school and the students?" This section was a very concise list of all the things we were asking of students, parents, and teachers so that everyone was clear about their responsibilities. If they read nothing else in the plan, this would at least make sure they were alerted to what the most important things to know were. It included encouragement for everyone to get a flu shot and people to stay home if they were ill. It gave them concise directives as to how to select a proper mask and how to wear it properly.

Then, I included a section that I have never seen in an operating plan before: "Before the school day begins." This section provided instructions for parents, including how to ensure their child has a clean face mask and a backup in case the mask is dropped on the floor or becomes soiled. It outlined for them how to check their child's temperature and ask them about any COVID-related symptoms, and encouraged them to consistently remind their child of the importance of wearing their mask and physical distancing.

The next section gave instructions on measures to take when sending children to school, including precautions to take if their child would be riding the school bus. That was followed by instructions on additional precautions to take upon arrival at school. The plan continued to provide instructions for the logical sequence of events once their child arrives at school—precautions to take in the hallways, followed by instructions for the classroom.

The plan went on to cover the precautions to be taken at recess, in the cafeteria, and during physical education classes, as well as instructions for the safe dismissal of students at the end of the day. The plan also gave guidance for parent-teacher conferences.

I repeatedly highlighted in bold the same key phrases—wearing proper masks properly, maintaining a safe physical distance of at least six feet, and frequent handwashing or sanitizing—throughout the plan to reinforce these most fundamental and important of all measures.

I then provided guidance on dealing with a sick teacher or student, on how to deal with an exposure, and on recommended contact tracing procedures and precautions for special education, sports, choir, band and orchestra, cheerleading and clubs. These items were organized into appendices to keep the overall plan short, especially since not everyone needs to read these additional materials.

After reconstructing the plan in this way, the next step was to get the school board's approval and then to circulate it and review it with staff, teachers, and parents. Part of this process were webinars that I held with parents and teachers to answer questions about SARS-CoV-2, COVID-19, and the operating plan. We received positive feedback about these Q&As and we recorded them and posted them to the school district's website so that those who were unable to listen to the live webinar could listen to them later when convenient for them.

Although revising the plan was the priority, I also indicated to the team that it was essential to work to regain the trust of teachers and parents. This would require enhanced communication and transparency. Whereas data on what was happening in the schools had before been closely guarded, I instead stressed the importance of sharing all the data publicly (with the proper privacy protections for individuals). I indicated that instead of asking attorneys how we can protect as much of the data as possible, we should ask attorneys how we can share the most data possible.

The operating plan was well received, the enhanced communication was welcomed, and posting data publicly on the website about cases in schools presented a good narrative on how we were able to operate schools safely.

The final step was to begin conducting public school walk-throughs to see how well the operating plan was being implemented and what barriers remained.

Recommendation #106
School Communications
Schools should communicate clearly and frequently with teachers and parents and ensure that they keep these important stakeholders updated. Communication and transparency are key to maintaining the trust of stakeholders. Schools should post publicly as much data as is meaningful and practical to give teachers and parents an understanding of how well the school is keeping students and staff safe.

Lessons for School Boards

I attended or watched remotely more than my share of school board meetings, especially during the fall and winter of 2020–2021. These were often long, drawn-out meetings with random musings and expressions of opinions. The meetings were characterized by unstructured decision-making, culminating in a vote based on an unclear decision path. This meandering often left either parents or teachers (and not infrequently both) bewildered and frustrated. More confusing was the fact that decisions made within a short interval of time sometimes seemed internally inconsistent. As an example, one week, a school board decided that the community transmission and case rates were so high that all students should receive remote online instruction. The following week, this same board decided that despite all classes being held remotely, athletics could resume in person as normal. This led to a lot of head-scratching, as the board offered no explanation as to how they arrived at this decision.

I do feel sorry for these board members, to an extent. The ones I dealt with were volunteers and generally had little understanding or expertise in public health. Few, if any, had ever served in a top leadership position or sat on the board of a large organization that must make trade-offs while dealing with huge risks and complexities. These school board members were being vigorously lobbied by multiple stakeholders with disparate views. In some cases, recall initiatives were discussed or launched. They clearly were under great pressure, but it did not have to be this way.

School boards were not the first boards to have to deal with a rapidly evolving situation involving significant risk. Unfortunately, these local boards did not avail themselves of the governance expertise that resided in our communities—namely, retired leaders who had run large, complex companies; companies that often dealt with high-risk environments. Instead, there were some cases of infighting on boards that led to further dysfunction, up to and including resignations from the boards.

What was missing was an overarching decision-making framework. This explains why school board meetings seemed to wander aimlessly. The discussions consisted of more opinions than real data or expert guidance, and some decisions made by the boards seemed inexplicable, further contributing to the stakeholders' mistrust.

So, how could public school boards have done things differently? For that, we must go back to the spring of 2020, when the pandemic was taking hold in the United States and schools were going remote or closing for the rest of the school year. At that time, there was debate about whether SARS-CoV-2 activity might be seasonal and thus ease up or even go away over the summer (it wasn't and it didn't). However, almost all experts agreed that even if a seasonal reduction were the case, the virus would be back in the fall and very likely with higher rates of infection cases. Spring and summer should have been the opportunity for school boards to begin planning for the fall, while they had the time to create a thoughtful decision-making framework.

To do this, school boards should have first identified their stakeholders and the experts available to the boards. Instead of disenfranchising teachers and parents and losing their trust, parents and teachers could have been brought into the process right from the beginning so that they could provide input. This would have given parents and teachers the benefit of understanding how decisions would be made.

Boards would then set out their overarching goal—something like this: "Our objective is to have as many students physically present in school in the fall as possible while still allowing us to keep staff, teachers, students, and their families safe. Furthermore, our goal is to make sure that schools are not contributing to community spread." Instead, many schools did little planning over the summer, and those that did often started problem solving without identifying the goals.

Boards could then select parents and teachers who were open-minded, willing to be guided by evidence in their decision-making, willing to be ambassadors and communicators to other teachers or parents, willing to make the necessary commitment of time to attend meetings and participate on committees, and who expressed agreement with the overarching goals.

The board would then solicit from the administration, teachers, and parents what factors should be considered in arriving at decisions in the new school year. It would institute strategies on when and how schools should be operated full-time and in-person or by using a hybrid model. Beyond that, it would determine whether or when schools must go to remote learning, and what factors should be considered when deciding whether sports and other extracurricular events should or should not be held.

This process would also respond to concerns I have heard raised about going remote that include the lack of effectiveness of online learning, the impact on mental health issues in children who cannot attend school, the problems of kids going hungry because they would not get adequate meals at home that are provided at school, the increase in child abuse and the inability to provide the necessary level of support at home to special needs students according to their IEP (Individualized Educational Plan) or 504 (section 504 of the Rehabilitation Act) plan.

In general, this approach would help planners contend with the balancing act required between implementing full, in-person classroom attendance, which would tamp down stay-at-home problems versus the possibility of in-school transmission between teachers and students, the contribution to community spread from infections occurring in school, and the risk to teachers' and students' families of bringing the infection home from school.

There may very well be additional concerns, but the main objective is to get the stakeholders to put all the concerns out on the table. Then, the board should determine whether the concerns raised affect any decision they would make that would tip the balance between reopening schools or going to remote learning.

Once the universe of concerns material to the board's future decision-making are identified, a large group of stakeholders can then be convened consisting of board members, school administrators, teachers, parents, and possibly even some high school students. The next task is to appoint co-chairs or a chair and vice-chair (it is important to identify two people in case one becomes ill or otherwise is unable to attend one or more meetings so that the momentum and progress can be maintained). Then, a timeline needs to be established for the committee to complete its work in time to prepare the school board to make decisions about if and how school will reopen in the fall.

The charter of this committee is to review and understand concerns that are identified as material to the board's decision-making. The committee can then put these concerns into perspective and determine whether there are ways to mitigate them, whether they can be monitored, and whether there are ways to rank and prioritize them. This will be done by inviting experts to educate and advise the committee as a whole or through subcommittees if the co-chairs decide to divide up the work. I suggest recording as many of these meetings as possible and posting them on the school website so that all stakeholders not on the committee can understand the work and the issues.

As an example, let us say that the board decides that the issue of food insecurity would tend to cause the board to be less willing to shift to remote learning if disease activity increased during the fall. The committee, or a subcommittee if one is constituted, would want to understand from experts and from the school's data how many of their students' families are food insecure. They would also want to understand how this problem is addressed during school breaks, holidays, and over the summer recess. If classes are fully remote, I should think they would also want to explore what alternatives there are to get meals to these children's homes (food banks, meals on wheels, volunteers, and so forth), or whether it is feasible for parents to swing by the school during a certain time of day to pick up meals. These questions are aimed at determining whether the concern of food insecurity can be dealt with should schools have to go remote.

Let us take another example and assume that the board determines that the mental health of students is a material factor in their decision-making and might cause them to resist moving students to remote instruction, even in the face of worsening community spread of disease. Again, the committee or subcommittee would want to hear from experts as to how big a problem this is. I would think that they would also want to know if there are ways to identify those who would be at higher risk and ways to intervene to maintain those student's mental health. Furthermore, I would think that the committee would want to understand ways to monitor students' mental health, perhaps with the use of technology. One example: there is emerging technology that can determine whether a student's interaction with the program is slow, perhaps signaling depression. It can examine word choices and apply algorithms that may suggest the student is depressed or even suicidal. It could be that there are ways to monitor students' mental health through these means, along with periodic calls to high-risk students by school counselors. It may also be possible to track visits to mental health professionals, log calls from parents to school counselors for help for their child, and monitor suicide attempts. Of course, the committee or subcommittee will also want to understand various options to reduce these problems.

In addition, when mental health is raised as a reason why kids must be in school, there never seems to be debate about the other side of the coin: what are the residual mental health effects on students who get COVID-19? What is the frequency of those effects? What is the psychological injury to an older child who realizes that they likely infected a family member, who then requires hospitalization or dies? It is important that the committee attempts to evaluate all sides of an issue and resists leaning on biases or preconceived notions.

Finally, with respect to the mental health of students, it seems that we lost an opportunity to teach families and students about coping mechanisms and developing resilience. More and more, we have realized that a large factor in whether individuals in all kinds of work develop burnout later in life can be tied in large part to resilience. Without appearing to be insensitive to the stress caused by remote learning, we must acknowledge that this is unlikely to be the greatest challenge that these children will ever face in their lives. This was a golden opportunity to teach this skill and help students through the current challenge, while also preparing them for the future challenges they are likely to face. It also would have benefited many parents to cope with the stress and model positive behaviors for their children. No doubt, in many cases, it was the stressed parents who contributed more to the child's stress than the remote learning. We often saw parents bringing young children to protests or school board meetings, where the parent got up to speak and yelled or cried.

After the committee has developed an understanding of all these concerns from school administrators and experts, they will want to weigh these issues to assist the board in its decision-making. For example, the committee might very well decide after reviewing data on how many of their students live in multigenerational homes with older individuals at high risk for severe disease or death and on how many students live in homes where one or both parents or a sibling has a severe medical condition that would place them at high risk, that the risk of students falling behind in their learning with online classes should be weighed less than the risk of children infecting high-risk family members.

Once factors that would go into the board's decision-making have been identified and weighed, the committee would then determine how those factors can be assessed, measured, updated, and reported to the board through the school year. A dashboard can be created with the factors listed in descending order according to the weighting.

The beauty of this approach is that it engages stakeholders. The dashboard can be regularly updated and posted to the website for transparency. As a result, everyone will understand how decisions are being made. The board will now have a decision framework to use to make these difficult decisions, and board meetings can be much more streamlined and focused on metrics. If the board uses the provided decision-making framework faithfully, it can avoid a multitude of internally inconsistent decisions and all stakeholders can understand what the board considered and how they came to decisions made during the school year.

The result should be more objective decision-making and less infighting on boards, fewer resignations, less pressure on board members from lobbying or protesting stakeholders, and more trust from the stakeholders. There is clearly much to be gained by including stakeholders in the process, giving them respected input into creating the decision-making framework.

Recommendation #107

Decision-Making Framework

School boards need to establish a decision-making framework to focus their decision making, to promote transparency as to how they are making decisions, to streamline board meetings, to ensure internal consistency of their decisions, to reduce the stress and pressure on board members, and to reduce in-fighting among board members. Stakeholders should be engaged in the process of creating the decision-making framework.

How a School Board Lost Trust

The following passage is reproduced from a Facebook posting by WAEA—West Ada Education Association—dated February 7, 2021.

> Soon the West Ada School Board will be voting to move our secondary schools to 100% in-person instruction. This decision will likely affect thousands of families' lives and routines in profound ways. They are doing this without listening to or asking the opinion of teachers, staff members, students or parents in the district.
>
> By eliminating social distancing from our plan, we are ignoring warnings coming to us from around the world. Dr. Pate and other medical professionals have indicated great concern about the variants of COVID

currently being spread through the U.S. Specifically the B.1.1.7 variant that has forced school in the U.K. back into full remote instruction.

Recommendations to avoid the need for fully remote instruction focus on the importance of physical distancing. Adopting the current recommendation dismisses the risk of widespread outbreaks, and provides no reason for doing so.

The School Board, and many community members, have made the claim that the hybrid schedule has been bad for learning. They do so with nothing more than anecdotal data, most of which dates back to last spring. While no one would deny that synchronous instruction has introduced new challenges, many teachers have communicated success in learning this year due to the benefits of lowered class sizes, and increased access to instructors and digital content. The disruption to learning caused by bounding between instructional strategies could be far worse than simply maintaining the hybrid schedule. A schedule that teachers and students have been able to adjust to, and one that they can thrive in if only they are given some sort of stability.

It is unprincipled to make such a large decision for so many people, without regard for what they think, with no evidence that they will be safe and with no guarantee learning will be improved.

As a district we have adopted the High Reliability schools model. The foundation of HRS is the safe supportive and collaborative schools for all students and staff. These criteria give no considerations for the safety of students, staff or our community at large. Input from students, teachers and community members was not sought. Many teachers and students are being left unsupported. The school board requires educators and staff to adhere to HRS guidelines, why is this important decision being made without adhering to these same ideals?

CHAPTER 15

Leadership Lessons from the Pandemic

You can't tweet change.

ANGELA BLANCHARD

The COVID-19 pandemic has taught us many things but arguably none more important than lessons in leadership.

We coauthors fought incessantly throughout the pandemic to keep politics out of it. We both believe that politics should have no part in managing and responding to a pandemic. But despite this, we witnessed politicization by others that antagonized our public health efforts, contributed to more disease and deaths, and prolonged the pandemic. It is even creating a barrier to our efforts to vaccinate a sufficient percentage of the population to bring the spread of SARS-CoV-2 to an end, or at least to sufficiently low levels of transmission that the virus will not threaten to overwhelm our health care system and produce more variants of concern.

But, as the cliché goes, leadership starts at the top. We cannot avoid the fact that a Republican was president, and that president was Donald Trump, during the initial response to the pandemic. No doubt we would have uncovered leadership lessons and provided constructive criticism, or at least opportunities for improvement, no matter who was in office and no matter what their politics were. No president could be expected to flawlessly oversee a pandemic with a novel virus for such a long period of time. There would be mistakes.

However, since Donald Trump was the president, we must learn from his particular mistakes. This is not to attack the Republican Party in general or the president specifically, but rather we want to ensure that when the next pandemic strikes, whoever is president and no matter which party the president represents, we have done all we can not to repeat the errors of the past. In fact, this is the entire purpose of our book and the very reason why the first epigraph of our book comes from thinker George Santayana: "Those who cannot remember the past are condemned to repeat it."

The leadership lessons learned from this pandemic derive from more than just the president. The vice president, members of the president's cabinet, leaders of agencies, legislators, governors, public health leaders, county commissioners, mayors, school board members, the press and media, and religious leaders all offer many lessons.

Lesson 1: Risk and Threat Assessment

"Some risks that are thought to be unknown, are not unknown," wrote Daniel Wagner. "With some foresight and critical thought, some risks that at first glance may seem unforeseen, can in fact be foreseen. Armed with the right set of tools, procedures, knowledge and insight, light can be shed on variables that lead to risk, allowing us to manage them."

Every organization and every government face risks and threats. It is important for leaders to work with their teams to seek out and identify all the material risks and threats they can think of. Those teams then need to prioritize the risks and threats by asking themselves three questions:

1. How likely is a particular threat compared to other identified risks and threats?
2. How damaging to the organization or the government would the risk or threat be if it materialized?
3. If the risk or threat cannot be eliminated, can it be reduced or mitigated?

Once these questions are answered, it is possible to take the list of risks and threats and prioritize them from the most severe to the least. The leader and team can then determine where to draw a cutoff line, below which the team is not going to allocate time, efforts, and attention at the highest organizational or governmental levels. It is not that you ignore the risks or threats below the cutoff line; on the contrary, these are delegated downward to departments or agencies within the organization or government, who are then charged to devise plans to address and monitor these items.

For the risks and threats above the cutoff line, the leader and the team can now plot them on the x-axis according to the likelihood of the event occurring and on the y-axis according to the severity of the impact if the event does occur. If one were to divide the resulting graph, like that depicted in figure 15.1, into four quadrants, the leader now has a framework for identifying the risks to focus on the most. This graph can also be updated as new risks emerge or old risks diminish.

Imagine that a leader and advisors have identified risks of priority by the likelihood the risk could materialize and by the harm that would occur to the organization if the risk became manifest. In this example, the top risks that the leadership team decided to address are plotted in the graph of figure 15.1. The risks in the right upper quadrant will be

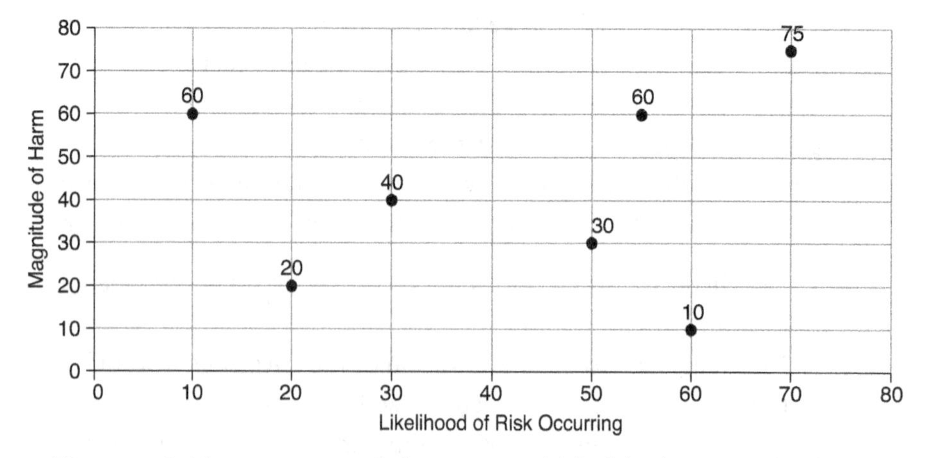

Figure 15.1. A risk assessment graph that measures risk both by the magnitude of harmful outcome and by the likelihood of it occurring.

the ones they will most aggressively seek to address. For example, the risks associated with the coordinates 55 and 60 and 70 and 75 are among the top three risks most likely to occur and among those most damaging to the organization if they do. On the other hand, the risks associated with other coordinates, (50, 30) and (60, 10) in the right lower quadrant, are less deserving of the team's time and attention. Although they are among the top four risks most likely to materialize, they are among the bottom three risks in terms of the degree of harm they might cause to the organization. These are risks that a business's leaders might decide are better addressed by purchasing insurance rather than devoting a lot of organizational resources to trying to reduce the risk. Finally, the leadership team will likely decide that the risk associated with the coordinates 10 and 60 deserves a review for possible mitigation measures. Although it is the least likely to occur among the team's prioritized risks, it is among the top three risks with respect to the amount of harm to the organization should the risk actually materialize.

Part of the process would be for the leader and team to understand why the risks and threats exist, what might be done to reduce the likelihood of the risks occurring and what could be done to mitigate the harm to the organization if they were to occur. To understand the risks, scenario planning or mock drills may be helpful. The Department of Defense does this frequently with threat assessments and war planning. The federal government has done this on several occasions around the threat of a pandemic. Though we don't have detailed reports, one can surmise that since they were doing this scenario planning and mock drills, the White House must have previously assessed the likelihood of a pandemic as at least high enough to raise this to the level of engagement of the senior team. Unfortunately, it does not appear to follow that they fully appreciated the harm to the country that could ensue from a pandemic and thus did not take adequate mitigation steps.

Recommendation #108

Risk Assessment

The best leaders conduct a threat or enterprise risk assessment. All leaders need to know as best they can what threats are possible, how likely those threats are, what the extent of harm would be if the threat materialized, and how to mitigate the threats or risks.

Lesson 2: Understand Vulnerabilities and Devise Mitigation Plans

A pandemic was identified by the government as a substantial threat. Scenario planning and mock simulations were done to identify the vulnerabilities. While the report of the most recent drill prior to the SARS-CoV-2 pandemic is not publicly available, there have been various reports that it was recognized that the Strategic National Stockpile did not have enough supplies and equipment if a large part of the country was affected all at once, though this was certainly conceivable in the setting of a pandemic. It was also revealed that there was a lack of clarity of roles within the federal government between agencies and poor coordination between the federal government and states.

Both of these vulnerabilities were recognized during the management of the SARS-CoV-2 pandemic during 2020. Unfortunately, the president and his senior team had not then put in place mitigation plans to address these vulnerabilities.

Recommendation #109

Risk Mitigation

Once material risks and threats are identified, great leaders conduct a thorough evaluation of the vulnerabilities and create mitigation plans.

Lesson 3: Create Teams with Expertise, Different Backgrounds, and a Willingness to Speak Up in Disagreement

Great leaders abhor group-think. These leaders know that they make the best decisions when those decisions are made following intense review and robust debate among the team. Difficult decisions are difficult usually because there is no clear answer and because the stakes are high if the wrong decision is made. Both of us either are or have been CEOs of complex organizations that operate in an environment of high risk. We know that the least helpful thing for us in making a difficult decision is to have people politely agreeing with us who don't actually agree, but who themselves feel no ownership of the problem or accountability for the decision. One of the great values we get from our teams is having them voice differing points of views and pointing out different perspectives on the matter. We do not seek disagreement among our teams to have conflict; we seek it to ensure that we have thought of all sides of an issue before making a difficult decision.

A danger of being a leader is having everyone perfunctorily reinforce your biases, making you even more committed to them. As described in chapter 11, this happened broadly in the country when many in the public reinforced their biases by reading or listening only to news sources or people who shared their views. This can also happen to leaders.

We saw this play out with President Trump, who became increasingly frustrated with his medical leaders and advisors that would not play down the virus as much as he wanted. He felt stymied by their unwillingness to agree with his prediction of a rapid end to the pandemic and by their reluctance to agree with his unsupported views on prevention and treatment strategies. In reaction, the president hired a neuroradiologist with no recognized expertise in infectious diseases, virology, or public health to be an advisor to his administration after he watched this physician espouse views on Fox News about the SARS-CoV-2 virus, COVID-19, and the pandemic. While these views were quite consistent with those of President Trump, they were strikingly out of the mainstream of medical and public health experts.[1] Unfortunately, in the end, surrounding himself only with people who faithfully shared his views resulted in the president not taking the proper steps to contain the spread of the virus and ultimately led to his own serious infection, followed by his loss in the 2020 presidential election.

Even if a leader encourages an environment that nourishes expertise and a variety of perspectives, if this leader does not invite intelligent debate and does not provide the opportunity for it, it may not happen. Worse, in the case of President Trump, he retaliated against those who offered different views with methods including intimidation, removing those who disagreed with him from meetings and press conferences, and even termination.

Dr. Deborah Birx, a member of the White House Coronavirus Task Force for the Trump administration, recalled the very difficult position she found herself in when during a press conference, President Trump, while speaking from the platform, turned to her and suggested that medical experts should explore how we could inject light or disinfectants into the human body to cure COVID-19. Of course, Dr. Birx knew, as do most physicians, that these are dangerous theories that could harm or kill people. Drs. Birx and Anthony Fauci have both explained the challenges associated with disagreeing with President Trump. Their quandary was that expressing too much disagreement, too publicly, could result in their firing and the fear that their replacements might be picked primarily for supporting the president's views in lockstep rather than for expertise in managing a pandemic.

We also saw this dynamic play out in the Idaho legislature, as well as in one of the public health district boards, where physicians were selected because they promoted debunked medical positions that supported the biases of the legislators and board members selecting them. So, too, we saw a school district in Idaho dismiss physician advisors when they would not support and endorse the plans that the board members had preemptively made.

When a leader is in fact wrong, any of these behaviors—hiring or inviting advice from people without expertise because they support your views, dismissing or terminating advisors or teammates because they do not, engaging in opinion-shopping, creating an environment where people are afraid to express differing views—merely facilitates the leader's desire to pursue the wrong course of action.

Recommendation #110
Teams Should Reflect Different Backgrounds, Experiences, and Points of View

Great leaders should surround themselves with team members who are recognized experts in their fields, who come from diverse backgrounds and have diverse experiences, who often think about things differently than the leader does, and who are not hesitant to offer contrary thoughts and opinions to, or even correct, the leader.

Lesson 4: Honesty Is the Best Policy

This is an axiom that remains true even to this day. Far more leaders have suffered undesired consequences from lying or concealing the truth than from telling it. It should be pointed out that telling the truth in leadership is not the same as telling the truth in a court of law, where a witness is sworn to tell the truth, the whole truth, and nothing but the truth. Leaders often do not need to tell the whole truth, and sometimes they cannot, whether because of restrictions resulting from security or confidentiality laws or a need to safeguard company or governmental competitive information and secrets. There will also be times when a leader has information the public or employees do not benefit from knowing. In such instances, disclosure may not be advised if doing so will only promote anxiety and no productive actions. There may also be times when less than full disclosure of the whole truth is necessary for national security purposes. Imagine if the president was holding a press conference about an egregious act carried out by a foreign power. While the president should tell the truth and nothing but the truth, that does not mean that the president must or even should disclose the whole truth, including military actions he or she may be contemplating. It also does not mean that the president must answer every question asked. But when the president does answer a question, it should be truthful as the president understands it at that time.

As we discussed in chapter 11, when there is a significant and unexpected event, it is important for leaders to get their messages out quickly. The goal should be to explain to employees and the public what is happening, how it happened, and why it is happening. For many, it is anxiety-provoking to not understand how unexpected events that may impact their lives happened. In the absence of information and an explanation, they will fill those gaps with rumors, conspiracy theories, or alternative explanations.

Further, if a company needs the help of its employees to address an unexpected event or the government needs to enlist aid from the public, then lying, concealing important information, blocking transparency, or minimizing or denying a problem undermines the faith, confidence, and trust in leaders. This, in turn, discourages people from following these leaders. Furthermore, should the time come when the leader must after all admit the problem and ask for employees' or the public's help, it will be much more difficult to enlist that support and assistance.

Recommendation #111

Honesty Is Still the Best Policy

Leaders should tell the truth. The trust and confidence of those you are privileged to lead depend on this. In a time of emergency or crisis, the American people are best served by understanding the truth as we know it, so that they can make informed decisions about whether and how to change their behavior to adjust to the new threat.

Lesson 5: Focus

We saw many examples of dysfunction when leaders failed to focus. Of course, it is also possible to create a dysfunctional response when you focus too narrowly on a problem. For example, Operation Warp Speed had many successes. It also had some failures. The leadership was so consumed with developing, testing, manufacturing, and distributing vaccines, they failed to assess whether states had the resources and capabilities to administer the vaccines effectively and efficiently. This reminds us of the common refrain that vaccines do not save lives; vaccinations do. Thus, Operation Warp Speed was a huge success in getting vaccines developed in a short timeline and getting them manufactured, but it was a huge failure, even by its own targets, in getting vaccine doses into the arms of Americans.

In the Idaho legislature, we saw a parade of examples of the dysfunction that can happen due to lack of focus on the real problem. In the current legislative session, lawmakers have debated and promoted bills that aim to weaken the available public health measures to control the spread of disease—taking away the authority of the governor to declare an emergency, prohibiting limits on size of gatherings, prohibiting mask mandates, and so on. The legislature has not held one hearing to explore lessons learned from this pandemic or proposed one bill to better prepare our state for the next pandemic.

In addition, as we discussed in chapter 14, Idaho school boards often lost focus and became easily distracted, failing to develop a decision-making framework to allow them to target data and monitoring that would inform their decisions.

Recommendation #112

Focus

During a time of impending threat, great leaders need to focus. These leaders redirect their attention, and that of their team, away from distractions and non-pressing matters toward the need for planning, monitoring, and responding to the threat.

Lesson 6: Accountability

A great leader takes accountability for mistakes, mishaps, and bad outcomes, even when they are not personally responsible for the event. These leaders certainly do not blame others publicly for mistakes that happen within their organization. When a reporter asked President Trump in March 2020 whether he took responsibility for the delay in making COVID-19 testing available to the public, he replied, "No. I don't take responsibility at all."

Now, we think that the public, in general, understands that not everything goes well or as intended all the time, even more so during an emergency and under new circumstances. But we also suspect that the public expects our leaders to be in charge, to be accountable for the team's response to an emergency. It seems unlikely that anyone would expect that President Trump was directly involved in developing the COVID-19 tests, so taking accountability would not have reflected President Trump's personal failure, but rather that he was invested and accepted ownership for the overall response. As Dr. Pate often tells developing leaders: you will get credit as the leader for many things that go well, even though you had little to do personally with the success, but with that comes accepting blame for the things that do not go as intended, even though you personally had little to do that outcome either.

Recommendation #113
Accountability
Great leaders take end-to-end accountability for everything that happens within their organization, their agency, or their government, even when they are not personally responsible for causing the undesired outcome.

Lesson 7: Create a Vision, Develop a Strategy to Achieve It, and Inspire People

Great leaders need to create a clear and compelling vision of what they are trying to achieve. This vision must be communicated in a way that inspires others to action. The communication about the vision needs to answer the question of *why* it needs to be achieved. A compelling vision for the COVID-19 pandemic that could have been developed in the early days of the pandemic might have sounded like this: "We will sacrifice now to preserve our lives and our economy so that we can return to normal sooner."

The message supporting this vision would state that the COVID-19 pandemic is a real and serious threat to our country that will test the mettle of our nation and each of us individually. However, if we all join together and protect each other, we can control the spread of this virus, by following public health guidelines, such as physical distancing, restrictions on size of gatherings, frequent handwashing, and the use of masks when around those we don't live with. Slowing the spread of this disease will not only make all of us safer, but it will also allow us time to develop a vaccine that can protect us and allow us to return to some sense of normalcy in our lives.

While many reading this messaging a year into the pandemic might scoff at this suggestion, keep in mind that your reaction is likely tainted by messages that were inconsistent, not supported by science or evidence, and were laced with misinformation, disinformation, and conspiracy theories. A year later, all the opportunities for that vision, planning, and messaging had been squandered, and one cannot undo that damage. Had President Trump embraced this approach back in February and March of 2020, it should be clear now that the tone and rhetoric of his regard for public health recommendations would almost certainly have been much better.

A vision of this sort serves several purposes. It states clearly that the attainment of the vision requires sacrifice. The sacrifice and the goal of saving lives speaks to the need to promote cooperative collectivism and not inwardly focused individualism. Finally, for those that would be asked to sacrifice, but aren't themselves at high-risk, it holds out the promise of the preservation of our economy and a sooner return to normal in exchange for that sacrifice.

If there was any doubt about the power and influence of the president and his words as we entered 2020, it should now be clear that President Trump would have strongly influenced a significant percentage of the American people. Had he been honest, he could have promoted the need to take public health precautions, urged the public to follow public health leaders' science-based advice, and role-modelled those behaviors himself. He would have then consistently communicated this vision to the public and relentlessly stayed on script, reinforcing these public health messages throughout the pandemic.

Finally, while doing so is important, it is not sufficient to set out a vision and inspire those who one leads. There must be a strategy and a plan to achieve the vision. A major failing of the Trump administration was that there never was a pandemic plan. Certainly there were pieces of a plan, such as Operation Warp Speed. But what the country, states, and public health officials needed was a comprehensive plan.

Recommendation #114

A Vision and a Strategic Plan Are Essential

In times of uncertainty, leaders need to set out a compelling vision, develop a comprehensive strategic and operating plan as to how to achieve that vision, communicate and distribute those plans, and speak often, consistently, and passionately about the vision and the plans to inspire others to embrace the vision and assist in executing the plans.

Lesson 8: Maintain Perspective

For good reason, we are programmed to focus very narrowly on a threat and not to be distracted by other things while facing danger. This is part of our fight-or-flight response. On a beautiful, peaceful day, we might observe the beauty of the stars in the night sky or the colors of leaves in the fall. However, if a danger presented itself, we would become focused on the threat and no longer have any conscious awareness of those stars or colorful trees. Obviously, this is good and important for our self-preservation.

However, during a prolonged crisis or danger lasting months, that kind of response is not healthy. We will become physically and emotionally exhausted. It will also affect our mood and outlook. This is where leaders must step in to express appreciation, to encourage people to take care of themselves, and to offer hope and optimism.

Part of helping to gain more compliance with public health measures is reminding people that these are temporary. Some of the resistance we saw was from people who believed that mask mandates would last into perpetuity. Of course, none of the medical and public health experts expected that to be the case, so leaders needed to help the public put these measures into perspective—they would only be necessary until such time that we can get the disease transmission under good control.

Recommendation #115

Maintain and Help Others Maintain Perspective

Leaders should help the public maintain a proper sense of perspective during the public health crisis. In an effort to promote compliance with public health guidance, leaders should frequently remind the public that the compliance measures are temporary and only needed until such time that the transmission of infection and disease can be controlled and contained.

Lesson 9: Flexibility and Nimbleness

It should not be surprising that there will be unexpected developments during a pandemic with a novel organism. As we previously mentioned, communications early on in a pandemic with a novel pathogen must emphasize that leaders will share what we know with the public. However, the American people should expect that what we know will evolve with ongoing study of the organism and the disease it causes. Leaders will update the public on the evolving state of our understanding, but as we see more cases and learn more from studies, our knowledge will increase and things that we thought we knew might be proved wrong. Leaders must be flexible enough to adapt to these changing circumstances and nimble enough to adjust their messaging and plans to fit the new information learned.

When new developments occur, it is important for the leader to carefully communicate what the developments are and what the implications of the new situation are. If this calls for new or different actions on behalf of the public, the leader needs a well-defined message describing what the new actions are, why they are needed, and how our fight to end the pandemic will benefit from these new actions.

Leaders should also augment their message with concise communication from relevant experts and leaders in their fields concerning the developments they are sharing with the public. These experts and leaders can be critical to maintaining public trust and understanding, as well as answering questions from the press and media, who can then further disseminate these important messages to their audiences.

Recommendation #116

Flexibility through Communication

Leaders must be flexible enough to adapt to changing circumstances and nimble enough to adjust their messaging and plans to account for new developments. Leaders should also be reinforcing to the public early on in a pandemic with a novel organism that there is much that is unknown, but more will become clear as we gain experience with more cases and insights from more clinical studies. Therefore, the public should expect updates and, on occasion, that new information may indicate that what we previously thought to be true no longer is.

Lesson 10: Empathy

We have been surprised by many things during the current COVID-19 pandemic. Among the most shocking of them has been how many leaders and elected officials have demonstrated callousness, a lack of empathy, and an utter disregard for the well-being of those they are hired or elected to serve.

John C. Maxwell arguably said it best: "People do not care how much you know until they know how much you care." Empathy and caring create a connection between leaders and those they lead. It is very difficult to trust someone who you don't believe understands the position you find yourself in or cares what happens to you. It also seems that the public is more forgiving of missteps by leaders they connect with and trust.

It was certainly not endearing to those families and friends who had lost loved ones to listen to President Trump respond to reporters who questioned him about the lives lost during the pandemic with "It is what it is," while insisting that the pandemic was "under control."[2]

While we propose that caring and empathy are important characteristics of the best leaders, even without those traits, one would still hope that pragmatism would drive leaders to do everything possible to combat a crisis. The popularity of leaders who do not handle crises well tends to dip significantly and reelection prospects generally dim when the public does not perceive that an elected leader has managed a crisis well. Even a completely indifferent president or governor should want to control the spread of a disease for their own benefit—a disease that will threaten seniors (an important voting block), raise health care costs and harm businesses. As pointed out by reporters for the New York Times of President Trump: "Since World War II, no American president has shown greater disdain for science—or more lack of awareness of its likely costs."[3]

Of course, the president was not the only elected leader to exhibit this fundamental lack of caring or empathy, along with a strong tendency to abandon science. We know the outcome for the president. It will be most interesting to see how broadly voters were perturbed by these traits and how long the public's memory is when it comes time for voters to determine the fate of local elected officials who they perceived neither cared about them nor followed science.

Recommendation #117

Leaders Need to Demonstrate Empathy

Leaders who care and have empathy for those they lead need to demonstrate it. Leaders who do not have these traits would be well served to have their staff members and speech writers help them try to compensate for these deficiencies.

Lesson 11: Humility

Oftentimes, those in leadership roles believe that it is important to project strength, confidence, and control. We don't disagree. We certainly would not want our president, or the leader of any group, to be projecting weakness, insecurity, a lack of confidence, or a sense of hopelessness when speaking to the country during a pandemic or other national threat. The key is for the leader to balance strength, confidence, and control with humility.

While humility might seem inconsistent or incompatible with strength, confidence, and control, it is not. What would this look like? It would be the president or leader expressing a plan to confront the threat, the confidence that, together, we can overcome the threat, and a promise that the president will marshal all the resources of the federal government to assist in combating the threat, but also asserting that he or she doesn't know all the answers, will surround him or herself with the best experts our country has, will listen to the experts and will adjust his or her plans as we learn more about the threat and how to combat it. In essence, it is a simple acknowledgement that the president doesn't know everything, but knows where to look for answers. When leaders do all the talking, create the impression that they have all the answers, and take all the credit, then the public is likely to attribute all the blame to the leader for anything that goes wrong. The public is much more likely to give a leader the benefit of the doubt when they express the humility that they don't know all the answers, but will seek out the best advice available and will do their best, realizing that a pandemic with a novel virus is likely to present never-before-seen problems and challenges.

In addition to admitting that the leader does not know everything or have it all figured out, humility involves admitting when mistakes are made and taking accountability for them, which serves to promote trust with the public. When leaders indicate that they have made no mistakes, have handled everything perfectly, and refuse to take accountability for mistakes, the focus of many will be on building the evidence that the leader did, in fact, err, serving only to draw out the focus on the errors with resulting loss of trust.

Trust is critical for any leader to successfully lead through a crisis or prolonged difficult challenge. Unfortunately, given the intensely partisan divide in recent years, trust is hard to come by. It can be earned by being transparent, communicating clearly and openly, demonstrating integrity, and matching your actions with your words. Humility is key to engendering and maintaining trust. Humility is evidence of an authentic leader, the kind of leader most people want to follow.

CHAPTER 16

Recommendation Checklists

To assist leaders as they reflect on lessons learned from the current pandemic and plan for the future, we have organized all of our recommendations into a set of checklists. These checklists are directed at those who are responsible for creating pandemic preparedness plans, at those revising and updating such plans, at those who will oversee portions of the federal or state government's response to a future pandemic, at those who lead these government agencies, at public health departments, at health care providers, and at school boards.

We realize that at this point in the pandemic, some people will look at particular recommendations and think that they are obvious. But keep in mind that almost every recommendation addresses an actual failure during this pandemic. Understand that our memories are short, and by the time we face our next pandemic, we are likely to fall back into old behaviors unless we recall these mistakes or missed opportunities and purposefully act on them.

Another criticism may be that some recommendations are not practical, and others—for example, teaching people skills to evaluate the reliability of online and social media sources—would take too long to implement. While we don't know how much time we have until our next pandemic, the previous pandemic preceded this one by a decade. That is plenty of time to incorporate such a skill in schools at all levels of education. We should not wait for the next pandemic to put some of these recommendations into action.

Federal Government

Prepare for the Next Pandemic Now (Recommendation #1)

The US government and its agencies must acknowledge the risk of future pandemics and plan for them.

We have had four formally declared pandemics in the past 70 years. We have had many more close calls. We must better prepare for future pandemics, which are certain to come and could be even more severe than the SARS-CoV-2 pandemic. This should include a critical review of the federal government's handling of this pandemic, revising our pandemic plans to reflect lessons learned, improved disease outbreak surveillance with the use of artificial intelligence, greatly enhanced communication plans, funding for research into vaccines and therapeutics for organisms with pandemic potential, addressing supply chain threats, recommitting to adequately stocking the National Strategic Stockpiles, working with the global community to develop new strategies to disease containment anywhere in the world where there is an outbreak of a suspected or confirmed novel organism, and annual multi-agency tabletop exercises, as well as the recommendations below.

Establish Public Health Presence in Foreign Countries (Recommendation #2)

Future administrations should recommit and invest sufficiently in establishing a public health presence in certain foreign countries to assist in the early identification of novel viruses (and other pathogens) and their containment.

We have learned from this pandemic that budget cuts that downsized our number of experts embedded in China significantly hampered us in getting real-time, reliable information sooner about the initial outbreak in Wuhan. We should recommit to this presence of our public health experts in foreign countries that would allow this, particularly in developing countries where populations are encroaching on wildlife habitats and in those countries that have been sites of previous epidemic or pandemic outbreaks, and especially those countries that are less transparent and less likely to be forthcoming about a disease outbreak. These embedded public health experts and scientists can gain a better understanding of the potential pandemic threats in that county and can forge collaborative and trusting relationships with local scientists and public health officials that may increase the likelihood that we will learn of a threat or outbreak before the information is suppressed.

Establish Infection Control Measures in Wet Markets (Recommendation #3)

The United States and the world's leaders must place pressure on China and those Asian countries that have wet markets to develop and enforce public health measures to prevent the high-risk activities that create significant threats for zoonotic infections and the transmission of novel viruses.

While we still don't know the origin of the SARS-CoV-2 pandemic, there appears to be little question that even if the wet markets in Wuhan were not the original site of spillover, they played a significant role in the transmission of SARS-CoV-2. As a precursor, the association of the wet markets with SARS-CoV in 2003 seems clear, and the risks for a novel avian influenza virus seem to be undeniable. Therefore, these threats must be mitigated.

Defense Production Act (Recommendation #8)

The president should be prepared to implement the Defense Production Act to address supply shortages, realizing that the normal supply chains are not designed for a sudden, sharp worldwide increase in demand and are likely not to function as needed if there is no government intervention.

We must understand that normal supply chains can fail when a pandemic drives a huge, sudden worldwide increase in demand. We must ensure adequate inventory levels for the Strategic National Stockpile; avoid dependence on a single country for supplies, equipment and pharmaceuticals; create manufacturing redundancies for critical supplies, equipment and pharmaceuticals in the United States, and the president must be prepared and willing to implement the Defense Production Act early when a threat is anticipated to be long-lasting. The federal government should use its leverage in buying supplies, equipment, and medications for the states during the time of a public emergency, rather than having states have to compete with each other and the federal government for these items.

The Administration Must Promote Public Health (Recommendation #19)

The role of the president, vice president and senior administration officials during a pandemic is to give accurate and timely information to the public and to stress the importance of public health measures to thwart the pandemic's spread. These leaders need to provide a "call to action" to motivate the populace to actively participate for the "good of the country" and for fellow citizens.

Efforts to downplay a public health threat may succeed in avoiding panic, but will result in much lower compliance with public health recommendations and endanger the public. Such efforts also lead to conflicting public messages, loss of trust in leaders, and large portions of the public obtaining their information from untrustworthy and unreliable sources. Leaders must communicate truthfully, frequently, and consistently.

Personal Protective Equipment and Supplies (Recommendation #27)

The federal government and states need a plan to be able to provide PPE to first responders promptly at the very beginning of a public health emergency with a contagious pathogen.

This recommendation addresses inadequate reserves in the Strategic National Stockpile, the failure of normal supply chains during sudden increases for products from countries worldwide, and President Trump's reluctance to implement the Defense Production Act. Given that China has often been the site of outbreaks of novel pathogens and is also one of the leading producers of PPE, we need other sources for PPE in the event of a pandemic, as China will understandably meet its own needs first, but also may have diminished manufacturing capacity if many of its workers are ill.

Protect Jobs, Pay, and Housing (Recommendation #39)

During an epidemic, pandemic, or other public health emergency, we cannot expect low-wage workers to isolate and quarantine if there is not protection of their income and jobs. Congress must act quickly to provide for these protections, as well as preventing evictions.

This speaks to the important role that non-profit organizations play during a public health emergency. It is critical that state and local governments include shelters, food banks, organizations that assist the poor and homeless with housing, and other such nongovernmental organizations in their pandemic planning and communications.

Act Early to Minimize the Severity and Duration of Non-pharmaceutical Interventions (Recommendation #40)

For future pandemics or other public health emergencies, it is important to keep in mind that public health measures will be better embraced if implemented early, when they can be milder in terms of the restrictions imposed. Delays in efforts to contain the spread of illness will allow the threat to increase, and this may require more severe restrictions that are not only less likely to be adopted by the general public, but in fact may be met with organized resistance.

This recommendation addresses the need to identify outbreaks caused by an organism with pandemic potential promptly and to focus efforts on containing the outbreak through isolation, quarantine, and restricting travel in and out of the area in hopes of avoiding introducing the infection into other countries, or at least slowing it down to allow for time to learn more about how to contain and treat the infection and to allow other countries to launch their preparations.

We saw that many countries struggled with implementing and maintaining non-pharmaceutical interventions due to the impacts on businesses, schools, and people's perception that this was infringing on their personal liberties. Unless something were to change to cause us to believe non-pharmaceutical interventions will be better embraced in the future, we authors believe that the only hope to control the spread of a novel, highly contagious respiratory virus in the future is to try to contain it at the site of the initial outbreak with a lockdown of that area. We realize that cases may have already leaked out of the area by the time the threat is recognized, but locking down the site of the outbreak may be the only hope for containing its spread or at least slowing it down as we race to develop therapeutics and vaccines.

Develop and Communicate the National Pandemic Response Plan (Recommendation #41)

In a time of a pandemic or other public health emergency, it is critical that there is a national plan, and that plan must be clearly communicated to the states so that there is a clear understanding of what the federal government will do and what the states will need to do, with or without support from the federal government.

It is imperative that the United States update and revise its pandemic plan and response based on the lessons from this current pandemic. Especially important will be determining what the federal commitment will be to the National Strategic Stockpile so that states can make decisions as to whether they need their own stockpiles, as well as better delineating the roles of the federal government and its agencies and those of the states.

Bipartisan Disdain for Misinformation and Disinformation (Recommendation #44)

Misinformation and untruths must become a common enemy for all Americans, and especially our leaders. In a time of a pandemic or other public health crisis, leaders of all parties must determine and agree on facts and actively refute misinformation and untruths. We then should have vigorous debate on how the country should respond to those facts, by persuasive arguments rather than personal attacks.

Communicating to the Public (Recommendation #45)

Leaders should be clear as to the role we all play in protecting our families and neighbors and in containing the spread of the infection. When we learn new information that is in conflict with what we previously thought and communicated, we must be clear that we were mistaken and now have better information, explain why, and explain what we need the public to do with the information. Leaders must model the desired behaviors, or they will undermine them.

In the future, we must do a better job communicating the need for people who are believed to be at lower risk for severe disease or death to engage in the public health measures to contain the spread of the disease, and we must do this as early as possible into the epidemic or pandemic. We found that the focus of too many messages was on the risk for death. We must be clear from the start that the reason to avoid transmission of the virus is not simply to prevent deaths, but to prevent known and as of yet unknown morbidity, keep schools and businesses open, avoid development of variants that may become more contagious or cause more severe illness, and relieve the pressures on our health care delivery system.

Coordinated, Unified National Response (Recommendation #49)

A coordinated, unified national response is essential to managing the next pandemic in order to ensure a successful rollout of testing, PPE, and vaccines.

Communicate Truthfully to Establish and Maintain Trust (Recommendation #50)

In a time of a national public health emergency, the president should be truthful with the American people. That does not mean that a president must tell the public all that he or she knows, but efforts to mislead the public or downplay the threat may give the public a false sense of reassurance and undermine efforts by public health officials to get the public to adopt their guidance. Maintaining the trust and confidence of the American people is critical to leading them through a crisis.

Be a Role Model for Desired Behaviors (Recommendation #52)

Leaders must model the desired behaviors they want the public to adopt. Even if the leaders have the benefit of additional protections not available to the general public, it is still important to reinforce these behaviors. The failure to do so will greatly undermine public health efforts.

President Trump often argued that he did not need to wear a mask because he was tested every day and those with whom he came into contact were regularly tested. That may or may not be the case, but even if it was so, the strategy was ineffective. The president became infected, as did at least two other members of his family and others in his inner circle. The words and actions of any leader, but especially the president, have a huge impact on those they are privileged to lead; the decision by the president and others not to follow the guidance that was being issued to the public undoubtedly undermined the public's compliance with the guidance.

Federal Role in Procuring and Distributing Supplies (Recommendation #54)

In the event of a public health emergency, purchasing of supplies, equipment, and medications should be done by the federal government on behalf of the states and their health care infrastructure. This contrasts with creating an uncontrolled purchasing free-for-all within the marketplace between the federal government and the individual states and territories, hospitals, and medical practices. In the end, such an uncoordinated strategy, where the federal government does not take a leadership role, most often causes these lower-level entities to lose out to, or at very least pay more than, other countries competing for the same supplies.

Defense Production Act (Recommendation #55)

In a public health emergency that is expected to last for months, and where shortages of supplies and equipment are already being experienced, the president should be quick to implement the Defense Production Act to ensure that the United States' needs can be met by production within the country by US companies and where the supply can be assured to be distributed to meet the United States' needs.

Create Redundancies in the Supply Chain (Recommendation #56)

We must identify critical supplies, equipment, and medications to ensure that we are not overly reliant on any one country, that would, in the case of a public health emergency, internal political instability or a war, be challenged in their ability to maintain the supply of these critical resources or for which a sudden increase in world demand would threaten the supply to the United States.

Vulnerabilities were exposed during this pandemic where countries that were the major manufacturers and distributers of PPE, such as China, or the major manufacturer and distributer of ingredients for medications and vaccines, such as India, were themselves significantly impacted by the pandemic, causing difficulty in maintaining manufacturing plant operations and production lines. We must examine the entire supply chain for critical equipment, supplies, and medications to ensure that there are redundancies and alternative sources for our needs during a worldwide emergency or an event directly impacting those countries that might affect production or shipping, along with a backup plan of how we would start up production in the United States in the event of a prolonged disruption to the supply chain.

Health Care Workforce Development (Recommendation #66)

Health care workforce policies and incentives need to be developed that will promote an increase in the numbers of physicians and nurses in both ambulatory and hospital settings. The plan should be especially directed at medically underserved areas and health professional shortage areas to address their needs for primary care and specialty care, including mental health. Furthermore, the plan should be directed at increasing the diversity of the health care workforce to better match the communities they serve.

Of course, this problem predates the onset of the pandemic, and like many other inherent weaknesses of the American health care delivery system, it merely became amplified and more visible during the pandemic. This recommendation is made in the hopes of spurring the US Congress and state legislatures to take this issue on during their next legislative sessions to address this chronic problem for the present, as well as in preparation for the next pandemic.

Health Care Professional Geographic Shortages (Recommendation #67)

A federal strategic plan must be developed for the geographic disparities and shortages in physician and nursing workforces across this country. Shortages of physicians and nurses in disadvantaged and rural communities and communities of color lead to a reduction in timely access to health care and worse outcomes for these at-risk populations. We see this even more clearly during a public health emergency, such as an epidemic or pandemic.

As was the case for Recommendation #66, this problem predates the onset of the pandemic, and like many other inherent weaknesses of the American health care delivery system, it also merely became amplified and more visible during the pandemic. This recommendation, too, is made in the hopes of spurring the US Congress and state legislatures to take this issue on during their next legislative sessions to address this chronic problem for the present, as well as in preparation for the next pandemic.

Expand the Medical Reserve Corps (Recommendation #70)

A greater effort should be made to inform physicians, nurses, and other health care professionals about the Medical Reserve Corps and to encourage their enlistment. The current focus on local health initiatives should be expanded to preparation for deployment anywhere in the country in the event of a public health emergency. Congress needs to make a greater commitment to sufficiently fund this effort and to ensure that, in the event of an emergency, proper laws are enacted to allow the practice of medicine, nursing, and other health professions in a state in which the professionals are not licensed, as well as providing the appropriate liability protections for these volunteers.

Virtual Care Reimbursement (Recommendation #72)

As long as health care reimbursement systems in the United States remain largely fee for service, we need those systems to cover and properly reimburse providers for their time and effort to manage the health of their patients without an in-person visit, such as telehealth, telephone, email, and text communications. To encourage providers to offer telehealth services for the safety and convenience of patients, these virtual visits should be reimbursed at parity with in-person visits.

Increase Funding for Public Health (Recommendation #77)

Appropriate levels of funding of the public health infrastructure should be established by the federal government and each state, as well as locally by county, driven by the creation of national benchmarks. This funding should be sufficient to allow for all the functions *of public health, but also with a sufficient investment for planning and preparation for future public health emergencies. A practical benchmark would be to move this funding from $100 per person per year to $300 per person per year.*

We have seen the costs that result from an uncontrolled pandemic. For the United States, in economic costs alone, it has been trillions of dollars. We hope that this can in itself justify greater investment in public health infrastructure and that during the times when we are not fighting a pandemic, this infrastructure can be utilized to help remedy health care disparities.

Protect Low-Wage Earners (Recommendation #85)

It is critical for lawmakers to understand the financial impacts that may cause people to resist complying with critical public health procedures aimed at isolating those who are sick and quarantining those who are close contacts. To control the spread of a pandemic disease, it is critical that those who are asked to isolate or quarantine do not have to fear loss of employment, income, or housing.

A great deal of support was provided by the United States government to businesses and individuals during the pandemic. However, much of the support to individuals was targeted at the jobless and lower-income individuals and was referred to variously as 2020 recovery rebates, economic impact payments, or stimulus payments. While very helpful, these payments did not ease the burden on those who retained employment, but would need to isolate or quarantine when their employers did not offer benefits of sick or leave pay and the individuals were living paycheck to paycheck. It is difficult to quantify how many people thus avoided getting tested or staying home when sick or exposed, and therefore may have sickened others.

Improved and Automated Reporting (Recommendation #86)

Federal, state, and local governments should pursue an integrated and interconnected public health data system that allows for data to be shared instantaneously. This data needs to be aggregated, reported, and examined with analytic tools to give governments, public health agencies, and health care providers real-time information and data as to the emergence and control of transmissible diseases.

Many hospitals were challenged by the reporting requirements, especially when different authorities had different requirements or those requirements kept changing. Furthermore, in most cases, the reporting was not automated, so there were data reporting delays that occurred over weekends and holidays that made interpretation of the data challenging. It should also be noted that in the case of a contagious disease such as COVID-19 that does not make most people sick enough to require hospitalization, public health agencies may not have early and complete information if there is no reporting from large medical practices and urgent care providers.

Leaders Must Inform the Public Truthfully and Factually (Recommendation #88)

Leaders are more likely to be politically successful if they tell the American public the truth. They need to communicate clearly and often with the public, embracing science and allowing scientists and public health officials to stand before the people at press conferences to provide guidance and answer questions. Leaders need to develop a strategy for dealing with the emergency and then effectively communicate that strategy to the public.

Combat Disinformation with Proactive Communication (Recommendation #89)

Speaking clearly, openly, truthfully, and often to the public helps to decrease anxiety and fill the information gaps so that others do not plug those gaps with misinformation, disinformation, and conspiracy theories.

Preempt Unhealthy Psychological Responses with Clear and Frequent Communication (Recommendation #92)

Fear, anxiety, and the need for humans to make sense of serious, unexpected events can lead to several unhealthy psychological responses, including denial, rationalization, and conspiracy theories. Governments, public health agencies, and physicians with expertise in the area must make the effort and devote the time to communicate openly and frequently about what we know so as not to leave gaps that can be filled with misinformation and disinformation. Experts must refute the misinformation and disinformation clearly and strongly.

Controlling the Pandemic Is Key to Protecting the Economy (Recommendation #96)

The best way to preserve the economy is to control the spread of infection; to make people, particularly those who feel at greatest risk, feel safe; and clearly communicate the successes in preventing infection through the adoption of public health guidance. Inevitably, if efforts to control spread are not successful, consumer confidence will suffer; governments are then invariably left with few options other than restrictions and closures, and employee productivity will decline along with a surge in employer health costs.

Public-Private Partnership for Vaccine Development (Recommendation #97)

In future pandemics, as was done in the current one, the United States should consider providing advance funding to the leading vaccine candidate manufacturers that get their vaccines to phase 3 clinical trials so that they can ramp up production and supply of vaccine in anticipation of authorization by the Food and Drug Administration and so begin shipping as soon as that authorization is given.

Develop Multiple Types of Vaccines Concurrently (Recommendation #98)

The United States should encourage the simultaneous development of different vaccine types when faced with the next pandemic with a novel contagion, so as to increase the chances that at least one of the vaccines will be safe and effective. The goal should be to have at least several manufacturers' vaccines authorized to allow for greater vaccine production and distribution on a rapid basis.

Computer-Assisted Vaccine Scheduling (Recommendation #99)

For future pandemics, when people must be assigned to priority groups due to limited vaccine, the federal government should create a website for each state's use that will allow people in that state to indicate that they wish to receive the vaccine, how far they are willing to drive for the vaccine, what days and times they are available for a vaccine appointment, the demographic and clinical information that will allow them to be prioritized, and whether they wish to be placed on a waiting list if a provider has vaccine left over at the end of the day. The system should not allow double-booking of appointments and should automatically cancel an existing appointment if the person is on a waiting list and has called in prior to their appointment.

Risk Mitigation (Recommendation #109)

Once material risks and threats are identified, great leaders conduct a thorough evaluation of the vulnerabilities and create mitigation plans.

Teams Should Reflect Different Backgrounds, Experiences, and Points of View (Recommendation #110)

Great leaders should surround themselves with team members who are recognized experts in their fields, who come from diverse backgrounds and have diverse experiences, who often think about things differently than the leader does, and who are not hesitant to offer contrary thoughts and opinions to, or even correct, the leader.

When dealing with high-risk, complex issues for which answers are not clear, it is essential that leaders seek out accurate data and expert opinion. This does not mean that a leader must automatically defer to expert opinion, and oftentimes there may be a difference of opinion among experts. However, leaders must have the benefit of objective data and the best thinking among those with the greatest experience and expertise in order to come to the best possible decisions. Unfortunately, we saw that when efforts were made to select or modify data in such a way as to present a more favorable picture and when those in the innermost circle of advisors to a leader are selected on the basis of loyalty rather than experience and expertise, the natural inclinations of the leader are reinforced rather than challenged.

Honesty Is Still the Best Policy (Recommendation #111)
Leaders should tell the truth. The trust and confidence of those you are privileged to lead depend on this. In a time of emergency or crisis, the American people are best served by understanding the truth as we know it, so that they can make informed decisions about whether and how to change their behavior to adjust to the new threat.

Focus (Recommendation #112)
During a time of impending threat, great leaders need to focus. These leaders redirect their attention, and that of their team, away from distractions and non-pressing matters toward the need for planning, monitoring, and responding to the threat.

Accountability (Recommendation #113)
Great leaders take end-to-end accountability for everything that happens within their organization, their agency, or their government, even when they are not personally responsible for causing the undesired outcome.

A Vision and a Strategic Plan Are Essential (Recommendation #114)

In times of uncertainty, leaders need to set out a compelling vision, develop a comprehensive strategic and operating plan as to how to achieve that vision, communicate and distribute those plans, and speak often, consistently, and passionately about the vision and the plans to inspire others to embrace the vision and assist in executing the plans.

Maintain and Help Others Maintain Perspective (Recommendation #115)

Leaders should help the public maintain a proper sense of perspective during the public health crisis. In an effort to promote compliance with public health guidance, leaders should frequently remind the public that the compliance measures are temporary and only needed until such time that the transmission of infection and disease can be controlled and contained.

Leaders Need to Demonstrate Empathy (Recommendation #117)

Leaders who care and have empathy for those they lead need to demonstrate it. Leaders who do not have these traits would be well served to have their staff members and speech writers help them try to compensate for these deficiencies.

World Health Organization, Centers for Disease Control and Prevention, and Public Health Agencies

Presume Contagiousness Until Proven Otherwise (Recommendation #4)

With a novel virus that causes respiratory illness, especially one belonging to a family of viruses known to be infectious, we should presume human-to-human transmission is possible until proven otherwise.

While in some areas we need our public health organizations to delay guidance as they await evidence—for example, in recommending therapies and vaccines—there are times that we need these agencies to issue preliminary guidance before all the evidence is in. Failing to do so may compromise our ability to contain the spread of disease, as happened with the SARS-CoV-2 virus. Such is the case with transmission modes. Instead of relying on statements from the Chinese government or awaiting firm evidence of human-to-human transmission, such transmission should have been presumed given that every other virus in the coronaviridae family that causes infection in humans is spread from person to person. Unfortunately, statements to the contrary created a lack of an urgent and intense response on the part of the United States government and various public health and medical communities. This impaired our ability to contain the entry of the virus into the United States and to slow or stop the spread once it was here.

Immediate Targeted Lockdowns (Recommendation #5)

With an estimated 4 million international travelers per day, health officials must act swiftly to lock down travel in and out of any area of the world with an outbreak of a novel virus. We must seek agreement from the world's leaders to cooperate in instituting travel restrictions as soon an outbreak with a novel virus is detected.

Efforts to restrict the entry of potentially infectious persons into other countries were largely unsuccessful. Without an understanding of the signs and symptoms of the disease, without an understanding of its incubation period and whether individuals can be contagious while asymptomatic or pre-symptomatic, and without a developed and available test for the infection, controlling inward and outward flow of infected individuals throughout the world is difficult to implement and will likely be ineffective. A far better solution, until we can answer these questions and have testing available, is to lock down the site of the outbreak.

Travel Restrictions Must Apply to All (Recommendation #6)

If a travel restriction is to be used, United States citizens returning home from a country where there has been an outbreak of infection must either be tested prior to entry, if a reliable test is available, or they should be quarantined for an appropriate amount of time prior to returning to their homes, families, friends, and work.

If a lockdown of the site of an outbreak is not possible, or if an additional travel restriction is put in place to augment the lockdown at the outbreak location, then we must not create exceptions to the restrictions based on citizenship or residency, since the virus does not make such a distinction in its targets of infection.

Promote Rapid Test Development (Recommendation #7)

The regulatory scheme must be modified to allow for rapid testing development in the private and academic setting under the direction of the CDC. If the WHO should develop a test prior to the CDC, we must be willing to employ the WHO's test until such time as we develop a test with greater sensitivity or specificity, with more rapid turnaround, or at a lower cost.

Such flexibility stands for the proposition that we do not want to have a single point of failure—in this case, in testing—that can jeopardize or delay our response to a novel pathogen. This is especially important since testing is absolutely critical to our containment strategies and our monitoring of disease transmission.

Improve Communication and Coordination (Recommendation #9)

Safeguards against the transmission and spread of a novel virus require coordination of efforts across the globe. There must be strong information sharing among the WHO member countries and the public health organizations of those countries, and strong mitigation measures must be put in place swiftly.

Rapid, Coordinated Responses to a Novel Virus are Necessary (Recommendation #13)

The world's leaders must be quick to respond to an outbreak of a novel virus. Locking down travel into and out of the site of an outbreak of a novel virus infection is likely to be more effective than other countries implementing travel restrictions.

The World Health Organization must work in conjunction with the member countries' representatives and public health organizations to stress the importance of alerting the WHO promptly upon the identification of a potential threat and sharing information transparently. History has taught us that efforts to conceal the transmission of a health threat are never successful and, in the end, will only result in greater spread of the disease, more deaths, and more embarrassment or resentment towards the country that concealed the information.

Expand the WHO's Authority (Recommendation #14)

The organizational documents of the WHO should be amended to allow the WHO to initiate a request for a site visit and investigation in coordination with the host country.

This recommendation is made to allow the WHO to initiate a site visit, rather than having to wait for an invitation. This will help to more quickly identify whether the outbreak is a novel organism and whether an immediate lockdown should be implemented.

The CDC Must Be the Independent, Trusted Voice of Science (Recommendation #15)

The CDC must regain the public's trust. It must be the voice of science and its leaders must speak out often and with clarity during a public health emergency, even when the information, guidance, and predictions conflict with the president and his or her administration.

As with the WHO above, it is critical that the American people retain trust in the CDC and its guidance. It is therefore incumbent on every president and administration to ensure that the CDC remains protected from political influence and that medical and public health experts from the CDC and other government agencies are able to speak directly and freely to the American people at press conferences without censoring or restrictions by the administration.

Multi-agency Review of the Pandemic Response (Recommendation #16)

The CDC must conduct a full, multi-agency, retrospective review of mistakes and lessons from the pandemic.

Revisions to Pandemic Plans and to CDC Competencies (Recommendation #17)

The CDC should revise and update its pandemic plans based on the lessons from this pandemic to include, at a minimum, needed investments in public health infrastructure, the positioning of CDC staff in certain foreign countries, the adoption of machine learning for enhanced surveillance, new strategies focusing on containment, and strengthening of disease reporting in the United States The CDC of the future will need social scientists, science communications experts, political scientists, experts in combating misinformation and disinformation, cultural anthropologists, and social media experts.

Combating the epidemics and pandemics of the future will rely not just on establishing the science, but in communicating it clearly, widely, and frequently for people of different ages, races, and cultural groups, while simultaneously combating misinformation and disinformation.

Increase in Research Funding (Recommendation #18)

We must increase our investment in research of novel organisms that are candidates for future pandemics. This should at least be a collaboration among our US medical and public health research agencies, if not a collaboration among the international community.

We must increase our research on the prevention and treatment of illness caused by organisms that pose the risk of pandemic threat based on our surveillance of these pathogens and any associated outbreaks. Ideally, focusing on the search for antivirals that are effective against entire families of viruses would allow us to roll out therapies much more quickly in response to the emergence of a novel virus.

Disinformation (Recommendation #22)

The CDC and NIH must combat disinformation that is gaining traction on social media or cable networks. They should use experts in science communication to explain clearly why these messages are incorrect.

Enforcement of Public Health Orders (Recommendation #29)

It is a best practice for public health officials to consult with law enforcement leaders about the penalties and enforcement of a public health before issuing that order.

Reevaluate the Qualifications of Public Health Board Members (Recommendation #33)

A best practice would be to require board members to have at least a basic understanding of public health and a commitment to its fundamental principles.

As some states are taking legislative action to strip powers of state officials and public health agencies to order non-pharmaceutical interventions, it will be even more critical for public health boards to provide their communities with good advice so that those who want to take steps to protect themselves and their families can be well informed. This can only be accomplished when board members embrace evidence-based public health measures and do not undermine those messages.

Providing Personal Protective Equipment and Testing to Vulnerable Workers (Recommendation #37)

We must identify those businesses with low-paid or skilled workers who must work in proximity to one another and may not have access to PPE, so that we can deliver PPE to them. Furthermore, we must make testing available on site since these workers may be unable to take time off to visit a testing center.

Communication and Education (Recommendation #42)

Effective and timely education, communication, and messaging with the assistance of social scientists and professional communications and marketing experts are essential to helping the public understand the threat to them, what they are being asked to do—and most importantly—why it is critical to do it.

Communication Must Be Customized (Recommendation #47)

It is important to try to understand people's thought processes when it comes to their behaviors and choices. Effective communication, education, and messaging campaigns must be developed that will target different groups of people with messages that will resonate with their thinking. The goal should be to encourage them to make the right individual choices to protect the overall community's health, economy, schools, and businesses.

A one-size-fits-all message will not be effective when the virus does not impact the population uniformly. When a virus such as SARS-CoV-2 disproportionately kills the elderly and those with underlying chronic medical conditions, we cannot expect young, healthy adults to be persuaded to comply with unpopular non-pharmaceutical interventions and to get vaccinated if the messages are all based on mortality. We must explain each person's role in the containment of spread of the virus and, unfortunately, in a time when substantial numbers of people cannot be persuaded simply to comply in order to protect others, we must explain why it is in their best interests to participate in controlling the virus's spread.

Use Trusted Spokespersons (Recommendation #48)

It will be important to find appropriate individuals that are respected by each specific group so that they will be accepted messengers and spokespersons for these groups. These respected individuals would be charged with having an impact on these groups by helping them to trust the message. This would facilitate people pulling together in one direction instead of polarizing into factions.

The Evolving Nature of Scientific Discovery (Recommendation #51)

It is critical during briefings to the American people to emphasize that the information and guidance being provided to them is the best information that we know as of that time, but it is entirely possible that, as we gain more knowledge and experience with the virus and the disease it causes, this information or guidance may change.

We must aim at retaining the trust of the American public as we learn more and, consequently, may need to modify the information or guidance previously issued.

Mobilize Public and Private Partners to Develop Tests (Recommendation #57)

The CDC should work with the Food and Drug Administration to modify existing rules or, alternatively, propose legislation, if necessary, that would allow our large, trusted commercial laboratories and US academic laboratories, under the direction of the CDC, to develop tests for the detection of a new pathogen that poses a threat to the health of US citizens.

It is critical that we develop reliable tests quickly in order to monitor the spread of disease and to contain the disease by isolating those who are infected and quarantining those who have been exposed. We cannot afford to place all of our hopes on the development of a single test, as limitations or a failure in the test cause an unacceptable delay that hampers our public health efforts to contain the disease, as we experienced in the current pandemic.

States' Public Health Communications Plans (Recommendation #61)

State and local public health agencies should review their communications plans. They should review their current capabilities and particularly address social media capabilities. They also need a "surge" plan to help expand communications capabilities during the next pandemic or public health emergency.

Optimize State Data Reporting Systems (Recommendation #62)

State and local public health agencies should identify the learnings from receiving, compiling, and reporting data so that these systems are in place and ready to go in the event of an epidemic, pandemic, or other public health emergency.

Automated Data Reporting (Recommendation #63)

State and local public health agencies should work with hospitals to determine what options exist to automate reporting, so that data continues to flow to the state on weekends and holidays and the reporting burden on hospitals is lessened.

Expand Data Reporting Sources (Recommendation #64)

To produce a more complete picture of disease activity, state and local public health agencies should explore options for urgent care and large medical group practices to report data during an epidemic, pandemic, or other public health emergency.

Keep Clinicians Updated (Recommendation #73)

To keep clinicians updated in the face of rapidly developing information about a new health threat, the CDC and professional associations should provide libraries of important articles on their websites, offer weekly podcasts to summarize and explain the latest developments, and send out weekly email summaries of important information and updates.

Combat Bad Behaviors (Recommendation #74)

It is up to elected leaders, public health officials and board members, the medical and nursing communities, professional associations, licensing boards and other health care workers, and each of us to combat the inequity, incivility, incoherence, inhumanity, and ignorance that emerged during the COVID-19 pandemic and that will likely recur in future pandemics. All must speak truth, model desired behaviors, and speak out to correct misinformation and disinformation. Health care professionals must help disseminate the best evidence, facts, and data to better inform the public and advise decision makers.

It cannot be overstated the amount of harm that that was done to our efforts to contain the spread of this disease by those who undermined public health efforts and those who spread disinformation. We must get out in front of this with the next pandemic, and it is essential that all speak out to correct misinformation and condemn those who spread disinformation. Arguably, it was a relatively few number of doctors who themselves did the most harm by perpetuating disinformation, and our profession, state medical boards, professional associations and colleges, and organizations that confer board certification must all respond and stand up to those who repeatedly spread false medical and public health information.

More discussion of how disinformation hugely undermined the management of the COVID-19 pandemic is available in chapter 11.

Inform the Public about the Role of Public Health (Recommendation #76)

There should be organized and targeted messaging and a communication plan that educates the public, health care providers, and social organizations about the roles and functions of the public health departments under normal conditions as well as during times of emergency.

Appointments to Public Health Boards (Recommendation #78)

The boards of public health departments in the future should be made up largely of physicians, nurses, social workers, educators, people who work to provide shelter for the homeless, and those who run food banks. We must have people who are serving the health and social well-being of the citizens of the counties and will use evidence, data, and deference to expertise in their decision-making.

Qualifications of Public Health Board Members (Recommendation #79)

Public health boards should not be primarily comprised of elected officials. Like other fiduciary boards, board members should not have conflicts of interest—political, ideological, or financial—that conflict with the mission and essential function of the public health board. Members of these boards should embrace foundational public health and infection control principles.

We would add that with efforts under way by some states to strip authority from public health boards, Recommendations #78 and #79 are even more important. Without the authority to implement orders or close schools or businesses, these boards become advisory in nature. In doing this, the public is left on its own to take the appropriate public health precautions. It is thus imperative that they receive correct, evidence-based information if they are to be properly informed. As a result, it is important that experts provide this guidance and not elected officials who may be swayed by the political nature of their positions.

Education of Public Health Board Members (Recommendation #80)

Public health department board members should undergo an extensive orientation and complete a curriculum and training in public health principles, infection control, social determinants of health, and public health emergencies.

Range of Interventions by Public Health Boards (Recommendation #81)

All public health board of directors must be educated about the differences between and implications of public health recommendations, advisories, and orders. If a public health order is issued, it is essential that mayors, police officers, and sheriffs are willing and committed to enforcing the order, or the order is unlikely to be effective.

Contact Tracing Surge Staffing (Recommendation #84)

Public health departments need the flexibility to rapidly ramp up (and ramp down) the number of trained persons available for contact tracing. Considerations should be given to cross-training public health workers who have different responsibilities under normal conditions, so that they can rapidly be redeployed. It would also be useful to create a volunteer corps of individuals who can be called on from their regular jobs or retirement to help when needed, along with a focus on cross-training community health workers who can be redirected to contact tracing efforts in a time of need.

Public Health Organizations Must Revise and Update Their Pandemic Plans (Recommendation #87)

The very first action for public health organizations as they prepare for the future is to learn from the past. They must review the entire course of the current pandemic and reflect on what went well and what did not. As they review and update their public health emergency history, they must capture the lessons learned and incorporate these lessons into their future pandemic plans.

Combat Disinformation with Proactive Communication (Recommendation #89)

Speaking clearly, openly, truthfully, and often to the public helps to decrease anxiety and fill the information gaps so that others do not plug those gaps with misinformation, disinformation, and conspiracy theories.

Public Health Measures (Recommendation #95)

As happened with COVID-19, it is likely that the elderly will have the highest risk for severe illness and death in a future pandemic with another pathogen. We must remember that when there are not yet effective therapies and vaccines, and when the strategy to preserve life and minimize the impact on hospitals is to sequester the elderly, young adults must abide by public health mitigation measures because the elderly will inevitably come into contact with them. Young people can pose a significant threat to the elderly, especially when they belong to an age group with a high rate of infection.

Promote Vaccines within Disadvantaged Communities (Recommendation #100)

When vaccines become available, public health departments must make vaccines available to socioeconomically disadvantaged communities and communities with barriers to accessing care, including low English fluency, low levels of health insurance, and employers that do not provide time off from work for vaccination, using persons fluent in the languages spoken in that community and who live in the community. Efforts to leverage people much trusted in those communities to help bring folks out for vaccination—trusted people such as teachers, coaches, clergy, doctors, nurses, community health workers, social workers, and pharmacists—should be made to the greatest extent possible.

Concern for the Development of Variants (Recommendation #101)

In future pandemics, the public and its leaders must be better educated about the dangers and risks of variants that can result if every reasonable effort is not made to control the transmission of the infection, especially when dealing with an RNA virus. The efforts of lower-risk persons to get infected to obtain immunity or for a population to intentionally try to achieve herd immunity are dangerous and risk the promotion of the development of variants.

It was very unfortunate that much of the public discussion around COVID-19 was its mortality rate, whether arguments were on the side of avoiding unnecessary deaths or on the side of arguing that the mortality rate was not so high as to warrant the public health measures that were put in place. Lost in all of this debate were the long-term health impacts to those who survived COVID-19 and the risks to all created by the emergence of variants resulting from uncontrolled disease transmission among those who did not die.

State and Local Governments

Avoid Strategies to Achieve Herd Immunity through Natural Infection (Recommendation #10)

Communicate clearly to the public the unintended consequences of prematurely returning to normal activities with the intent of developing herd immunity through natural infection.

Protect High-Risk Individuals (Recommendation #11)

Communication of public health measures must also include additional guidance for those who are at high risk, including those who are immunocompromised. Communication to the general public must explain the importance of compliance with public health measures among those believed not to be at high risk, in order to protect those who are at high risk.

Accelerate Trials of Therapeutics and the Development of Vaccines (Recommendation #12)

Begin the trials of convalescent plasma, monoclonal antibodies, and antivirals as soon as possible. Provide incentives for pharmaceutical companies to develop a wide variety of potential vaccines, and get those vaccines into clinical trials as soon as possible.

State Leaders Must Promote Public Health Measures (Recommendation #20)

In a public health emergency, such as a pandemic, the governor, lieutenant governor, and legislative leaders must put partisan politics aside and speak together as one voice to support public health measures to address the emergency. During a public health emergency that threatens the welfare and lives of people, there is no political base to be played to; these leaders must protect all their state's citizens.

Public Health is Good for Business (Recommendation #21)

During a public health emergency, especially a pandemic, elected leaders must lead, even when the public is divided and there is no politically safe decision. Educating their citizens about the importance of public health measures to contain the spread of the virus and protect the lives and welfare of their communities and citizens is paramount, but it is also the way to keep businesses open, people employed, and schools open.

It should be clear by now that attempts to politicize a pandemic do not have a long-term beneficent payoff. A virus will act in the same manner whether we choose to take it seriously or not. A failure to adopt public health advice resulted in many leaders themselves becoming infected, resulted in more illness and deaths among the public, and affected businesses and the economy more negatively. Arguably, mishandling the pandemic cost the president of the United States his reelection, and it remains to be seen if other leaders will pay a political price for bungling disease outbreaks.

Emotional and Psychological Support (Recommendation #28)

We urge cities, counties, and states to consider options to provide necessary emotional and psychological support to first responders.

Reevaluate State Public Health Structures and Infrastructure (Recommendation #32)

Each state should reevaluate their public health structure and infrastructure to determine what worked and what didn't work, and what changes should be made, anticipating that we will go through more epidemics and pandemics in the future.

Health Care Disparities (Recommendation #36)

State and local public health agencies should partner with local social service organizations, schools, churches, libraries, and food banks to provide education relative to a public health crisis, screening, testing, and on-site or mobile health care services in a culturally sensitive manner.

Of course, the issue of health care disparities is not limited to pandemics. Health care disparities have played out in health outcomes for decades. Ultimately, this issue must be addressed through health care reform and social policies. However, during a pandemic, we saw how lack of access to health care, close working conditions, lack of PPE, lack of access to testing during work hours, and the inability to take time off from work caused the disproportionate spread of infection among minority and socioeconomically disadvantaged populations. If we are to avoid this in future pandemics, we must take our screening procedures, testing, and vaccinations to these communities and workplaces.

Protect Jobs, Pay, and Housing (Recommendation #39)

During an epidemic, pandemic, or other public health emergency, we cannot expect low-wage earners to isolate and quarantine if there is no protection of their income and jobs. Congress must act quickly to provide these protections, as well as preventing evictions.

This speaks to the important role that nonprofit organizations play during a public health emergency. It is critical that state and local governments include shelters, food banks, organizations that assist the poor and homeless with housing, and other such nongovernmental organizations in their pandemic planning and communications.

Personal Responsibility (Recommendation #46)

We must stress the need for individual responsibility and accountability for our actions and the risks we pose to ourselves and others during the time of a pandemic. We must be clear about what is needed for each American and the consequences and risks posed by those who do not adopt our public health guidance. Furthermore, we must expect leaders to be role models for responsible behaviors.

States Must Secure a Supply Source for a Future Pandemic (Recommendation #53)

States must be able to count on a quickly accessible, dependable source of emergency supplies for their hospitals, long-term care facilities, medical practices, and first responders. Unless the federal government can commit to this with adequate funding by Congress, each state should consider whether it will rely on the SNS or create its own stockpile.

Update State Emergency Operations Plans (Recommendation #58)

States should update the section of their emergency operations plans that deals with pandemics, epidemics, and other public health emergencies to reflect the lessons learned from the COVID-19 pandemic.

Reevaluate the Public Health Structure (Recommendation #59)

As appropriate, states should reconsider whether they were well served by a decentralized public health system if that structure led to a patchwork of inconsistent public health measures, conflicting messages, different degrees of control of disease transmission, and people moving their activities to avail themselves of weaker restrictions.

Public Health Board Composition (Recommendation #60)
States should review the composition of their boards or decision-making bodies to determine whether these boards are comprised of people who can, without conflicts of interest, put the public's health and safety at the forefront of their decision-making process. States should seek out board members that have well-suited backgrounds, experience, and knowledge to serve in roles where they will be making public health guidance or policy for the public.

State Medical Supply Stockpile (Recommendation #65)
States should consider whether they should operate their own stockpile and, if so, whether cost savings are available by partnering with a distributor or health system in the state.

Combat Bad Behaviors (Recommendation #74)
It is up to elected leaders, public health officials and board members, the medical and nursing communities, professional associations, licensing boards and other health care workers, and each of us to combat the inequity, incivility, incoherence, inhumanity, and ignorance that emerged during the COVID-19 pandemic and that will likely recur in future pandemics. All must speak truth, model desired behaviors, and speak out to correct misinformation and disinformation. Health care professionals must help disseminate the best evidence, facts, and data to better inform the public and advise decision makers.

Realignment of Public Health Districts (Recommendation #82)
Functional and geographical alignment of counties into health districts by size, population density, and resource distribution will

better ensure that similar issues that nevertheless impact populations differently are more effectively addressed, with the goal of achieving consistency of effort and outcome.

Coordinated, Unified Approach to Statewide Public Health Emergency (Recommendation #83)

While local public health districts or agencies can function well during normal times and times of localized outbreaks of disease, in a time of an epidemic, pandemic, or other statewide public health emergency, state legislators should authorize the governor and state health department by law to lead the public health efforts in a coordinated manner across the state.

Essential Workers (Recommendation #94)

For future public health emergencies, avoid the phrase "essential workers." In reaction to such a designation, some workers not falling into the state's definition of "essential" will take offense, incorrectly assuming that "essential" means important and, by extension, "non-essential" means not important. Furthermore, politicians and protestors who opposed restrictions will be tempted to take up the rallying cry that all *jobs are essential. This can prove to be a huge distraction. While there is unlikely any categorization that completely escapes criticism, perhaps a designation such as "critical infrastructure" or "critical public infrastructure" might be less prone to attack.*

Controlling the Pandemic is Key to Protecting the Economy (Recommendation #96)

The choice between taking aggressive measures to fight a pandemic and saving the economy is a false dichotomy.

When consumers are fearful of the risks of infection, they will restrict their activities and avoid events and certain businesses. If governments and public health authorities do not take action to control the spread of disease, businesses without subsidization will reduce hours, lay off or furlough employees, or close down, driving increasing unemployment. Unemployment will then further reduce consumer spending.

Risk Mitigation (Recommendation #109)

Once material risks and threats are identified, great leaders conduct a thorough evaluation of the vulnerabilities and create mitigation plans.

Teams Should Reflect Different Backgrounds, Experiences, and Points of View (Recommendation #110)

Great leaders should surround themselves with team members who are recognized experts in their fields, who come from diverse backgrounds and have diverse experiences, who often think about things differently than the leader, and who are not hesitant to offer contrary thoughts and opinions to, or even correct, the leader.

Focus (Recommendation #112)

During a time of impending threat, great leaders need to focus. These leaders redirect their attention, and that of their team, away from distractions and non-pressing matters towards the need for planning, monitoring, and responding to the threat.

Accountability (Recommendation #113)

Great leaders need to take end-to-end accountability for everything that happens within their organization, their agency, or their government, even when they are not personally responsible for causing the undesired outcome.

Maintain and Help Others Maintain Perspective (Recommendation #115)

Leaders should help the public maintain a proper sense of perspective during the public health crisis. In an effort to promote compliance with public health guidance, leaders should frequently remind the public that the compliance measures are temporary and only needed until such time that the transmission of infection and disease can be controlled and contained.

Flexibility through Communication (Recommendation #116)
Leaders must be flexible enough to adapt to changing circumstances and nimble enough to adjust their messaging and plans to account for new developments. Leaders should also be reinforcing to the public early on in a pandemic with a novel organism that there is much that is unknown, but more will become clear as we gain experience with more cases and insights from more clinical studies. Therefore, the public should expect updates and, on occasion, new information may indicate that what we previously thought to be true no longer is.

State Licensing Boards

Disciplinary Action (Recommendation #26)
Health care professionals of all types have the great privilege to care for patients, but also the weighty responsibility to ensure their health, safety, and welfare. Health care professionals have an obligation to study the science of disease and to provide their patients with the best recommendations available based on the science. Health care professionals can do special harm to patients when they disregard the standard of care and the prevailing authoritative guidance due to the special trust patients place in their caregivers. Licensing boards should establish expectations for behavior and practices of their licensees and then discipline those licensees that disregard the rules, the practices, and the science and place the public at risk.

We call on the Federation of State Medical Boards to create model rules to address the professional responsibility of physicians for providing public health guidance and the disciplinary provisions for physicians that refuse to adopt public health guidance in their practices or who encourage the public to disregard public health guidance in the press or media or in their testimony before public health boards.

State Boards Must Be More Active (Recommendation #93)

State boards of health care professionals need to play a more active role in ensuring that their licensees are following the CDC's and their state's public health guidance and that providers who are promoting disinformation in the press, on media outlets, or on social media are disciplined. Unfortunately, these health care professionals, though few, have played into the public's distrust and the denial, rationalization, and conspiracy theories of some of the public.

Health Care Providers

Hospitals (Recommendation #24)

Hospital leaders, physicians, and nurses understandably do not want to unnecessarily scare the public. On the other hand, if they do not send clear messages to state and local leaders and the public about the potential for the hospital to be overwhelmed—and what that would mean for the people of that community—they lose the opportunity to engage the public in taking greater precautions in support of their hospitals. If they fail to communicate this message to the public, as well as define the steps they have taken to prevent this situation, they also risk being blamed for the consequences of rationing decisions that would have to be made in the event of overwhelmed resources.

State Pandemic Reporting (Recommendation #25)

States that report hospital bed capacity generally report the number of beds or the percent occupancy. These are misleading numbers that tend to overstate hospital capacity because they do not account for limitations in staffing, which may be particularly acute during a pandemic with a highly contagious virus. These numbers often include beds that cannot be used for adult patients, such as when neonatal or pediatric intensive care beds are included in the numbers of ICU beds. Therefore, hospitals or hospital associations need to work with their states to understand these limitations in the data and to come up with appropriate language to include on the website where bed capacity is reported to explain this so as not to mislead the public.

Access to Care (Recommendation #38)

We must increase timely access to health care in racial and ethnic minority communities. This should be accomplished by having culturally appropriate health care clinics located in these neighborhoods with employees that reflect the diversity of the communities and who are able to take care of children, pregnant and nursing mothers, adults, and seniors. Arrangements must be in place to allow for a sliding scale fee schedule according to the family's income so that the care is affordable or provided at no cost.

Evidence-Based Visitation Policies (Recommendation #69)

Hospitals should review their visitation policies in light of what we have learned from this pandemic in preparation for the next. Visitor policies should be evidence-based and internally consistent.

While policies do need to protect patients and staff, many policies included restrictions that were overly harsh and not supported by the evidence and may have compromised patient safety. There needs to be a balancing of the harms and benefits of having someone stay with a patient, especially those patients who might be prone to confusion or may be slightly impaired due to medications. A family member is often critical to reducing patient falls and medication errors and improving understanding and compliance with post-discharge instructions.

Furthermore, there needs to be an acknowledgment of the increased anxiety of family members if their loved one is hospitalized but they cannot be with them and if, in return, the ill family member cannot provide regular updates to the family. We also need to acknowledge the psychological harms that have remained with families who were unable to talk to or be with loved ones who died.

Few would question the need for tighter restrictions on hospital visitation during a pandemic. However, the tremendous differences in hospital visitation policies across the country reflected the arbitrariness of many of such policies. Additionally, internal inconsistencies created significant frustration for family members. If a father is permitted to attend the delivery of his child, why would a husband not be able to be at the bedside of his dying wife, even if his wife did not have COVID-19? One local health system allowed a visitor for a bone marrow transplant recipient but would not allow a family member to spend the night with a patient recovering from surgery and anesthesia, even if the family member was willing to go through the same COVID-19 testing conducted on the patient preoperatively. The failure to follow science in designing visitor policies not only put staff in conflict with families, but also undermined those hospitals' pleas to the public to follow the science in their personal responses to the pandemic. We call on the American Hospital Association to work with experts to design evidence-based visitation policies in anticipation of the next pandemic.

Risk Assessment (Recommendation #108)

The best leaders conduct a threat or enterprise risk assessment. All leaders need to know as best they can what threats are possible, how likely those threats are, what the extent of harm would be if the threat materialized, and how to mitigate the threats or risks.

This would be applicable to leaders of hospitals, health systems, and large physician groups.

Risk Mitigation (Recommendation #109)

Once material risks and threats are identified, great leaders conduct a thorough evaluation of the vulnerabilities and create mitigation plans.

Medical and Nursing Schools

Medical and Nursing Education (Recommendation #68)

Medical and nursing school curricula need to address training and preparation for public health emergencies, such as epidemics and pandemics. Education and training must also promote inter-professional teamwork and communication, professionalism, respect, and trust.

Physicians must also be trained on medical informatics, data analytics, and how to critically evaluate clinical studies as our understanding of a novel pathogen during an epidemic or pandemic evolves.

Education, Training, and Services to Support Health Care Workers (Recommendation #71)

Education, training, and continuing education programs should address stress reduction, mindfulness, resilience, behavioral therapy, and incident debriefing to help prevent or address anxiety, depression, burnout, and post-traumatic stress disorder. During a time of increased and prolonged stress, leaders must be proactive in reaching out to their workforce and offering services to them.

Social Determinants of Health (Recommendation #75)

It is imperative that we educate health care professionals in all phases of their education, training, and continuing education about the social determinants of health and strategies to address them. Students and trainees should be involved in community projects or initiatives to address and mitigate health care disparities.

The Press and Media

Combat Disinformation with Proactive Communication (Recommendation #89)

Clear and truthful communication is the best way to engage Americans in public health measures that will bring an end to a pandemic sooner and so minimize loss of life, added health care costs, and negative impact on the economy. Reporters are an asset to help disseminate the information that the American public needs to know. Speaking and writing openly and often to the public helps to decrease anxiety and fill the information gaps so that others do not plug those gaps with misinformation, disinformation, and conspiracy theories.

The press and media have a huge role to play in helping us combat misinformation and disinformation, which caused immense harm to our efforts to teach the public how to protect themselves and others from SARS-CoV-2. It was not uncommon for people who had been deceived to request vaccination only after being admitted to a hospital and realizing they had been duped. In other cases, the deception was so extensive that patients or family members refused to acknowledge that the patient could have COVID, even as preparations were being made to place the patient on a ventilator. Unfortunately, in some cases, the disinformation spawned such distrust of health care workers that family members assaulted staff or made threats of violence against them.

It is critical that the press and media evaluate the qualifications of experts that they are going to interview or whose advice they are going to promote. It is also important that the news agency not promote information that has already been debunked or is inconsistent with the consensus of the medical and scientific communities. Fact checking and questions solicited from the public and answered by experts can be particularly helpful.

Religious Leaders

The Role of Religious Leaders (Recommendation #34)

We urge religious leaders to work more closely with public health experts to understand health threats, minimize risks to their congregants, and amplify the public health messages that will help protect members of their faith.

Religious leaders have special relationships with their communities and positions of trust. That provides a huge opportunity for religious leaders to help promote public health messages and encourage their worshippers to care for others by adopting non-pharmaceutical interventions, as well as getting vaccinated when vaccines are available.

Schools

Critical Thinking and Assessing Reliability (Recommendation #23)

Schools, colleges, and universities should teach students digital media literacy, how to distinguish high-quality information sources from low-quality sources, and how to develop critical thinking. For adults who have already completed school, Facebook's "Tips to Spot False News" can be a useful resource. The public should also be directed to websites that end with .gov, .edu and .org as likely trustworthy sites.

This becomes even more important in the future as some state legislatures, like Idaho, are rescinding the powers and authorities of state public health departments to issue orders or close schools. If these bills pass into law, increasingly the public will be on its own to decide what actions they will take to protect themselves and others. It is important that they are able to identify reliable sources of information in order to make informed decisions.

School Boards Must Begin Planning Early (Recommendation #30)

School boards and superintendents need to engage physicians, public health experts, and business leaders or governance experts early on in a public health crisis to assist them with planning and mitigation efforts. That planning should include clear, frequent, and transparent communications with stakeholders and provide for their engagement in the planning process.

School Boards Need a Decision-Making Framework (Recommendation #31)

School boards need a structured process with a decision framework and dashboard to guide their decision-making so that board discussions are focused, objective, transparent, and internally consistent.

For a detailed discussion about how boards can do this, see chapter 14.

Preparing Our Children for the Next Pandemic (Recommendation #35)

In preparation for the next pandemic, educators must find ways to teach students methods for assessing the reliability and trustworthiness of news and information. We must also instill in our children that as members of a society, we must realize that in those situations where the consequences of our choices do not solely affect ourselves, but can harm others, we must make responsible actions that protect others.

Civics and Social Responsibility (Recommendation #43)

People of all ages need a better understanding of social contracts, particularly the US Constitution and the rights and liberties it confers, along with the limitations on those rights and liberties in the interest of promoting the well-being of our country's inhabitants. This education should begin in elementary school.

There were many personal rights asserted to be guaranteed under the Constitution, which are not. The misunderstanding as to proper restraints on personal freedoms led to conflict with local and state governments that imposed such restrictions. It appears that more education in civics is needed.

Schools Must Teach Students How to Assess the Credibility of Sources (Recommendation #90)

We need to reevaluate our educational curriculums to ensure that we are teaching children and young adults the critical thinking skills they need in an age of social media. We must teach students how discern the truth, how to evaluate the veracity and reliability of sites they may go to for information, and how to evaluate the credentials of those they are looking to for information. They need to be educated in the importance of peer review in medical and scientific literature, in the role political bias and financial conflicts of interest can play in shaping someone's opinions, and in the importance of looking at multiple sources for confirmation.

Promote Science Literacy (Recommendation #91)

We must promote science literacy among students. All students should have a working knowledge of the scientific method and how to judge the strength or weakness of scientific studies, as well as the limitations of such studies.

Too often with SARS-CoV-2, we saw even physicians and public health board members point to anecdotes as scientific evidence.

Include Experts in Pandemic Planning Early (Recommendation #102)

School administration and boards should engage a broad array of experts early to advise them on planning during an epidemic, pandemic, or other public health emergency.

A Robust Operating Plan Is Essential (Recommendation #103)

A robust operating plan is essential to operating schools safely during an epidemic or pandemic. It is critical to have the input of physicians and public health experts in creating and reviewing the plan.

The operating plans must be clearly written to help everyone understand the actions that are called for. These plans must also cover all aspects of school activities and programs (see Recommendation #104), and be clear and concise to help ensure the target audiences will read them.

Operating Plans Need to Be Comprehensive (Recommendation #104)

School pandemic operations plans should address all risks from the time students and staff arrive on campus until the time they depart, and not focus solely on traditional classroom risks. As examples, plans should address the cafeteria, physical education, sports, special education, and extracurricular activities. These plans should also contain mitigation strategies for all modes of transmission of the disease.

School Walk-throughs (Recommendation #105)

School and public health officials should consider implementing walk-throughs of schools after developing the pandemic operations plan in order to assess staff knowledge of the plan, how effectively the plan is being implemented in the school, risks that might have been missed in creating the operations plan, and barriers to the implementation of the plan.

School Communications (Recommendation #106)

Schools should communicate clearly and frequently with teachers and parents and ensure that they keep these important stakeholders updated. Communication and transparency are key to maintaining the trust of stakeholders. Schools should post publicly as much data as is meaningful and practical to give teachers and parents an understanding of how well the school is keeping students and staff safe.

Decision-Making Framework (Recommendation #107)

School boards need to establish a decision-making framework to focus their decision making, to promote transparency as to how they are making decisions, to streamline board meetings, to ensure internal consistency of their decisions, to reduce the stress and pressure on board members, and to reduce in-fighting among board members. Stakeholders should be engaged in the process of creating the decision-making framework.

For a detailed explanation about what a decision-making framework is and how to go about developing one, see chapter 14.

Conclusion

We recognize that the full story of the COVID-19 pandemic remains unknown. For example, we still do not know how or when this pandemic began, and we do not know how or when it will end. Nevertheless, we know a lot. We should not allow unanswered questions to prevent us from applying the lessons learned from this pandemic.

The pandemic has provided many examples of triumphs: the rapid identification and sequencing of the novel virus by Chinese scientists; the rapid development of new and best practices for the management of the most severely ill patients with COVID-19 by physician experts in pulmonary and critical care medicine; the global collaboration of scientists to abandon current research projects and focus on research that contributed to our knowledge and understanding of the SARS-CoV-2 virus and the disease that it causes; the sharing of new research by preprint servers and journals that took down paywalls to provide free and open access to these new studies; the development of new, safe, and incredibly effective vaccines in less than a year; and the dedication and sacrifices of our public health and health care workers.

On the other hand, we also witnessed an alarmingly high frequency of failed leadership among the world's leaders and, in the United States, among leaders at all levels of government. While we certainly don't lay all the blame for the missteps during this pandemic at the feet of leaders in all levels of government, it is clear that failures in leadership negatively impacted the public's compliance with public health guidance, and in many cases helped to fuel disinformation and conspiracy theories—no doubt resulting in many more infections and deaths than we otherwise would have incurred, some of which involved those very leaders.

We are reminded of a quote from Walt Kelly: "We have met the ene my and he is us." We lament the fact that just as President Trump compared the pandemic to a war, Americans did not rally against this common enemy but rather turned against one another.

We should all be clear on one thing: this was not our first pandemic, and it will not be our last. Just as each of the pandemics of the past century—in 1918, influenza A(H1N1); in 1957, influenza A(H2N2); in 1968, influenza A(N3H2); in 2009, influenza A(H1N1pdm09); and in 2019, betacoronavirus (SARS-CoV-2)—differed in terms of which age ranges were most susceptible, which countries were most severely impacted, and what demographics saw higher mortality rates, our next pandemic will too. The next pandemic may be more or less deadly; may, like the pandemic of 2009, impact children and young adults disproportionately; may be transmitted to a much greater extent in schools than was this current infection; and may have different modes of transmission. The next pandemic could occur in a year's time, or in ten years' time.

We must prepare now. We must improve our surveillance of pathogens capable of epidemic or pandemic spread, and we must continue research on these infectious threats, including developing therapeutics that can target entire families of viruses. And, equally importantly, we must prepare and improve our response to the next pandemic. That is the purpose of our book. We implore leaders at all levels of government, local public health agencies, health care providers, and schools to revise their pandemic plans with the lessons from this pandemic in mind.

We have attempted to capture many of these lessons to assist in the revision of pandemic plans and in preparation for the next pandemic. For some who have been on the forefront of fighting this pandemic, many of the recommendations we captured will seem obvious. To them, we point out that these recommendations address shortcomings and mistakes that were made during the pandemic, even if the advice seems clear now in retrospect. We find it critical to capture and document the lessons learned in this book because we are reminded of the truism stated by Georg Wilhelm Friedrich Hegel: "We learn from history that we do not learn from history."

GLOSSARY

ACE-2 (angiotensin-converting enzyme-2) receptor. This protein receptor resides on many cell types, including those that line the respiratory and gastrointestinal tracts and the blood vessels. This receptor is the attachment site for part of the spike protein of the SARS-CoV-2 virus; attachment causes a cell to ingest the virus, resulting in infection and allowing the virus to use the cellular machinery to reproduce itself.

acute respiratory distress syndrome (ARDS). A rapidly developing condition in which fluids build up in the lungs, making it difficult for a patient to get adequate oxygen into the blood from breathing. It often occurs in critically ill patients with significant injuries or a serious underlying infection. Patients with ARDS require intensive care in a hospital and most often need assistance with breathing, from mechanical ventilation, for instance. ARDS is associated with a high mortality rate, especially in those of advanced age or with an underlying advanced illness.

aerosols. Suspensions of biologic secretions exiting the nose or mouth while breathing, talking, yelling, singing, sneezing, or coughing that are smaller in size than respiratory droplets. Because these suspensions are smaller and lighter than respiratory droplets, they can travel across an entire a room, not just the six feet typically advised for social distancing. If a person is infected with a virus, that virus, in suspension, can travel on an airstream and infect a person who is a considerable distance away.

airborne transmission. This describes the mode of transmission of infection by aerosols (as opposed to respiratory droplets) to one or more persons from someone who is infected, usually occupying the same indoor space. Super-spreader events are generally thought to be related to this mode of transmission.

antibodies. Proteins, also known as immunoglobulins, that are produced by the body in response to something that the body's immune system perceives to be an intruder or an anomaly. Antibodies are only one part of the body's immune system, referred to as humoral immunity. An infectious organism, such as SARS-CoV-2, triggers the production of an array of antibodies, only some of which are effective in preventing the virus from entering a cell. These latter antibodies are referred to as neutralizing antibodies. Most often, neutralizing antibodies bind to a part of the virus that is critical to its attaching to a receptor on a cell—in the case of the SARS-CoV-2 virus, the ACE-2 receptor. When an antibody forms a strong attachment to the part of the virus necessary for binding to a cell receptor, it will often impair binding or even block it entirely, thus preventing the virus from infecting the cell.

asymptomatic. The state of being without symptoms.

cellular immunity. One of the three main parts of the body's immune system, cellular immunity is mediated by specific types of white blood cells called T lymphocytes. While antibodies have a key role in preventing a virus from attaching to a receptor and entering a cell, antibodies are of little use once a virus has already infected a cell. Certain triggered T cells can identify infected cells and destroy them, which most often also kills the virus. Cellular immunity contributes importantly to long-term immunity to certain infections.

Centers for Disease Control and Prevention (CDC). An agency of the US Department of Health and Human Services charged with protecting public health and safety through the control and prevention of disease, injury, and disability. Located in Atlanta, Georgia, the CDC, short for Communicable Disease Center when it opened on July 1, 1946, was founded in large part to address the then-major threat of malaria.

close contacts. A phrase referring to persons who spent time near someone with a confirmed infection, which warrants identifying, testing, and isolating those exposed persons. For the SARS-CoV-2 virus, the guidelines currently used for close contact are a distance of six feet or less for a cumulative period of 15 minutes a day.

cluster. An aggregation of cases that are associated in time (usually occurring within days of one another) and by a common source of exposure—for example, a high school cheerleading practice.

community spread. A frequency of transmission in a given community (for SARS-CoV-2, generally when the average daily number of new cases is 1–9 per 100,000 in the population) at which it is no longer possible to reliably identify the risk (recent travel, say) or the source (a particular person who tested positive) of new infections through contact tracing.

contact tracing. A process used by public health authorities and schools to stop the spread of disease. Contact tracing begins when a person is confirmed to be infected with the disease. All close contacts of the infected person within the period of presumed infectivity are identified, and those persons are asked to quarantine and be tested. If a close contact tests positive, then that person's close contacts are also identified. By isolating those infected and quarantining their close contacts, contact tracing aims to break the chain of transmission.

coronavirus. Any virus belonging to the family of viruses named *Coronaviridae*. These viruses share similar features, including a large single strand of RNA surrounded by an envelope with club-shaped spike proteins that give the viruses the appearance of a crown when viewed under an electron microscope.

COVID, or COVID-19. The disease caused by infection with the SARS-CoV-2 virus. The name is a contraction of corona (CO) virus (VI) disease (D) with the addition of 19 in reference to the year of its discovery, 2019.

COVID fatigue. A yearning to return to "normalcy" marked by resenting or defying public health advice asking people to wash or sanitize their hands frequently, clean frequently touched surfaces, maintain a physical distance of six feet from others when outside the home, wear a face covering whenever possible in enclosed public places, and avoid large gatherings.

crisis standards of care. A set of standards by which health care resources, such as ventilators or beds in an intensive care unit, are in short supply relative to demand and therefore are rationed, usually according to patients' likelihood of survival. Such crisis standards are pursuant to an order by a state's governor or the director of the state's department of health and welfare, in conjunction with an emergency declaration or order. The standards include liability protections for health care providers.

Defense Production Act. A federal law passed in 1950 during the Korean War. It authorizes the president to require that private businesses in the United States manufacture items necessary for national defense.

disinformation. Incorrect information spread with the intent to harm, confuse, mislead, or otherwise sway people's hearts and minds toward accepting or supporting the stance of those spreading the false information.

droplets, or respiratory droplets. Particles expelled through the mouth and nose when breathing, talking, yelling, singing, cheering, coughing, or sneezing. These particles can be a mixture of saliva, secretions, and, if the person is infected, virus. Droplets are larger and denser than aerosols, which are also emitted along with droplets. Whereas aerosols can remain suspended in airstreams for a longer time and so travel the length of a room, droplets tend to land within six feet of someone who is breathing or talking normally. Louder vocalizing or coughing and sneezing can propel droplets as far as 13 feet.

efficacy. The success of a vaccine or medication in achieving a desired outcome, such as the prevention of infection, in a clinical trial under defined study conditions. This is in contrast to the term *effectiveness*, which indicates success in achieving a desired outcome in a non-controlled setting, such as real-world clinical practice.

emergency use authorization (**EUA**). The result of an expedited review of a test, vaccine, or medication by the US Food and Drug Administration (FDA), based on early, preliminary results of clinical trials, when there is an urgent need for the product to address a health threat to Americans. The manufacturer of the test, vaccine, or medication is expected to update the FDA with data as the product gets used in practice. When enough data is accumulated over a sufficient length of time to allow the FDA to make conclusions as to the safety and effectiveness of the product, the FDA can then formally approve it.

epidemic. An unexpected increase in the number of cases of infection or disease in a specific geographic area.

epidemic curve, or epidemiological curve or epi curve. A graph of case counts associated with an outbreak over time. The graph can show the onset of an outbreak, whether the outbreak is accelerating or contracting, and whether mitigation measures are having a positive impact.

epidemiology. The study of the determinants and distribution of health states in a population.

field hospitals. Temporary hospitals using large tents or converted non-hospital facilities, such as convention centers, as sites for treating less acutely ill patients when hospitals are overwhelmed in a civilian context. During the COVID-19 pandemic in the United States, field hospitals were often supplied with equipment from the Department of Defense and in many cases staffed by health care professionals who traveled from across the country to volunteer their assistance.

fitness advantage. A transmission advantage that one virus or variant may gain over another, often through mutation that has made it more contagious. In some cases, where a significant amount of immunity in a population has been acquired by natural infection or vaccination, a variant may gain a fitness advantage through mutation that gives it the capability of immune escape or evasion. In either case, whether more contagious or more evasive, the virus or variant has a fitness advantage, which may become apparent when a growing proportion of infections are caused by it.

Food and Drug Administration (**FDA**). An agency of the US Department of Health and Human Services that was established by the Federal Food, Drug, and Cosmetic Act of 1938. The FDA is responsible for protecting the public and promoting public health through the regulation of food safety, medications, vaccines, and medical devices.

frontier areas. Sparsely populated areas that are geographically isolated from population centers, with fewer than six people per square mile.

genomic sequencing. A technique for analyzing an organism's full genetic code. With SARS-CoV-2, genomic sequencing allowed scientists to analyze virus samples obtained over time to determine changes to the virus, particularly the acquisition of mutations that might enhance its transmissibility or virulence. Genomic sequencing can also be used to compare virus samples taken from people in a population who were infected around the same time to determine which persons were infected with a variant of concern, the proportion of cases caused by different variants, and the acquisition of a fitness advantage by a variant.

herd immunity. A level of immunity within a population, either from natural infection or immunization, that is high enough to result in an infectious agent (usually a virus) no longer being able to transmit efficiently in that population. With herd immunity, the rate of infection has become quite low in the population, and that low incidence will protect the vulnerable (those too young to be vaccinated, those with a contraindication to vaccines, those who refuse to be vaccinated, those who are immunocompromised by disease or medications, and those whose immunity is waning) because their chances of encountering someone whose infection is contagious are greatly reduced.

host. A larger organism that harbors a smaller organism. A host may be a carrier or transmitter of an infectious organism and thus serves as an intermediary or the host may be the destination wherein the organism causes symptoms of infection and coopts cells of the host for its replication.

IgG (immunoglobulin G) antibody. The body produces a variety of immunoglobulins in response to infection, which serve different roles. IgG is the most common type of antibody; it circulates in the blood and protects the body from bacterial or viral infection.

immune escape/evasion. A capability that a virus may acquire through mutation in its genetic code, resulting in a change to its structure that diminishes or even overcomes a potential host's immune response acquired through prior infection or immunization, thereby making the host more susceptible to the strain or variant with this new capability.

isolation. When someone infected or potentially infected with a pathogen has no close contact with others for the duration of time the infection is thought to be contagious, in order not to spread it.

long COVID. *See* **post-acute sequelae of SARS-CoV-2 infection (PASC).**

long haulers. A popular name for those individuals with long COVID. *See* **post-acute sequelae of SARS-CoV-2 infection (PASC).**

mechanical ventilation. A form of life support in which a machine—a ventilator—delivers breathing support to a patient to raise that person's blood oxygen concentration.

messenger RNA (mRNA). A single-stranded molecule of RNA (ribonucleic acid) that carries the genetic sequence of a gene to the cellular machinery that then synthesizes proteins using the instructions from the mRNA code. One vaccine technology utilizes mRNA to carry a message for cells to make the spike protein that is part of SARS-CoV-2. That spike protein will, in turn, stimulate an immune response that will protect vaccinated persons from infection with the SARS-CoV-2 virus.

Middle East respiratory syndrome (MERS). A respiratory illness caused by a novel coronavirus first reported in Saudi Arabia in 2012. It spread to 27 other countries, including the United States. It was on the brink of becoming a pandemic before it was successfully contained.

misinformation. Incorrect information spread by a person who believed it to be true at the time of communicating it. *See also* **disinformation.**

monoclonal antibody. An identical antibody that can be produced in a laboratory and used as a therapy in someone who is early in the course of an infection, before the body has had a chance to make its own antibodies.

morbidity. The adverse effects of an illness short of death.

mortality rate. The rate at which people die from any cause or from a specific cause. In epidemiology, there are different ways to look at the rate of mortality from an infection. One is to quantify the case fatality rate, which is the number of deaths caused by the infection divided by the number of people with confirmed infection. Another method is to estimate the infection fatality rate, which is the number of deaths caused by the infection divided by the estimated total number of people who have been infected. In the case of COVID-19, where many infections are mild or asymptomatic and people may not get tested to confirm infection, it has been common to estimate the total number of people infected, often by using seroprevalence studies that identify the percentage of people who have antibody evidence of past infection. Researchers can then compare the number of people with antibodies to the number of confirmed cases of infection to estimate the percentage of people who get infected and are asymptomatic. This step lets researchers arrive at a denominator used to calculate the infection fatality rate.

multisystem inflammatory syndrome in adults (MIS-A). A hyperinflammatory illness in adults, ranging in age from 21 to 50 years, similar to multisystem inflammatory syndrome in children, but first recognized in the fall of 2020.

multisystem inflammatory syndrome in children (MIS-C). A peculiar illness in children, found two to four weeks following a COVID-19 illness, which resembles a combination of Kawasaki disease and toxic shock syndrome. Signs and symptoms include fever, abdominal (stomach) pain, a rash, bloodshot eyes, vomiting, diarrhea, and profound weakness. The illness generally requires hospitalization and may prove fatal.

mutation. A change to the structure of a gene caused by the substitution, deletion, or addition of one of the letters of the genetic code sequence. Most mutations are of little concern, but some mutations create a fitness advantage for a pathogenic organism that can make it more contagious, more virulent, more resistant to treatments, or provide it with the ability to partially or completely escape the immunity of someone who was previously infected by it or was vaccinated for it.

natural infection. A reference, generally, to antibodies produced in response to being infected with an organism naturally, rather than to antibodies produced in reaction to immunization.

neutralizing antibodies. *See* **antibodies.**

N95 face mask. A mask commonly referred to as a N95 respirator. It meets the classification standards of the US National Institute for Occupational Safety and Health, meaning that it filters at least 95 percent of airborne particles.

novel virus. A new virus or new strain of a virus for which no one in the world can be expected to have immunity.

Operation Warp Speed. A program set up under the Trump administration within the US Department of Defense for the purpose of partnering with private industry to accelerate the development, testing, supply, and distribution of safe and effective COVID-19 vaccines by the end of 2020.

pandemic. The worldwide spread of an infection or disease.

pathogen. An organism that causes a disease.

pauci-symptomatic. Literally "few symptoms." In the context of COVID-19, this term describes people with COVID-19 who are not asymptomatic but who have a mild illness with few symptoms, which often are mistakenly attributed to allergies or fatigue rather than to COVID-19.

PCR (polymerase chain reaction). This is a testing method of nucleic acid amplification in which a small sample is taken from a patient and then millions or billions of copies of the genetic material of a pathogen, if one is present, are reproduced, which allows a laboratory to identify the presence of portions of the genetic material that match the genetic material of the pathogen tested for.

personal protective equipment (PPE). Equipment used to protect individuals from the transmission of a disease. PPE includes gowns, gloves, face masks, face shields, goggles, and N95 respirators.

phase 3 clinical trials. The last step in clinical trials prior to the authorization or approval of a new medical product by the Food and Drug Administration. The first step in clinical trials usually takes place in a laboratory with cells grown in a petri dish or test tube. The next step in testing a new drug or vaccine is often done in animals. Phase 1 clinical trials are generally done with small numbers of humans to find out whether the product is safe. The next step, phase 2, also involves humans and is designed to find out whether the product is effective. Finally comes phase 3, where safety and efficacy are tested in much larger numbers of humans, often comparing the product to a placebo or another existing therapy.

physical distancing. Also referred to as social distancing, this is a public health mitigation measure for separating people at a distance that lessens the likelihood of transmitting an infection by respiratory droplets. In controlling the spread of COVID-19, the physical distancing recommendation in the United States has been six feet, but some other countries have recommended only three feet.

pneumonia. An inflammation of the lungs, most often caused by a bacterial or viral infection. Pneumonia can be characterized by fever, pressure or tightness in the chest, shortness of breath, and coughing, sometimes ejecting phlegm. In many cases, the inflammation and attendant accumulation of pus and fluid will create abnormalities that can be seen on chest X-rays or scans of the lungs.

post-acute sequelae of SARS-CoV-2 infection (PASC). Also referred to as long COVID, chronic COVID, post-acute COVID, or long hauler's syndrome, it is characterized by wide-ranging symptoms that persist for months following COVID-19 infection (sometimes even after a mild case) with disabling effects in adults who were previously active and healthy but now find themselves unable to do everyday things without overwhelming symptoms. It is just now being recognized that a similar disorder can occur in children. The pathophysiology for this disorder is unknown but hypothesized to be the result of ongoing stimulation of the immune system either from persistent viral RNA or from the virus itself (for example, residual virus in the gastrointestinal tract). On the other hand, it could be due to the effects of immune-mediated damage caused by the original infection. It may even be the case that both mechanisms could contribute to this disorder.

pre-symptomatic. A reference to those who are currently asymptomatic but will soon develop symptoms.

quarantine. To prevent further spread of infection, a person who has been around someone with a documented infection is isolated so as to avoid close contact with others for the time necessary to determine whether that person too will become infected.

reproduction number (R-naught or R_0). The number of other people that someone infected at the beginning of an outbreak can be expected to infect in turn, when no one has preexisting immunity and no mitigation measures are in place.

respiratory droplets. *See* **droplets.**

SARS-associated coronavirus (SARS-CoV). The novel coronavirus that caused severe acute respiratory syndrome (SARS) in an outbreak in 2003.

SARS-CoV-2, 2019 novel coronavirus (2019-nCoV). The novel coronavirus, considered to be related to the SARS-associated coronavirus, or SARS-CoV, that causes COVID-19, beginning with an outbreak in China in December 2019. At the time of this writing, there have been 127 million cases of COVID-19 and 2.8 million deaths worldwide in 192 countries. The case fatality rate varies but is typically 2 to 3 percent.

sepsis. An extreme response by the body to an overwhelming infection. Septic shock impairs the blood flow to important organs and can result in death.

sequester. An effort to limit an individual's close contacts to a small number of people (often just members of the same household) to minimize chances of exposure to a contagion.

seronegative. A negative test result for antibodies in the blood.

seroprevalence. The frequency of positive antibody tests within a population.

severe acute respiratory syndrome (SARS). The respiratory syndrome caused by a novel coronavirus outbreak first reported in Asia in 2003. This disease spread to more than two dozen countries before it was contained. The case fatality rate was 11 percent.

social determinants of health. A variety of environmental factors that affect as much as 80 percent of health and health outcomes. These factors include income, health insurance, access to health care, safe homes, safe neighborhoods, safe communities, safe workplaces, clean water, sufficient food, healthy food, reliable transportation, quality education, and others.

spike protein. A protein on the surface of the SARS-CoV-2 virus that gives it a crown-like appearance under an electron microscope. This protein is critical to the virus's ability to infect human cells, and it is also an effective target for antibodies in preventing infection.

strain. A genetic subtype of a species of microorganism possessing similar properties such as transmissibility and virulence.

Strategic National Stockpile. Twelve secret locations across the United States where medical supplies, equipment, and medications are stored in the event of a national disaster or emergency.

test positivity rate. In the case of COVID-19, the number of positive tests for COVID-19 as a percentage of all tests done to rule out COVID-19, in a set time frame for a specific population.

transcription. The copying of genetic instructions for the production of proteins in a cell.

transmissibility. Transmissibility is how easily a virus spreads within a population. The reproduction number (R_0) and/or the secondary rates are often used to infer the transmissibility of a virus. Transmissibility is determined by the infectivity of the virus, the contagiousness of the infected person, the susceptibility of those who are exposed to the infected person, and environmental factors (such as population density or physical distancing of individuals in the case of airborne viruses or sanitation practices in the case of foodborne illnesses), as well as the degree of existing immunity in the population.

vaccine. A substance introduced into the body to stimulate an immune response that will protect the person from future infection without the need for them to have been infected.

vaccine hesitancy. Concerns or mistrust that cause people to put off getting vaccinated.

variant. In the context of disease, a variant is an identifiable subtype of a microorganism resulting from accumulated mutations. Viral variants often arise in situations of high disease transmission, when replication across many hosts produces a mutation that proves stable enough to transmit successfully as subsequent generations.

variants of concern. Variants that warrant study because the mutations acquired appear to make the microbe more contagious, more virulent, or more elusive to immunity.

viral dose. The amount of virus necessary to cause infection.

viral load. The amount of virus in a person's body, which often correlates with the contagiousness of the infected person and the severity of disease in that person.

virulence. The likelihood that a virus will cause severe disease or even death.

virus. An infectious agent too small to be seen under regular microscopes. A virus is made up of DNA or RNA and a protein coating but is incapable of replicating on its own. A virus must enter the cells of a host and use their cellular machinery to copy itself.

wild-type virus. Generally, the original, naturally occurring, and non-mutated strain of a virus. It can also refer, though, to the predominant strain of circulating virus prior to a new strain taking over in an infected population.

World Health Organization (WHO). An international agency established under the auspices of the United Nations with its own constitution adopted in 1946. It began operation in April 1948 and today has 194 member countries. The mission of the WHO is to promote health and control the spread of communicable diseases in all countries of the world.

zoonotic infection. An infection resulting from the spread of germs between animals and humans.

NOTES

Chapter 1. The SARS-CoV-2 Virus and the COVID-19 Pandemic

1. Aaron Blake, "Trump Keeps Saying 'Nobody' Could Have Foreseen Coronavirus. We Keep Finding Out about New Warning Signs," *Washington Post*, March 19, 2020, https://www.washingtonpost.com/politics/2020/03/19/trump-keeps-saying-nobody-could-have-foreseen-coronavirus-we-keep-finding-out-about-new-warning-signs/.
2. Marissa Taylor, "Exclusive: U.S. Slashed CDC Staff inside China prior to Coronavirus Outbreak," Reuters, March 25, 2020, https://www.reuters.com/article/us-health-coronavirus-china-cdc-exclusiv-idUSKBN21C3N5.
3. Taylor, "Exclusive: U.S. Slashed CDC Staff inside China."
4. S. Lock, "Number of U.S. Residents Travelling Overseas 2002–2019," Statistica, last updated February 21, 2020, https://www.statista.com/statistics/214774/number-of-outbound-tourists-from-the-us/.
5. Chaolin Huang et al., "Clinical Features of Patients Infected with 2019 Novel Coronavirus in Wuhan, China," *Lancet* 395, no. 10223 (2020): 497–506, https://doi.org/10.1016/S0140-6736(20)30183-5.
6. Robert G. Webster, "Wet Markets—a Continuing Source of Severe Acute Respiratory Syndrome and Influenza?," *Lancet* 363, no. 9404 (2004): 234–36, https://doi.org/10.1016/s0140-6736(03)15329-9.
7. Antonella Amendola et al., "Evidence of SARS-CoV-2 RNA in an Oropharyngeal Swab Specimen, Milan, Italy, Early December 2019," *Emerging Infectious Diseases* 27, no. 2 (2021): 648–50, https://doi.org/10.3201/eid2702.204632.
8. US Department of State, "Fact Sheet: Activity at the Wuhan Institute of Virology," last modified January 16, 2021, https://2017-2021.state.gov/fact-sheet-activity-at-the-wuhan-institute-of-virology/index.html.
9. Mingkun Zhan et al., "Death from Covid-19 of 23 Health Care Workers in China," *New England Journal of Medicine* 382, no. 23 (2020): 2267–68, https://doi.org/10.1056/nejmc2005696.
10. Shawna Williams, "Person-to-Person Spread of Novel Coronavirus Confirmed in China," *Scientist*, January 21, 2020, https://www.the-scientist.com/news-opinion/person-to-person-spread-of-novel-coronavirus-confirmed-in-china--66995.
11. Michelle L. Holshue et al., "First Case of 2019 Novel Coronavirus in the United States," *New England Journal of Medicine* 382, no. 10 (2020): 929–36, https://doi.org/10.1056/nejmoa2001191.
12. Amy Orciari Herman, "WHO Declares Public Health Emergency over Coronavirus; Person-to-Person Transmission Confirmed in U.S.," *NEJM Journal Watch*,

January 31, 2020, https://www.jwatch.org/fw116303/2020/01/31/who-declares-public-health-emergency-over-coronavirus.

13. Robert P. Baird, "What Went Wrong with Coronavirus Testing in the U.S.," *New Yorker*, March 16, 2020, https://www.newyorker.com/news/news-desk/what-went-wrong-with-coronavirus-testing-in-the-us.
14. Michael Lycklama, "Idaho Orders a Statewide Closure of Public Schools, One of the Last in the Country," *Idaho Statesman*, March 23, 2020, https://www.idahostatesman.com/news/coronavirus/article241449166.html.
15. Camilla Rothe et al., "Transmission of 2019-nCoV Infection from an Asymptomatic Contact in Germany," *New England Journal of Medicine* 382, no. 10 (2020): 970–71, https://doi.org/10.1056/nejmc2001468.
16. Daniel P. Oran and Eric J. Topol, "Prevalence of Asymptomatic SARS-CoV-2 Infection," *Annals of Internal Medicine* 173, no. 5 (2020): 362–67, https://doi.org/10.7326/M20-3012.
17. Officer of the Governor, "Idaho Leads in Economic Rebound, Gov. Little Highlights Steps Taken to Strengthen Economy," Government of Idaho, last updated September 18, 2020, https://gov.idaho.gov/pressrelease/idaho-leads-in-economic-rebound-gov-little-highlights-steps-taken-to-strengthen-economy/.
18. Matthew A. Winkler, "Idaho Defies Trump's Nationalism with Best U.S. Economy," *Bloomberg Opinion*, October 22, 2020, https://www.bloomberg.com/opinion/articles/2020-10-22/idaho-s-red-hot-economy-defies-trump-nationalism.
19. "People with Certain Medical Conditions," Centers for Disease Control and Prevention, last updated May 2, 2022, https://www.cdc.gov/coronavirus/2019-ncov/need-extra-precautions/people-with-medical-conditions.html.
20. Eli S. Rosenberg et al., "Cumulative Incidence and Diagnosis of SARS-CoV-2 Infection in New York," *Annals of Epidemiology*, 48 (2020): 23–29.e4, https://doi.org/10.1016/j.annepidem.2020.06.004.
21. BNO News, "COVID-19 Reinfection Tracker," last accessed July 2, 2021, https://bnonews.com/index.php/2020/08/covid-19-reinfection-tracker/.
22. Giacomo Grasselli et al., "Pathophysiology of COVID-19-Associated Acute Respiratory Distress Syndrome: A Multicentre Prospective Observational Study," *Lancet: Respiratory Medicine* 8, no. 12 (2020): 1201–8, https://doi.org/10.1016/S2213-2600(20)30370-2.
23. Sharon E. Fox et al., "Pulmonary and Cardiac Pathology in African American Patients with COVID-19: An Autopsy Series from New Orleans," *Lancet: Respiratory Medicine* 8, no. 7 (2020): 681–86, https://doi.org/10.1016/s2213-2600(20)30243-5.
24. Jacob Avila et al., "Thrombotic Complications of COVID-19," *American Journal of Emergency Medicine*, 39 (2021): 213–18, https://doi.org/10.1016/j.ajem.2020.09.065.
25. "Health Department–Reported Cases of Multisystem Inflammatory Syndrome in Children (MIS-C) in the United States," Centers for Disease Control and Prevention, last accessed July 2, 2021, https://www.cdc.gov/mis-c/cases/index.html.
26. Jia-Hui Zeng et al., "First Case of COVID-19 Complicated with Fulminant Myocarditis: A Case Report and Insights," *Infection* 48, no. 5 (2020): 773–77, https://doi.org/10.1007/s15010-020-01424-5.

27. Sanjay Kumar, Alfred Veldhuis, and Tina Malhotra, "Neuropsychiatric and Cognitive Sequelae of COVID-19," *Frontiers in Psychology,* 12 (2021), https://doi.org/10.3389/fpsyg.2021.577529.
28. Jeffrey E. Gold et al., "Investigation of Long COVID Prevalence and Its Relationship to Epstein-Barr Virus Reactivation," *Pathogens* 10, no. 6 (2021): 763, https://doi.org/10.3390/pathogens10060763.
29. Gold et al., "Investigation of Long COVID Prevalence."
30. Valentina O. Puntmann et al., "Outcomes of Cardiovascular Magnetic Resonance Imaging in Patients Recently Recovered from Coronavirus Disease 2019 (COVID-19)," *JAMA Cardiology* 5, no. 11 (2020): 1265–73, https://doi.org/10.1001/jamacardio.2020.3557.
31. Angelo Carfì et al., "Persistent Symptoms in Patients after Acute COVID-19," *Journal of the American Medical Association* 324, no. 6 (2020): 603–5, https://doi.org/10.1001/jama.2020.12603.
32. N. J. Lambert and Survivor Corps, "COVID-19 'Long Hauler' Symptoms Survey Report," Indiana University School of Medicine, 2020, https://dig.abclocal.go.com/wls/documents/2020/072720-wls-covid-symptom-study-doc.pdf.
33. Damian Paletta and Yasmeen Abutaleb, *Nightmare Scenario: Inside the Trump Administration's Response to the Pandemic That Changed History* (New York: HarperCollins, 2021).

Chapter 2. Pandemic Surveillance and Early Response in the Future

1. "Prioritizing Diseases for Research and Development in Emergency Contexts," World Health Organization, last accessed August 3, 2021, https://www.who.int/activities/prioritizing-diseases-for-research-and-development-in-emergency-contexts.

Chapter 3. The Intersection of COVID-19 and Society

1. Hannah Ritchie and Max Roser, "Urbanization," Our World in Data, revised November 2019, https://ourworldindata.org/urbanization.
2. United Nations Department of Economic and Social Affairs, Population Division, *World Population Ageing, 2019*, 2020, https://www.un.org/en/development/desa/population/publications/pdf/ageing/WorldPopulationAgeing2019-Report.pdf.
3. Jonathan Chait, "Trump: I Was Right, Coronavirus Cases 'Will Go Down to Zero, Ultimately,'" *New York Intelligencer,* April 28, 2020, https://nymag.com/intelligencer/2020/04/trump-coronavirus-cases-will-go-down-to-zero-ultimately.html.
4. Kevin Breuninger, "Trump Wants 'Packed Churches' and Economy Open Again on Easter despite the Deadly Threat of Coronavirus," CNBC, updated March 24, 2020, https://www.cnbc.com/2020/03/24/coronavirus-response-trump-wants-to-reopen-us-economy-by-easter.html.
5. Brian Holmes, "City of Eagle Holds Annual Tree Lighting Ceremony despite Ada County Public Health Order," KTVB7, December 7, 2020, https://www.ktvb.com/article/news/local/208/eagle-tree-lighting/277-35c2ffd8-23e2-4045-88a2-068601abc57e.

6. Nicolas Shanosky, Daniel McDermott, and Nisha Kurani, "How Do U.S. Health-care Resources Compare to Other Countries?," Peterson-KFF Health System Tracker, August 12, 2020, https://www.healthsystemtracker.org/chart-collection/u-s-health-care-resources-compare-countries/#item-start.
7. Jason Hoffman, "Trump Baselessly Claims Doctors Are Inflating Coronavirus Death Counts for Money as Cases Again Hit Record Levels," CNN Politics, updated October 31, 2020, https://www.cnn.com/2020/10/30/politics/trump-doctors-covid/index.html.
8. Oregon Medical Board, *Order of Emergency Suspension of License and Notice of Opportunity for Hearing*, December 4, 2020, https://omb.oregon.gov/Clients/ORMB/OrderDocuments/ff970292-5807-41ba-9c1e-c2b81de89cd1.pdf.
9. James Dawson, "Unmasked Protesters Push Past Police into Idaho Lawmakers' Session," NPR, August 25, 2020, https://www.npr.org/2020/08/25/905785548/unmasked-protesters-push-past-police-into-idaho-lawmakers-session.
10. AP News Wire, "Idaho Health Board Meeting Halted after 'Intense Protests,'" *Independent*, December 9, 2020, https://www.independent.co.uk/news/world/americas/idaho-health-board-meeting-halted-after-intense-protests-boise-safety-idaho-health-police-b1768433.html.
11. Nicole Blanchard, "Gov. Little Left Mask Mandates to Health Districts. Some Trustees Call COVID-19 a Hoax," *Idaho Statesman*, July 16, 2020, https://www.idahostatesman.com/news/coronavirus/article244219242.html.
12. Nicole Blanchard, "'That's Just Irresponsible': Inslee Says Idaho's COVID-19 Response Hurts Wash. Hospitals," *Moscow-Pullman Daily News*, November 16, 2020, https://dnews.com/coronavirus/that-s-just-irresponsible-inslee-says-idaho-s-covid-19-response-hurts-wash-hospitals/article_f250c68d-2cbc-5aea-9633-3b8c35a55dde.html.
13. Blanchard, "Gov. Little Left Mask Mandates to Health Districts."

Chapter 4. The Haves and the Have-Nots

1. CDC, "Disparities in COVID-19 Illness: Racial and Ethnic Health Disparities," last updated December 10, 2020, https://www.cdc.gov/coronavirus/2019-ncov/community/health-equity/racial-ethnic-disparities/increased-risk-illness.html.
2. Thomas Hubbard, "The Boston Paradox: Lots of Health Care, Not Enough Health," Boston Foundation, June 2007, https://folio.iupui.edu/bitstream/handle/10244/730/BostonParadoxReport.pdf?sequence=2.
3. CDC, "Disparities in COVID-19 Illness."
4. CDC, "Disparities in COVID-19 Illness."
5. CDC, "Disparities in COVID-19 Illness."
6. CDC, "Disparities in COVID-19 Illness."
7. CDC, "Disparities in COVID-19 Illness."
8. CDC, "Disparities in COVID-19 Illness."
9. CDC, "Disparities in COVID-19 Illness."
10. CDC, "Disparities in COVID-19 Illness."
11. CDC, "Disparities in COVID-19 Illness."

12. CDC, "Disparities in COVID-19 Illness."
13. CDC, "Disparities in COVID-19 Illness."
14. CDC, "Disparities in COVID-19 Illness."
15. CDC, "Disparities in COVID-19 Illness."
16. CDC, "Disparities in COVID-19 Illness."
17. Kim Parker, Rachel Minkin, and Jesse Bennett, "Economic Fallout from COVID-19 Continues to Hit Lower-Income Americans the Hardest," Pew Research Center, September 24, 2020, https://www.pewresearch.org/social-trends/2020/09/24/economic-fallout-from-covid-19-continues-to-hit-lower-income-americans-the-hardest/.
18. Parker, Minkin, and Bennett, "Economic Fallout from COVID-19."
19. CDC, "Disparities in COVID-19 Illness."
20. Alisha Coleman-Jensen et al., "Household Food Insecurity in the United States in 2016," US Department of Agriculture, Economic Research Service ERR-237, 2017, https://www.ers.usda.gov/webdocs/publications/84973/err-237.pdf?v=4025.1.
21. United States Census Bureau, "Household Pulse Survey Data Tables [Week 12 Household Pulse Survey: July 16–July 21 and Week 1 Household Pulse Survey: April 23–May 5]," August 27, 2020, https://census.gov/data/tables/2020/demo/hhp/hhp1.html#techdoc.
22. Mark É. Czeisler et al., "Delay or Avoidance of Medical Care Because of COVID-19-Related Concerns—United States, June 2020," *Morbidity and Mortality Weekly Report* 69, no. 36 (2020): 1250–57, http://dx.doi.org/10.15585/mmwr.mm6936a4.
23. CDC, "Disparities in COVID-19 Illness."
24. Ashton M. Verdery et al., "Tracking the Reach of COVID-19 Kin Loss with a Bereavement Multiplier Applied to the United States," *Proceedings of the National Academy of Sciences of the United States of America* 117, no. 30 (2020): 17695–701, https://doi.org/10.1073/pnas.2007476117.

Chapter 5. The Growing Fire

1. Aaron Blake, "Trump's Dumbfounding Refusal to Encourage Wearing Masks," *Washington Post*, June 25, 2020, https://www.washingtonpost.com/politics/2020/06/25/trumps-dumbfounding-refusal-encourage-wearing-masks/.
2. "Map: Coronavirus and School Closures in 2019–2020," Education Week, updated October 13, 2021, https://www.edweek.org/leadership/map-coronavirus-and-school-closures-in-2019-2020/2020/03.
3. CDC, "Risk for COVID-19 Infection, Hospitalization, and Death by Age Group," updated June 27, 2022, https://www.cdc.gov/coronavirus/2019-ncov/covid-data/investigations-discovery/hospitalization-death-by-age.html.
4. Scripps Research Institute, "Up to 45 Percent of SARS-CoV-2 Infections May Be Asymptomatic," *Science Daily*, June 12, 2020, https://www.sciencedaily.com/releases/2020/06/200612172208.htm.
5. Nicholas G. Davies et al., "Age-Dependent Effects in the Transmission and Control of COVID-19 Epidemics," *Nature Medicine*, 26 (2020): 1205–11, https://doi.org/10.1038/s41591-020-0962-9.

6. SPLC Southern Poverty Law Center, "Antigovernment Movement," last accessed July 14, 2022, https://www.splcenter.org/fighting-hate/extremist-files/ideology/antigovernment.
7. Matthew Rosenberg and Ainara Tiefenthäler, "Decoding the Far-Right Symbols at the Capitol Riot," *New York Times*, January 13, 2021, https://www.nytimes.com/2021/01/13/video/extremist-signs-symbols-capitol-riot.html.
8. Sheila Kennedy, "This Is Your Brain on Grievance," *Sheila Kennedy: A Jaundiced Look at the World We Live In* (blog), December 27, 2020, https://www.sheilakennedy.net/2020/12/this-is-your-brain-on-grievance/.
9. Kennedy, "This Is Your Brain on Grievance."
10. Maxine Bernstein, "Conspiracy Charge, Defendants' 'State of Mind' Proved Hurdles in Ammon Bundy Prosecution," *Oregonian*, October 30, 2016, https://www.oregonlive.com/oregon-standoff/2016/10/conspiracy_charge_defendants_s.html.
11. Michael Ames, "How Ammon Bundy Helped Foment an Anti-masker Rebellion in Idaho," *New Yorker*, December 21, 2020, https://www.newyorker.com/news/us-journal/how-ammon-bundy-helped-foment-an-anti-masker-rebellion-in-idaho.
12. Ames, "How Ammon Bundy Helped Foment an Anti-masker Rebellion in Idaho."
13. Ximena Bustillo, "Hundreds Rally at Idaho Capitol to Protest Gov. Little's Stay-Home Order," *Idaho Statesman*, April 17, 2020, https://www.idahostatesman.com/news/coronavirus/article242092321.html.
14. "Cheers & Jeers: Just the Facts," *Lewiston Tribune*, September 4, 2020, https://lmtribune.com/opinion/cheers-jeers-just-the-facts/article_3609ffb1-46c8-516d-a6d5-3580d04af4bd.html.
15. Mike Wehner, "Which States Are the Best and Worst at Wearing Masks?," BGR, October 29, 2020, https://bgr.com/2020/10/29/mask-wearing-by-state-survey/.
16. Hannah Allam, "Right-Wing Embrace of Conspiracy Is 'Mass Radicalization,' Experts Warn," NPR, December 15, 2020, https://www.npr.org/2020/12/15/946381523/right-wing-embrace-of-conspiracy-is-mass-radicalization-experts-warn.

Chapter 6. Man versus Virus

1. Victor Cha and Dana Kim, "A Timeline of South Korea's Response to COVID-19," Center for Strategic & International Studies, May 27, 2020, https://www.csis.org/analysis/timeline-south-koreas-response-covid-19.

Chapter 7. Needed Changes to the Federal Response

1. Brian Bennett and Tessa Berenson, "'Our Big War.' As Coronavirus Spreads, Trump Refashions Himself as a Wartime President," *Time*, March 19, 2020, https://time.com/5806657/donald-trump-coronavirus-war-china/.
2. Nahal Toosi, Daniel Lippman, and Dan Diamond, "Before Trump's Inauguration, a Warning: 'The Worst Influenza Pandemic since 1918,'" Politico, March 16, 2020, https://www.politico.com/news/2020/03/16/trump-inauguration-warning-scenario-pandemic-132797.
3. Jordan Fabian, "Trump Told Governors to Buy Their Own Virus Supplies, Then Outbid Them," Bloomberg Prognosis, March 19, 2020, https://www.bloomberg

.com/news/articles/2020-03-19/trump-told-governors-to-buy-own-virus-supplies -then-outbid-them.

4. Bob Woodward, *Rage* (New York: Simon & Schuster, 2020).
5. "Fast Facts on U.S. Hospitals, 2020," American Hospital Association; 2022 information available at https://www.aha.org/statistics/fast-facts-us-hospitals.
6. Jacob Pramuk and John W. Schoen, "This Timeline Shows How the US-China Trade War Led to the Latest Deal with Beijing," CNBC, December 13, 2019, https://www .cnbc.com/2019/12/13/timeline-of-trump-china-trade-war-and-trade-deal.html.
7. David Jackson and Michael Collins, "Trump to Mike Pence: 'Don't Call the Woman in Michigan,' aka Gov. Gretchen Whitmer," *USA Today*, April 2, 2020, https://www.usatoday.com/story/news/politics/2020/03/27/coronavirus-donald -trump-tells-pence-not-call-michigan-governor/2931251001/.
8. Ebony Bowden and Steven Nelson, "Trump Rips Cuomo, Says NY Won't Get COVID-19 Vaccine Until Gov OKs It," *New York Post*, November 13, 2020, https://nypost.com/2020/11/13/trump-says-covid-vaccine-wont-be-given-to-ny -until-cuomo-approves-it/.

Chapter 8. The Future Role of the States

1. Olivia Heersink, "Southwest District Health Hears Conflicting Information from Medical Practitioners," *Idaho Press*, November 17, 2020, https://www.idahopress .com/coronavirus/southwest-district-health-hears-conflicting-information-from -medical-practitioners/article_0e4f8a4d-8300-5c18-b7d3-311885efe2db.html.
2. Heersink, "Southwest District Health Hears Conflicting Information."

Chapter 9. Preparing Future Doctors, Nurses, and Public Health Workers for the Next Pandemic

1. Karen Gilchrist, "Covid Has Made It Harder to Be a Health-Care Worker. Now, Many Are Thinking of Quitting," CNBC, updated June 1, 2021, https://www.cnbc .com/2021/05/31/covid-is-driving-an-exodus-among-health-care-workers.html.
2. Data taken from StatSoft Europe, "Statistica," Nov 5, 2020, https://www.statistica .com.
3. Data taken from StatSoft Europe, "Statistica," Nov 6, 2020, https://www .statistica.com.
4. Victoria Simpson, "Countries with the Most Physicians Per Capita," World Atlas, accessed February 25, 2021, https://www.worldatlas.com/articles/countries-with -the-most-physicians-per-capita.html.
5. Ellen Kershner, "Countries with the Most Nurses and Midwives Per Capita," World Atlas, accessed February 25, 2021, https://www.worldatlas.com/articles /countries-with-the-most-nurses-and-midwives-per-capita.html.
6. US Department of Health and Human Services, Health Resources and Services Administration, National Center for Health Workforce Analysis, "Sex, Race, and Ethnic Diversity of U.S. Health Occupations (2011–2015)," August 2017, https:// bhw.hrsa.gov/sites/default/files/bureau-health-workforce/data-research/diversity -us-health-occupations.pdf.

7. US Department of Health and Human Services, "Sex, Race, and Ethnic Diversity of U.S. Health Occupations (2011–2015)."
8. National Center for Biotechnology Information, "Welcome to NCBI," National Library of Medicine, accessed March 9, 2021, https://www.ncbi.nlm.nih.gov/.
9. Rural Health Information Hub, "Your First Stop for Rural Health Information," accessed March 9, 2021, https://www.ruralhealthinfo.org.
10. Rural Health Information Hub, "Your First Stop for Rural Health Information."
11. T. W. Nasca, "Plenary Lecture at the Accreditation Council for Graduate Medical Education (ACGME) Annual Educational Conference" (lecture, virtual session, February 25, 2021).
12. D. M. Berwick, "Plenary Lecture at the Accreditation Council for Graduate Medical Education (ACGME) Annual Education Conference" (lecture, virtual session, February 26, 2021).
13. Jonathan Bryant-Genevier et al., "Symptoms of Depression, Anxiety, Post-traumatic Stress Disorder, and Suicidal Ideation among State, Tribal, Local, and Territorial Public Health Workers during the COVID-19 Pandemic—United States, March–April 2021," *Morbidity and Mortality Weekly Report* 70, no. 26 (2021): 947–52, 947, https://doi.org/10.15585/mmwr.mm7026e1.

Chapter 10. Preparing Public Health Departments for the Next Pandemic

1. Lauren Weber et al., "Hollowed-Out Public Health System Faces More Cuts amid Virus," Kaiser Health News, updated on August 24, 2020, https://khn.org/news/us-public-health-system-underfunded-under-threat-faces-more-cuts-amid-covid-pandemic/.
2. Weber et al., "Hollowed-Out Public Health System."
3. Susan R. Bailey, "Pandemic Exposes Dire Need to Rebuild Public Health Infrastructure," American Medical Association, February 10, 2021, https://www.ama-assn.org/about/leadership/pandemic-exposes-dire-need-rebuild-public-health-infrastructure.
4. Brian Castrucci, Chrissie Juliano, and Thomas V. Inglesby, "Four Steps to Building the Public Health System Needed to Cope with the Next Pandemic," *Journal of Public Health Management and Practice* 27, Suppl. 1 (2021): S98–S100, https://doi.org/10.1097/phh.0000000000001303.
5. Big Cities Health Coalition, *Building Resilient, Equitable, and Healthy Communities Post Pandemic and Always: Recommendations for the Next Administration and 117th Congress*, October 19, 2020, https://debeaumont.org/wp-content/uploads/2020/10/BCHCTransitionPaper.pdf.

Chapter 11. The Rejection of Science

1. Robert Glatter, "Calls to Poison Centers Spike after the President's Comments about Using Disinfectants to Treat Coronavirus," *Forbes*, April 25, 2020, https://www.forbes.com/sites/robertglatter/2020/04/25/calls-to-poison-centers

-spike--after-the-presidents-comments-about-using-disinfectants-to-treat -coronavirus/?sh=5819875e1157.

2. Burgess Everett and John Bresnahan, “Republicans Praise Trump’s Pandemic Response with Senate Majority at Risk,” Politico, May 6, 2020, https://www.politico.com/news/2020/05/06/senate-republicans-trump-coronavirus-response-240454.
3. Grant McCool and Mark Egan, “Giuliani and Bloomberg: NY Mayors Linked by Sept 11,” Reuters, September 6, 2011, https://www.reuters.com/article/us-sept11-mayors/giuliani-and-bloomberg-ny-mayors-linked-by-sept-11-idUSTRE7850YB20110906.
4. “Two-in-Three Critical of Bush’s Relief Efforts,” Pew Research Center, September 8, 2005, https://www.pewresearch.org/politics/2005/09/08/two-in-three-critical-of-bushs-relief-efforts/.
5. Natalie Colarossi, “11 Times Trump Has Lashed Out at Reporters and Called Them ‘Nasty’ during His Coronavirus Press Briefings,” Insider (business section), May 13, 2020, https://www.businessinsider.com/trump-lashes-out-at-reporters-during-coronavirus-press-briefings-2020-4.
6. Mathew Ingram, “White House revokes press passes for dozens of journalists,” *Columbia Journalism Review*, May 9, 2019, https://www.cjr.org/the_media_today/white-house-press-passes.php.
7. Nolan D. McCaskill, “Trump Accuses Cruz’s Father of Helping JKF’s Assassin,” Politico, May 3, 2016, https://www.politico.com/blogs/2016-gop-primary-live-updates-and-results/2016/05/trump-ted-cruz-father-222730.
8. Lia Eustachewich, “What Is QAnon? What We Know about the Conspiracy Theory,” *New York Post*, October 16, 2020, https://nypost.com/article/what-is-qanon-conspiracy-theory/.
9. Dora Mekouar, “Why Do People Embrace Conspiracy Theories?,” VOA News, February 20, 2021, https://www.voanews.com/usa/all-about-america/why-do-people-embrace-conspiracy-theories.
10. Oregon Medical Board, State of Oregon, “Order of Emergency Suspension of License and Notice of Opportunity for Hearing,” December 4, 2020, https://omb.oregon.gov/Clients/ORMB/OrderDocuments/ff970292-5807-41ba-9c1e-c2b81de89cd1.pdf.
11. Mia Jankowicz, “How a Rogue Doctor Who Called the Vaccine ‘Needle Rape’ Was Made an Idaho Public-Health Official in Its Worst COVID Crisis Yet,” Insider (business section), September 15, 2021, https://www.businessinsider.com/idaho-ryan-cole-public-health-board-anti-vaccine-2021-9.
12. Tony Green, “A Harsh Lesson in the Reality of COVID-19,” *Dallas Voice*, July 24, 2020, https://dallasvoice.com/a-harsh-lesson-in-the-reality-of-covid-19/.

Chapter 12. Dangerous and Erroneous Approaches

1. Centers for Disease Control and Prevention, “People with Certain Medical Conditions,” updated May 2, 2022, https://www.cdc.gov/coronavirus/2019-ncov/need-extra-precautions/people-with-medical-conditions.html.

2. World Health Organization, "WHO Coronavirus (COVID-19) Dashboard," accessed February 27, 2021, https://covid19.who.int/.
3. Summer E. Galloway et al., "Emergence of SARS-CoV-2 B.1.1.7 Lineage—United States, December 29, 2020–January 12, 2021," *Morbidity and Mortality Weekly Report* 70, no. 3 (2021): 95–99, https://doi.org/10.15585/mmwr.mm7003e2.
4. Eli S. Rosenberg et al., "Cumulative Incidence and diagnosis of SARS-CoV-2 Infection in New York," *Annals of Epidemiology*, 48 (2020): 23–29.e4, https://doi .org/10.1016/j.annepidem.2020.06.004.
5. BNO News, "COVID-19 Reinfection Tracker," updated November 26, 2021, https://bnonews.com/index.php/2020/08/covid-19-reinfection-tracker/.
6. "Fact Check: Sweden Has Not Achieved Herd Immunity, Is Not Proof That Lockdowns Are Useless," Reuters, December 2, 2020, https://www.reuters.com /article/uk-factcheck-prageru-sweden-herd-immunit/fact-check-sweden-has -not-achieved-herd-immunity-is-not-proof-that-lockdowns-are-useless -idUSKBN28C2R7.
7. Coronakommissionen, *Äldreomsorgen under Pandemin* [*Elderly Care during the Pandemic*], December 15, 2020, https://coronakommissionen.com/wp-content /uploads/2020/12/sou_2020_80_aldreomsorgen-under-pandemin_webb.pdf.
8. Steve Goldstein, "Sweden Didn't Impose a Lockdown, but Its Economy Is Just as Bad as Its Neighbors," MarketWatch, June 27, 2020, https://www.marketwatch .com/story/sweden-didnt-impose-a-lockdown-its-economy-is-just-as-bad-as-its -neighbors-who-did-2020-06-25.

Chapter 13. Vaccines and Variants

1. Jens-Peter Gregersen, "What History Tells Us about Vaccine Timetables," *Eureka*, June 9, 2020, https://www.criver.com/eureka/what-history-tells-us-about-vaccine -timetables.
2. United States Department of Health and Human Services, "Explaining Operation Warp Speed," August 2020, https://www.nihb.org/covid-19/wp-content/uploads /2020/08/Fact-sheet-operation-warp-speed.pdf.
3. City News Service, "House Panel Investigates One Medical for Allegedly Allowing Rich Clients to Cut Vaccine Line," ABC 10 News San Diego, March 3, 2021, https://www.10news.com/news/coronavirus/house-panel-investigates-one -medical-for-allegedly-allowing-rich-clients-to-cut-vaccine-line.
4. Will Feuer, "Florida Gov. DeSantis Accused of Favoritism in Distributing Covid Vaccine, Congress Urged to Investigate," CNBC, March 1, 2021, https://www.cnbc .com/2021/03/01/florida-gov-desantis-accused-of-favoritism-in-distributing-covid -vaccine.html.
5. Jeffrey V. Lazarus et al., "A Global Survey of Potential Acceptance of a COVID-19 Vaccine," *Nature Medicine* 27 (2021): 225–28, https://doi.org/10.1038/s41591-020 -1124-9.
6. Cary Funk and Alec Tyson, "Intent to Get a COVID-19 Vaccine Rises to 60% as Confidence in Research and Development Process Increases," Pew Research Center, December 3, 2020, https://www.pewresearch.org/science/2020/12/03/intent

-to-get-a-covid-19-vaccine-rises-to-60-as-confidence-in-research-and-development-process-increases/.
7. Johns Hopkins University of Medicine Coronavirus Resource Center, "Vaccines: Understanding Vaccination Progress," accessed July 3, 2021, https://coronavirus.jhu.edu/vaccines/international.
8. CBS News, "More Than Half of Americans Favor Vaccine Mandates at Work, Poll Finds," August 26, 2021, https://www.cbsnews.com/news/covid-vaccine-mandate-work-poll-americans-favor/.
9. Bridges et al. v. Houston Methodist et al. Civil Action H-21-1774. (S.D. Tex. 2021). Order on Dismissal, signed by Judge Lynn N. Hughes, June 12, p. 4, https://www.govinfo.gov/app/details/USCOURTS-txsd-4_21-cv-01774/context.

Chapter 14. Preparing Schools for the Next Pandemic

1. Victoria Kim, "Infected after 5 Minutes, from 20 Feet Away: South Korea Study Shows Coronavirus' Spread Indoors," *Los Angeles Times*, December 9, 2020, https://www.latimes.com/world-nation/story/2020-12-09/five-minutes-from-20-feet-away-south-korean-study-shows-perils-of-indoor-dining-for-covid-19.

Chapter 15. Leadership Lessons from the Pandemic

1. Matt Perez, "Who Is Dr. Scott Atlas? Trump's New Covid Health Adviser Seen as a Counter to Fauci and Birx," *Forbes*, August 12, 2020, https://www.forbes.com/sites/mattperez/2020/08/12/who-is-dr-scott-atlas-trumps-new-covid-health-adviser-seen-as-counter-to-fauci-and-birx/?sh=4532384620a4.
2. William Cummings and Courtney Subramanian, "'It Is What It Is,' Trump Says of Rising Coronavirus Death Toll as He Insists Outbreak Is 'Under Control,'" *USA Today*, August 4, 2020, https://www.usatoday.com/story/news/politics/2020/08/04/trump-tells-axios-rising-covid-19-death-toll-is-what-is/5579765002/.
3. Neal F. Lane and Michael Riordan, "The President's Disdain for Science," *New York Times*, January 4, 2018, https://www.nytimes.com/2018/01/04/opinion/trump-disdain-science.html.

INDEX